SCLERODERMA

A MEDICAL DICTIONARY, BIBLIOGRAPHY,
AND ANNOTATED RESEARCH GUIDE TO
INTERNET REFERENCES

JAMES N. PARKER, M.D.
AND PHILIP M. PARKER, PH.D., EDITORS

ICON Health Publications
ICON Group International, Inc.
4370 La Jolla Village Drive, 4th Floor
San Diego, CA 92122 USA

Printed in the United States of America.

Last digit indicates print number: 10 9 8 7 6 4 5 3 2 1

Publisher, Health Care: Philip Parker, Ph.D.
Editor(s): James Parker, M.D., Philip Parker, Ph.D.

Publisher's note: The ideas, procedures, and suggestions contained in this book are not intended for the diagnosis or treatment of a health problem. As new medical or scientific information becomes available from academic and clinical research, recommended treatments and drug therapies may undergo changes. The authors, editors, and publisher have attempted to make the information in this book up to date and accurate in accord with accepted standards at the time of publication. The authors, editors, and publisher are not responsible for errors or omissions or for consequences from application of the book, and make no warranty, expressed or implied, in regard to the contents of this book. Any practice described in this book should be applied by the reader in accordance with professional standards of care used in regard to the unique circumstances that may apply in each situation. The reader is advised to always check product information (package inserts) for changes and new information regarding dosage and contraindications before prescribing any drug or pharmacological product. Caution is especially urged when using new or infrequently ordered drugs, herbal remedies, vitamins and supplements, alternative therapies, complementary therapies and medicines, and integrative medical treatments.

Cataloging-in-Publication Data

Parker, James N., 1961-
Parker, Philip M., 1960-

Scleroderma: A Medical Dictionary, Bibliography, and Annotated Research Guide to Internet References / James N. Parker and Philip M. Parker, editors
        p.   cm.
Includes bibliographical references, glossary, and index.
ISBN: 0-597-84299-X
1. Scleroderma-Popular works.   I. Title.

Disclaimer

This publication is not intended to be used for the diagnosis or treatment of a health problem. It is sold with the understanding that the publisher, editors, and authors are not engaging in the rendering of medical, psychological, financial, legal, or other professional services.

References to any entity, product, service, or source of information that may be contained in this publication should not be considered an endorsement, either direct or implied, by the publisher, editors, or authors. ICON Group International, Inc., the editors, and the authors are not responsible for the content of any Web pages or publications referenced in this publication.

Copyright Notice

Acknowledgements

The collective knowledge generated from academic and applied research summarized in various references has been critical in the creation of this book which is best viewed as a comprehensive compilation and collection of information prepared by various official agencies which produce publications on scleroderma. Books in this series draw from various agencies and institutions associated with the United States Department of Health and Human Services, and in particular, the Office of the Secretary of Health and Human Services (OS), the Administration for Children and Families (ACF), the Administration on Aging (AOA), the Agency for Healthcare Research and Quality (AHRQ), the Agency for Toxic Substances and Disease Registry (ATSDR), the Centers for Disease Control and Prevention (CDC), the Food and Drug Administration (FDA), the Healthcare Financing Administration (HCFA), the Health Resources and Services Administration (HRSA), the Indian Health Service (IHS), the institutions of the National Institutes of Health (NIH), the Program Support Center (PSC), and the Substance Abuse and Mental Health Services Administration (SAMHSA). In addition to these sources, information gathered from the National Library of Medicine, the United States Patent Office, the European Union, and their related organizations has been invaluable in the creation of this book. Some of the work represented was financially supported by the Research and Development Committee at INSEAD. This support is gratefully acknowledged. Finally, special thanks are owed to Tiffany Freeman for her excellent editorial support.

About the Editors

James N. Parker, M.D.

Dr. James N. Parker received his Bachelor of Science degree in Psychobiology from the University of California, Riverside and his M.D. from the University of California, San Diego. In addition to authoring numerous research publications, he has lectured at various academic institutions. Dr. Parker is the medical editor for health books by ICON Health Publications.

Philip M. Parker, Ph.D.

Philip M. Parker is the Eli Lilly Chair Professor of Innovation, Business and Society at INSEAD (Fontainebleau, France and Singapore). Dr. Parker has also been Professor at the University of California, San Diego and has taught courses at Harvard University, the Hong Kong University of Science and Technology, the Massachusetts Institute of Technology, Stanford University, and UCLA. Dr. Parker is the associate editor for ICON Health Publications.

About ICON Health Publications

To discover more about ICON Health Publications, simply check with your preferred online booksellers, including Barnes&Noble.com and Amazon.com which currently carry all of our titles. Or, feel free to contact us directly for bulk purchases or institutional discounts:

ICON Group International, Inc.
4370 La Jolla Village Drive, Fourth Floor
San Diego, CA 92122 USA
Fax: 858-546-4341
Web site: **www.icongrouponline.com/health**

Table of Contents

FORWARD

In March 2001, the National Institutes of Health issued the following warning: "The number of Web sites offering health-related resources grows every day. Many sites provide valuable information, while others may have information that is unreliable or misleading."[1] Furthermore, because of the rapid increase in Internet-based information, many hours can be wasted searching, selecting, and printing. Since only the smallest fraction of information dealing with scleroderma is indexed in search engines, such as **www.google.com** or others, a non-systematic approach to Internet research can be not only time consuming, but also incomplete. This book was created for medical professionals, students, and members of the general public who want to know as much as possible about scleroderma, using the most advanced research tools available and spending the least amount of time doing so.

In addition to offering a structured and comprehensive bibliography, the pages that follow will tell you where and how to find reliable information covering virtually all topics related to scleroderma, from the essentials to the most advanced areas of research. Public, academic, government, and peer-reviewed research studies are emphasized. Various abstracts are reproduced to give you some of the latest official information available to date on scleroderma. Abundant guidance is given on how to obtain free-of-charge primary research results via the Internet. **While this book focuses on the field of medicine, when some sources provide access to non-medical information relating to scleroderma, these are noted in the text.**

E-book and electronic versions of this book are fully interactive with each of the Internet sites mentioned (clicking on a hyperlink automatically opens your browser to the site indicated). If you are using the hard copy version of this book, you can access a cited Web site by typing the provided Web address directly into your Internet browser. You may find it useful to refer to synonyms or related terms when accessing these Internet databases. **NOTE:** At the time of publication, the Web addresses were functional. However, some links may fail due to URL address changes, which is a common occurrence on the Internet.

For readers unfamiliar with the Internet, detailed instructions are offered on how to access electronic resources. For readers unfamiliar with medical terminology, a comprehensive glossary is provided. For readers without access to Internet resources, a directory of medical libraries, that have or can locate references cited here, is given. We hope these resources will prove useful to the widest possible audience seeking information on scleroderma.

The Editors

---

[1] From the NIH, National Cancer Institute (NCI): **http://www.cancer.gov/cancerinfo/ten-things-to-know**.

CHAPTER 1. STUDIES ON SCLERODERMA

Overview

In this chapter, we will show you how to locate peer-reviewed references and studies on scleroderma.

The Combined Health Information Database

The Combined Health Information Database summarizes studies across numerous federal agencies. To limit your investigation to research studies and scleroderma, you will need to use the advanced search options. First, go to **http://chid.nih.gov/index.html**. From there, select the "Detailed Search" option (or go directly to that page with the following hyperlink: **http://chid.nih.gov/detail/detail.html**). The trick in extracting studies is found in the drop boxes at the bottom of the search page where "You may refine your search by." Select the dates and language you prefer, and the format option "Journal Article." At the top of the search form, select the number of records you would like to see (we recommend 100) and check the box to display "whole records." We recommend that you type "scleroderma" (or synonyms) into the "For these words:" box. Consider using the option "anywhere in record" to make your search as broad as possible. If you want to limit the search to only a particular field, such as the title of the journal, then select this option in the "Search in these fields" drop box. The following is what you can expect from this type of search:

- **Long-Term Outcomes of Scleroderma Renal Crisis**

  Source: Annals of Internal Medicine. 133(8): 600-603. October 17, 2000.

  Contact: Available from American College of Physicians. American Society of Internal Medicine. 190 North Independence Mall West, Philadelphia, PA 19106-1572. Website: www.acponline.org.

  Summary: Although scleroderma renal (kidney) crisis, a complication of systemic sclerosis, can be treated with ACE (angiotensin converting enzyme) inhibitors, its long term outcomes are not known. This article reports on a study undertaken to determine outcomes, natural history, and risk factors in patients with systemic sclerosis and scleroderma renal crisis. The study included 145 patients with scleroderma renal crisis who received ACE inhibitors and 662 patients with scleroderma who did not have renal crisis. Among patients with renal crisis, 61 percent had good outcomes (55 received no dialysis, and 34 received temporary dialysis); only 4 (4 percent) of these patients progressed to chronic renal failure (CRF) and permanent dialysis. More than half of the patients who initially required dialysis could discontinue it 3 to 18 months later. Survival of patients in the good outcome group was similar to that of patients with diffuse scleroderma who did not have renal crisis. Some patients (39 percent) had bad outcomes (permanent dialysis or early death). The authors conclude that renal crisis can be effectively managed when hypertension is aggressively controlled with ACE inhibitors. Patients should continue taking ACE inhibitors even after beginning dialysis in hopes of discontinuing dialysis. 2 figures. 13 references.

- **Scleroderma Renal Crisis**

Source: Rheumatic Disease Clinics of North America. 22(4): 861-878. November 1996.

Contact: Available from W.B. Saunders Company. Periodicals Fulfillment Department, 6277 Sea Harbor Drive, Orlando, FL 32821-9816.

Summary: Kidney involvement in scleroderma can result in renal abnormalities including proteinuria, azotemia, and hypertension, outside of renal crisis; however, they may not always be attributed to the scleroderma. This article reviews the pathogenesis, clinical setting, therapy, outcome, and nonrenal crisis abnormalities in the kidney of people with systemic sclerosis. Renal crisis occurs in systemic sclerosis patients with rapidly progressive diffuse cutaneous thickening early in their disease. Scleroderma renal crisis (SRC) is characterized by malignant hypertension, hyperreninemia, azotemia, microangiopathic hemolytic anemia, and renal failure. This complication, which in the past has been almost uniformly fatal, is now successfully treated in most cases with ACE inhibitors. This therapy has improved survival, reduced requirement for dialysis, and, in those on dialysis, has often allowed discontinuation of dialysis 6 to 18 months later. The author stresses that prompt diagnosis and early, aggressive initiation of therapy with ACE inhibitors will result in the most optimal outcome. Chronic nonrenal crisis renal insufficiency is unusual and rarely progresses to significant renal dysfunction. 4 figures. 1 table. 72 references.

- **Mandibular Resorption Due to Progressive Systemic Sclerosis: A Case Report**

Source: Journal of Oral and Maxillofacial Surgery. 59(5): 565-567. May 2001.

Contact: Available from W.B. Saunders Company. Periodicals Department, P.O. Box 629239, Orlando, FL 32862-8239. (800) 654-2452. Website: www.harcourthealth.com.

Summary: Progressive systemic sclerosis (PSS), also known as scleroderma, is a connective tissue disorder of unknown origin, characterized by fibrosis of the skin and other visceral organs. The disease generally occurs between 30 and 50 years of age, and women are mostly affected. The disease progresses with the firmness of the skin leading to limitation of mobility of the fingers. The tight sclerotic skin causes extrinsic pressure and the overproduced collagen in the small arteries leads to the obliteration of the vessels and eventually induces destruction of the bone. This article reports a case of PSS with general and facial findings, and extensive mandibular (lower jaw) resorption. The patient, a 45 year old white woman, presented with a complaint of mobility of her anterior mandibular teeth. Her PSS had been diagnosed 21 years previously. The oral opening was reduced to 32 mm because of atrophy of the lip muscles and tightening of the skin. Intraoral examination revealed poor oral hygiene, loss of teeth, and periodontitis that was especially localized to the anterior mandibular region. After extensive evaluation, results revealed no other pathology, metabolic bone disease or neoplasia that could be causing her bone resorption. Esophageal involvement, with dysphasia (swallowing difficulty) and pulmonary (lung) involved were also diagnosed in this patient. 5 figures. 1 table. 18 references.

- **Scleroderma: Oral Manifestations and Treatment Challenges**

  Source: SCD. Special Care in Dentistry. 20(6): 240-244. November-December 2000.

  Contact: Available from Special Care Dentistry. 211 East Chicago Avenue, Chicago, IL 60611. (312) 440-2660.

  Summary: Scleroderma is a connective tissue disorder of excess collagen production characterized by intense fibrosis of the skin, with internal organ involvement. A wide range of oral sequelae complicate maintenance of oral health and dental treatment in patients with scleroderma. These sequelae can include microstomia (reduced mouth opening), oral mucosal or gingival fibrosis (development of fibrous connective tissue or scarring), xerostomia (dry mouth) and mandibular (lower jaw) bone resorption. In this article, the authors review the literature regarding oral health and scleroderma, and present two illustrative case studies. The authors stress that dental management of these patients requires a multidisciplinary approach. Mouth stretching and oral augmentation exercises have been proven successful in increasing mouth opening. Dry mouth symptoms can cause a high caries rate and an increased incidence of candida (thrush, a fungus) infections. Sugarless candies and mints and drug therapy (i.e., pilocarpine) may be used to stimulate salivary flow and saliva substitutes may improve comfort. Daily fluoride treatments with the use of custom fluoride trays are useful for caries control. Adaptive equipment may be used to assist in good oral hygiene. 6 figures. 37 references.

- **Oral-Facial Characteristics of Circumscribed Scleroderma: Case Report**

  Source: Journal of Clinical Pediatric Dentistry. 17(4): 239-242. Spring 1993.

  Summary: Scleroderma is a rare disorder of unknown etiology. Circumscribed scleroderma is a localized focal form. It may present as well defined elevated or depressed white or yellowish patches termed 'morphea' or linear bands made up of a furrow with elevated ridges on the margins. This article describes the oral-facial characteristics of circumscribed scleroderma in a ten year old female. The authors describe both extra-oral and intra-oral findings in this patient, the cephalometric analysis used, and psychological and social considerations. The patient in this care report exhibits root development defects of the maxillary central and lateral incisors on the affected side. A lesion on the left side of the face involves the eyebrows and eyelashes. During the period of time the patient has been seen by the authors, the lateral incisor on the affected side has erupted in spite of arrested root development. The dental problem may require stabilization or even extraction of the lateral incisor as further eruption occurs. 8 figures. 1 table. 9 references. (AA-M).

- **Scleroderma: Not One of the Usual Suspects**

  Source: Advance for Speech-Language Pathologists and Audiologists. 7(1): 11, 42. January 7, 1997.

  Contact: Available from Merion Publications, Inc. 650 Park Avenue, Box 61556, King of Prussia, PA 19406-0956. (800) 355-1088 or (610) 265-7812.

  Summary: This article, from a professional newsletter for speech language pathologists and audiologists, reviews the condition of scleroderma. Scleroderma is a rare autoimmune disease characterized by fibrosis of the skin and internal organs; the disease can affect the mouth, vocal cords, and larynx. The article interviews two clinicians. Topics include the speech problems associated with scleroderma; the effect of collagen infiltration in the vocal cords; Sjogren's syndrome; scleroderma treatment programs; swallowing impairments that may accompany scleroderma; risk factors for cancer in the oral cavity, vocal cords, and larynx; patient assessment considerations; staging of disease; and intervention options, ranging from conservative to aggressive treatments. The article concludes with a brief discussion of the importance of increasing physician and public awareness of scleroderma. The contact information for the two clinicians interviewed is provided. 2 figures.

- **Effective Intervention in Scleroderma Renal Crisis**

  Source: Journal of Musculoskeletal Medicine. 14(3): 25-28,34-36; March 1997.

  Summary: This journal article for health professionals discusses recent advances in aborting scleroderma renal crisis; however, these advances are possible only with early diagnosis and treatment with angiotensin converting enzyme (ACE) inhibitors. Once irreversible and invariably fatal, scleroderma renal crisis is now considered a treatable complication of systemic sclerosis. Patients with early, rapidly progressive diffuse systemic sclerosis and those with symptomatic pericardial disease and microangiopathic hemolytic anemia are at highest risk. Early recognition and immediate initiation of therapy with captopril or another short-acting ACE inhibitor may be lifesaving. One-year patient survival, once unheard of, has increased to approximately 75 percent. Patients at risk must be educated in self-monitoring of blood pressure and recognition of the early warning signs of renal crisis. If treatment of renal crisis is delayed, long-term dialysis may be required pending the possible return of renal function. 19 references, 2 figures, and 3 tables. (AA-M).

- **Cutaneous Manifestations of Rheumatic Diseases: Lupus Erythematosus, Dermatomyositis, Scleroderma**

  Source: Dermatology Nursing. 10(2): 81-95. April 1998.

  Summary: This journal article presents nurses and other health professionals with information, which is part of a continuing education series, on recognizing and managing the cutaneous manifestations of rheumatic diseases. It discusses the classification, diagnosis, clinical features, and management of skin disease seen in patients with lupus erythematosus (LE), dermatomyositis (DM), and scleroderma/systemic sclerosis. The cutaneous manifestations of LE can be divided into those that are histologically specific and those that are not. Each LE-specific skin disease produces a particular type of skin lesion. Patients with LE are photosensitive, so they should protect their skin from sun exposure. In addition, patients with LE may be treated with topical and intralesional corticosteroids, antimalarials, nonimmunosuppressive anti-inflammatory drugs, and immunosuppressives. A cautious approach should be used with regard to surgery. DM is characterized by skin lesions and a histopathologically specific pattern of skeletal muscle inflammation. Patients should use sunscreens, and they may be treated with topical antipruritics, antihistamines, antimalarials, prednisone, and other drugs. Scleroderma, which has two forms, is characterized by thickened, hardened, leather-like skin. The initial manifestation of localized scleroderma is asymmetrical circumscribed indurated plaques on the truck or proximal extremities that are often surrounded by a halo of violaceous skin. Systemic sclerosis, the second form, usually begins with Raynaud's phenomenon. The same moisturization and antipruritic measures described for DM should be used for scleroderma: that is systemic antibiotics, vasodilators, anticoagulants, immunosuppressive drugs, and various investigational approaches. 8 figures, 7 tables, and 21 references.

- **Association of Microsatellite Markers Near the Fibrillin 1 Gene on Human Chromosome 15q With Scleroderma in a Native American Population**

Source: Arthritis and Rheumatism. 41(10): 1729-1737. October 1998.

Summary: This journal article provides health professionals with information on a case control study that investigated the association of microsatellite alleles on human chromosome 15q and 2q with scleroderma in an American Indian population. Microsatellite alleles on these chromosomes, homologous to the murine tight skin 1 (tsk1) and tsk2 loci, respectively, were analyzed for possible disease association in 18 Choctaw patients with systemic sclerosis (SSc) and 77 normal Choctaw controls. Genotyping first-degree relatives of the cases identified potential disease haplotypes, and haplotype frequencies were obtained by expectation maximization and maximum likelihood estimation methods. Simultaneously, the ancestral origins of contemporary Choctaw SSc cases were ascertained using census and historical records. A multilocus 2 cM haplotype identified on human chromosome 15q homologous to the murine tsk1 region, which showed a significantly increased frequency in SSc cases compared with controls. This haplotype contains two intragenic markers from the fibrillin 1 (FBN1) gene. Genealogic studies demonstrate that the SSc cases were distantly related and that their ancestry could be traced back to five founding families in the eighteenth century. The probability that the SSc cases share this haplotype because of familial aggregation effects alone was calculated and found to be very low. There was no evidence of any microsatellite allele disturbances on chromosome 2q in the region homologous to the tsk2 locus of the region containing the interleukin 1 family. The article concludes that a 2 cM haplotype on chromosome 15q that contains FBN1 is associated with scleroderma in Choctaw Indians from Oklahoma. This haplotype may have been inherited from common founders about 10 generations ago and may contribute to the high prevalence of SSC that is now seen. 1 appendix, 1 figure, 3 tables, and 59 references. (AA-M).

- **Connective Tissue Disease Update: Focus on Scleroderma**

Source: Consultant. 39(7): 2071-2074,2077-2078,2081-2082. July 1999.

Summary: This journal article, the second in a three-part series on connective tissue diseases, provides health professionals with information on the manifestations, pathogenesis, diagnosis, and treatment of scleroderma. Scleroderma represents a group of diseases in which a general process of thickening and induration of the skin results from the excessive deposition of collagen and other matrix proteins. Localized scleroderma refers to asymmetric skin induration and thickening without internal organ involvement. Systemic scleroderma is characterized by fairly symmetric cutaneous induration and thickening, accompanied by visceral organ involvement that may lead to complications. The two major variants of localized scleroderma are morphea and linear scleroderma. Morphea is characterized by circumscribed, indurated, round or ill-defined patches of skin with varying degrees of pigmentary change. The linear variant affects the extremities more commonly than the trunk and is almost always asymmetric. There is no specific therapy for localized scleroderma, although topical corticosteroids, antimalarials, and vitamins D and E have been effective in treating morphea. Most patients require only an emollient for dry skin. Limited systemic scleroderma is characterized by disseminated telangiectasias and sclerodermatous skin changes limited to the hands, forearms, and face. In diffuse systemic scleroderma, Raynaud's phenomenon and systemic rheumatologic, cardiac, neurologic, gastrointestinal, and pulmonary symptoms are common. Treatment of systemic scleroderma is aimed at improving quality of life. Vasoactive therapy includes nicotinic acid, dipyridamole, and calcium channel blockers. Anti-inflammatory therapy consists mainly of oral corticosteroids. Agents used to influence connective tissue metabolism include immunosuppressives and D-penicillamine. Localized scleroderma is typically a self-limited disease that lasts between 3 and 5 years. Systemic scleroderma is chronic, with a slow course of progressive morbidity and disability in 70 to 90 percent of patients. 2 figures, 5 tables, and 15 references. (AA-M).

Federally Funded Research on Scleroderma

The U.S. Government supports a variety of research studies relating to scleroderma. These studies are tracked by the Office of Extramural Research at the National Institutes of Health.[2] CRISP (Computerized Retrieval of Information on Scientific Projects) is a searchable database of federally funded biomedical research projects conducted at universities, hospitals, and other institutions.

Search the CRISP Web site at **http://crisp.cit.nih.gov/crisp/crisp_query.generate_screen**. You will have the option to perform targeted searches by various criteria, including geography, date, and topics related to scleroderma.

For most of the studies, the agencies reporting into CRISP provide summaries or abstracts. As opposed to clinical trial research using patients, many federally funded studies use animals or simulated models to explore scleroderma. The following is typical of the type of information found when searching the CRISP database for scleroderma:

- **Project Title: ABI PRISM 7900HT SEQUENCE DETECTION SYSTEM**

  Principal Investigator & Institution: Teng, Ba-Bie; Associate Professor; Human Genetics Center; University of Texas Hlth Sci Ctr Houston Box 20036 Houston, Tx 77225

  Timing: Fiscal Year 2002; Project Start 01-MAY-2002; Project End 30-APR-2003

  Summary: We are requesting an ABI Prism 7900HT Sequence Detection System with the automation accessary. This instrument will be housed in the Vector Development Core Laboratory at the Institute of Molecular Medicine. The group of investigators participating in this grant application includes ten researchers with NIH-supported grant projects and three potential young investigators. The investigators are from the Institute of Molecular Medicine and the Medical School from UT- Houston and the Institute of Biosciences and Technology from Texas A&M University. The research projects involved are diverse, ranging from basic biology, cancer research, the identification of target genes in various diseases, gene therapy, and investigating differential gene expression in tissues from human and animals to clinical studies involving the genotyping of susceptibility to **Scleroderma** and stroke. We intend to use this instrument for the high-throughput real-time quantitative analysis of RNA transcripts and DNA targets in biological samples and for single nucleotide polymorphism genotyping. As indicated in the research project. from each investigator, the availability of the proposed instrument will significantly improve the scope of each

---

[2] Healthcare projects are funded by the National Institutes of Health (NIH), Substance Abuse and Mental Health Services (SAMHSA), Health Resources and Services Administration (HRSA), Food and Drug Administration (FDA), Centers for Disease Control and Prevention (CDCP), Agency for Healthcare Research and Quality (AHRQ), and Office of Assistant Secretary of Health (OASH).

one's study. It will allow us to rapidly follow up the exciting discoveries from our currently funded projects. The goal of this multidisciplinary collaborative effort is to develop and share the advanced technology resources needed to carry out the cutting-edge scientific work that will characterize medical research of the future. Most importantly, the established investigators will be able to provide exposure to students and medical fellows to this powerful instrument and to have an environment with new biological tools in which young potential investigators can develop his/her own scientific research. The requested instrument is a high-throughput real-time PCR system that detects and quantifies nucleic acid sequences. An automation accessory with a 96- or 384-well plate capacity facilitates 24-hour unattended operation. The integrated bar code readers simplify sample tracking. The 7900HT system is a remarkably simple instrument to operate. The entire RT-PCR run will be completed in 2 h and the individual can then retrieve his/her results and analyze the data using the software installed in his/her own computer. The ABI Prism Sequence Detection System has been proven to be a stable and easy to operate. The availability of this instrument is essential for improving our current funded projects.

Website: http://crisp.cit.nih.gov/crisp/Crisp_Query.Generate_Screen

• **Project Title: ALVEOLITIS AND FIBROSIS IN SCLERODERMA LUNG DISEASE**

Principal Investigator & Institution: Goldin, Jonathan G.; Acting Section Chief; Radiology; University of California Los Angeles 10920 Wilshire Blvd., Suite 1200 Los Angeles, Ca 90024

Timing: Fiscal Year 2002; Project Start 23-SEP-2002; Project End 31-JUL-2005

Summary: (provided by applicant): Currently bronchoalveolar lavage (Bal) evidence of alveolitis is used to diagnose active alveolitis in patients with **Scleroderma** Lung Disease (SLD). Detection of alveolitis may therefore have little prognostic or pathogenic relevance in the assessment of these cases. Preliminary novel quantitative image analysis (QIA) of HRCT data has been shown to correlate with BAL cellularity with the added ability of assessing regional heterogeneity of the entire lung not possible with BAL alone. CT Q!A can also identify manifestation of fibrosis, which is not possible with BAL or visual inspection of HRCT, thus, there is the potential for using this technique to investigate the relationship between alveolitis and fibrosis in the pathogenesis os SLD. Specifically if the progression of QIA-detected regional variation in fibrosis or alveolitis can be determined to be independent of each other the postulate that the fibrosis is due to pathways other than alveolitis can be implied. The hypothesis of this study is that the relationship of the extent and distribution of alveolitis to fibrosis in the progression of SLD can be further elucidated by the added ability of QIA techniques to assess alveolitis and fibrosis independently on a comprehensive and regional basis which is not possible with conventional techniques. The specific aims of this project are: (1) To assess the presence and severity of alveolitis and fibrosis in asymptomatic patients with mild or moderate SLD on a comprehensive (whole lung) and regional (portion of lung segment) basis; (2) to determine the interrelationship between alveolitis and fibrosis (as measured by QIA) in the progression of SLD; and (3) to determine whether interval changes of global and regional QIA features of fibrosis and alveolitis on follow up CT are predictive of outcome as assessed by symptoms (dyspnea index) and FVC in treated and untreated patients. Two experiments are proposed: Experiment 1: Comprehensive regional detection and quantitation of alveolitis and fibrosis (specific aim1); Experiment 2: Assessment of the relationship between alveolitis and fibrosis in the progression of SLD (specific aims 2 and 3). These findings will potentially improve our understanding of the relationship between alveolitis and fibrosis and to the pathogenesis of fibrosis in SLD.

Website: http://crisp.cit.nih.gov/crisp/Crisp_Query.Generate_Screen

- **Project Title: AUTOIMMUNITY CENTERS OF EXCELLENCE**

Principal Investigator & Institution: Chess, Leonard; Professor; Medicine; Columbia University Health Sciences New York, Ny 10032

Timing: Fiscal Year 2002; Project Start 28-SEP-1999; Project End 31-AUG-2003

Summary: The overall aim of this center proposal is to establish an interdisciplinary basic and clinical research program at Columbia primarily focused on the evaluation of novel therapeutic approaches to five autoimmune diseases; rheumatoid arthritis (RA), systemic lupus erythematosus (SLE), multiple sclerosis (MS), type one diabetes mellitus (TIDM) and **scleroderma**. In each of these diseases there are ongoing basic and clinical research programs involving pathophysiologic and/or clinical immunotherapeutic studies. We hypothesize that there are four principal events involved in the immunopathogenesis of these diseases: (1) predisposing genes establish a T-cell repertoire capable of recognizing self peptides intrinsic to the autoimmune process; (2) previously tolerant autoreactive effector T cells; (3) regulatory mechanisms, including the activation of TH1 and TH2 CD4+ T cell subsets as well as those involving CD8 T-cells fail, through processes such as clonal deletion or changes in the cytokine milieu and (4) pathogenic autoantibodies develop through cognitive T- cell B-cell interactions which effect tissue injury. In these diseases, one would predict that reducing the clonal expression of relevant autoreactive T cells by blockade of T cell receptor signaling or interruption of the CD40 ligand-dependent pathway could down-modulate disease activity. Moreover, interruption of the inflammatory effector functions of T cells mediated by TNF or CD40L would similarly reduce disease potential. We propose to test these hypotheses in the above patients during the natural history of disease and during specific immune intervention. In particular, we will study patients with SLE treated with anti-CD40L; MS patients receiving IFN-beta or anti-CD40L; T1DM patients receiving anti-CD3 and RA patients receiving the recombinant TNF receptor inhibitor (Embrel). During these studies we will: (1) identify by PCR based spectratyping techniques and TCR sequencing, oligoclonal and autoantigen-driven expansions in the CD4 alphabeta TCR repertoire; (2) Identify changes in the T cell functional response to autoantigens and (3) directly study the regulatory interactions of TH1, TH2 and CD8+ T cells in controlling the TCR repertoire. In select patients, we will directly study the function and repertoire of T cells at the site of inflammation (CNS, Joints) using HVS immortalization techniques.

Website: http://crisp.cit.nih.gov/crisp/Crisp_Query.Generate_Screen

- **Project Title: AUTOMATED, QUANTITATIVE IMMUNOFLUORESCENT ASSAY**

Principal Investigator & Institution: Newton, Kenneth R.; Hyperion, Inc. 14100 Sw 136Th St Miami, Fl 33186

Timing: Fiscal Year 2003; Project Start 01-JUL-2000; Project End 30-JUN-2005

Summary: (provided by applicant): Diagnosis of auto-immune and connective tissue diseases such as Systemic Lupus Erythematosus, Sjorgren syndrome and **scleroderma** often makes use of an Immunofluorescent assay (IFA) for antinuclear antibodies (ANA). More detailed diagnostic support may also utilize an IFA test for double-stranded DNA (dsDNA). IFA tests detecting Anti-Neutrophil Cytoplasmic Autoantibodies (ANCA) are diagnostic for systemic necrotizing vasculitis and glomerulonephritis. All these IFA tests require significant laboratory preparation time from highly trained technicians using current, manual techniques. The VisiQuant system developed as a prototype in Phase I, combined with Hyperion's Hyprep automated assay preparation system will automate both preparation and reading of the IFA tests, achieving significant cost savings and potential error reduction. During the Phase II project period, an updated VisiQuant Microscope will be introduced along with improved ANA assay and preparation procedure. The assay will be improved by applying results of a study of assay parameters and conditions. The Microscope will be upgraded by incorporating engineering enhancements to the optics and electronics, including features to optimize the joint operation of the Microscope with the HyPrep, and software improvements to the fluorescence intensity algorithm. New test kits for dsDNA based on Crithidia luciliae and for ANCA will be developed, tested and brought to market. Development work in automated image classification will lead to a complementary product that finds the best match to each sample image from a standard ANA image pattern library. Further development of the image classification software will be done based on input from the consultants. This will lead to an advanced Image Classification system to be brought to market at the end of the Phase II period. Image classification to support ANCA test will be started but is not expected to be ready for market until after completion of this project. These developments will result in Hyperion obtaining more than 18% share of the global market for autoimmune IFA based IVD tests by 2010. The development team includes personnel with many years of experience in dye chemistry, immunology in vitro device development, instrument development and image processing.

Website: http://crisp.cit.nih.gov/crisp/Crisp_Query.Generate_Screen

- **Project Title: BIOCHEMICAL AND VASCULAR ALTERATIONS IN SCLERODERMA**

Principal Investigator & Institution: Jimenez, Sergio A.; Professor; Medicine; Thomas Jefferson University Office of Research Administration Philadelphia, Pa 191075587

Timing: Fiscal Year 2002; Project Start 01-SEP-1987; Project End 31-MAR-2005

Summary: (Adapted from the applicant's abstract) - **Scleroderma** or **systemic sclerosis** (SSc) is a disease of unknown etiology characterized by the excessive deposition of collagen and other connective tissue components of the skin and multiple internal organs, prominent and often severe alterations in the microvasculature and humoral and cellular abnormalities. Although the mechanisms involved in the pathogenesis of SSc are not completely known, it is clear that cutaneous, visceral, and vascular fibrosis is responsible for most of the clinical manifestations of the disease. It has been previously demonstrated that fibroblasts from affected SSc skin cultured in vitro produce excessive amounts of a variety of extracellular proteins. The exaggerated extracellular matrix production by SSc fibroblasts is the result of increased collagen-gene expression that largely results from higher transcription rates of various collagen genes. Despite the recent advances in the understanding of collagen-gene expression under normal conditions, there is very little known regarding the intimate mechanisms responsible for the pathologic increase in the expression of collagen genes in SSc. The investigators propose to examine the hypothesis that excessive production of collagen in SSc fibroblasts is due to alterations in the mechanisms that regulate the rates of transcription of collagen genes and involves abnormalities in the interactions of cis-regulatory elements present in the promoter and first intron of these genes with specific trans-acting DNA-binding proteins. To test this hypothesis, the applicants will analyze sequences in the promoter and first intron of the 1 alpha (I) procollagen gene that are involved in up-regulation of its expression in SSc fibroblasts, identify DNA-binding proteins that recognize specific regulatory elements within these regions of the gene, and perform quantitative comparisons between normal and SSc cells of the amounts of DNA-binding proteins that interact with these regulatory elements. The applicants also will examine the effects of DNA-binding drugs which mimic transcription factors in their ability to interact with specific DNA sequences and of specific inhibitors of certain intracellular pathways, including those involving phospholipase C, protein kinase C gamma, and geranylgeranylprenylation which they have recently shown to exert potent modulation of collagen-gene expression. It is expected that the results from these studies will provide valuable clues towards the understanding of the pathogenesis of tissue fibrosis in SSc, and may provide new avenues of investigation towards the development of therapeutic agents for this incurable disease.

Website: http://crisp.cit.nih.gov/crisp/Crisp_Query.Generate_Screen

- **Project Title: BIOGENESIS AND FUNCTION OF CONNECTIVE TISSUE PROTEINS**

Principal Investigator & Institution: Bornstein, Paul; Professor; Biochemistry; University of Washington Grant & Contract Services Seattle, Wa 98105

Timing: Fiscal Year 2002; Project Start 01-FEB-1975; Project End 31-JAN-2005

Summary: The transcriptional regulation of the genes encoding the two type I collagen chains, alpha1(I) and alpha2(I), is one of special interest because these genes are expressed at widely different levels that correlate with the tissue specificity of collagen synthesis, and with development and maturation of the organism. Furthermore, the genes for alpha1(I) and alpha2(I) are responsive to cues generated by injury and repair, and by a variety of cytokines, hormones, and pharmacological agents. Finally, the expression of type I collagen genes is disturbed in orders such as pulmonary fibrosis and cirrhosis, and in diseases such as **scleroderma.** Although post-transcriptional mechanisms undoubtedly play an important role in regulating collagen synthesis, there is good evidence that transcriptional control represents the major means by which this regulation is achieved. A major goal of this grant is to determine how this astonishingly intricate pattern of expression is established and maintained, and how it is altered during development, in response to injury, and in disease. Current studies of gene regulation generally involve the evaluation of mutations in chimeric regulatory/reporter genes in transfection and transgenic experiments. While these approaches represent necessary preliminary steps, it is our contention that definitive results can best be achieved by testing such mutations in the context of the endogenous gene. Gene targeting techniques will therefore be used to create mutations in putative regulatory regions of the Collal gene in mice, and mutant mice will be evaluated for expression of the altered allele and for phenotypic changes. In particular, the proposed experiments will test the hypothesis that modular elements in the Collal gene direct the synthesis of type I collagen selectively to tissues such as skin and bone. It is anticipated that some of the mutations created in mice will generate useful models for human disorders of these tissues, specifically some of the Ehlers-Danlos syndromes and osteoporosis.

Website: http://crisp.cit.nih.gov/crisp/Crisp_Query.Generate_Screen

- **Project Title: CD40L/CD40 INTERACTIONS IN SCLERODERMA--POTENTIAL ANTI CD40L TRIAL**

Principal Investigator & Institution: Yellin, Michael J.; Columbia University Health Sciences New York, Ny 10032

Timing: Fiscal Year 2002

Summary: In this grant proposal we plan to study the role of CD154-CD40 interactions in orchestrating inflammation and fibrosis in scleroderma. Additional, we will utilize new technology to study the TCR repertoire and antigen specificity of T cells cloned from dermal lesions of patients with scleroderma. Scleroderma is an autoimmune disease characterized by endothelial cell and fibroblast activation resulting in obliterative vasculopathy and fibrosis. Antigen activated CD4+ T cells play central roles in orchestrating the inflammation and fibrosis characteristic of the disease. The identity of antigens driving the cellular immune response in tissues of patients are not known. Additionally, the T cell effector antigens driving the cellular immune response in tissues of patients are not known. Additionally, the T cell effector molecules regulating inflammation and tissue injury in scleroderma are not precisely known but it is likely that CD154 mediated signals participate in the process. In this regard, CD154 is an activation induced cell surface molecule predominantly expressed on antigen activated CD4+ T cells. The CD154 counter-receptor is CD40, expressed on a variety of cells, including endothelial cells and fibroblast. CD154-CD40 interactions play key roles in both humoral and cellular immune responses and blocking CD154 mediated signals in vivo inhibits murine models of systemic lupus erythematosis and rheumatoid arthritis. With regard to potential roles in regulating cellular immune responses, we have previously demonstrated that CD40 ligation induces endothelial cell and fibroblast activation. In more recent studies, we have demonstrated that CD154-CD40 interactions induce fibroblasts and endothelial cells to secrete prostaglandins and/or leukocyte chemoattractants. Moreover, CD154 mediated signals appear to regulate leukocyte migration in vivo because anti-CD154 mAB therapy prevents the perivascular accumulation of inflammatory cells in the murine bleomycin induced pulmonary fibrosis model. Evidence for CD154-CD40 interactions playing pathogenic roles in scleroderma is provided by our observation of infiltrating CD154+ lymphocytes in dermal biopsy specimens from patients with scleroderma. Because T cells and T cell effector molecules in particular CD154, are likely key mediators of scleroderma pathogenesis, we plan the following studies: 1) characterize the functional role of CD40 on scleroderma fibroblasts in vitro. In particular, we will determine if CD154-CD40 interactions modulate fibroblast growth, extracellular matrix production or chemokine secretion. 2) Utilize the technology provided in Core Laboratories A and B of this project to clone T cells from dermal lesions and characterize the TCR repertoire and antigen specificity of the cells. In particular, T cells will be immortalized with herpes virus saimairi (HVS). HVS immortalized cells grow indefinitely in culture and retain there antigen specificity. 3) pilot a study of anti-CD154 mAb in treating early diffuse scleroderma. We plan to study the efficacy of a humanized anti-CD154 mAb, initially developed at Columbia, in modulating the cellular performance and humoral immune responses and clinical outcome in patients.

Website: http://crisp.cit.nih.gov/crisp/Crisp_Query.Generate_Screen

- **Project Title: CHARACTERIZING MICROFIBRIL ABNORMALITIES IN SCLERODERMA**

Principal Investigator & Institution: Milewicz, Dianna M.; Associate Professor; Internal Medicine; University of Texas Hlth Sci Ctr Houston Box 20036 Houston, Tx 77225

Timing: Fiscal Year 2002; Project Start 27-SEP-1999; Project End 31-AUG-2004

Summary: Progressive fibrosis of the skin and internal organs is the pathologic hallmark of scleroderma or systemic sclerosis (SSc). The etiology of SSc is unknown but both genetic and environmental factors have been proposed. Based on the genetic evidence that defects in the gene for fibrillin-1 may contribute to the etiology of SSc, we studied the cellular metabolism and matrix incorporation of fibrillin-1 using dermal fibroblasts explanted from both Choctaw and non-Choctaw patients with SSc. These studies demonstrated that the SSc cells assembled fibrillin-1 into microfibrils, but that these microfibrils were unstable to biochemical manipulation. These preliminary results are the basis of the hypotheses to be tested in this grant proposal. We hypothesize that patients with SSc have a genetic defect that leads to degradation of fibrillin-1-containing microfibrils in tissues. The degradation of microfibrils causes release of TGF-beta from sites of sequestration in microfibrils. In addition, the release of microfibril fragments leads to an autoimmune response and the generation of antifibrillin-1 antibodies. The long-term goal of the proposed research is to understand the contribution of microfibril defects to the etiology of SSc. The specific aims are the following: (1) characterize microfibril abnormalities in fibroblast cell strains from ethnically diverse individuals with SSc and related disorders; (2) determine if fibroblast cell strains of first-degree relatives of SSc patients have microfibril abnormalities similar to those observed in the SSc patients' cells; (3) determine if the microfibrils assembled by SSc fibroblasts are turned over more rapidly, are more sensitive to proteolytic degradation, and release more microfibril fragments into the media of the cultures than microfibrils made by normal fibroblasts; (4) confirm that TGF-beta1 is associated with fibrillin-1-containing microfibrils in dermal fibroblast cultures, and determine if there is more TGF-beta1 released from the microfibrils in the cultures of SSc cells than in control cells; (5) determine if SSc patients have anti-fibrillin-1 autoantibodies in the serum and if the presence of these autoantibodies correlates with the clinical disease. The research proposed in this grant will determine the contribution of abnormalities in fibrillin-1-containing microfibrils to the activation of fibroblasts, which leads to the fibrosis that characterizes SSc.

Website: http://crisp.cit.nih.gov/crisp/Crisp_Query.Generate_Screen

- **Project Title: CHEMOKINE REGULATION OF NKT CELLS, AND ACAID**

Principal Investigator & Institution: Stein-Streilein, Joan E.; Senior Scientist; Schepens Eye Research Institute Boston, Ma 02114

Timing: Fiscal Year 2002; Project Start 01-AUG-2000; Project End 31-JUL-2004

Summary: Chemokines are associated with a variety of inflammatory and autoimmune diseases for their role in recruitment of cells to the sites of immune induction and inflammation. However, few studies have explored a role for chemokines in peripheral tolerance induction and no studies are reported for specific chemokines for NKT cells. This research plan will explore the role of specific chemokines in negative regulation of an immune inflammatory response and specifically in the recruitment of NKT cells to the site of tolerance induction. Anterior Chamber Associated Immune Deviation (ACAID) is associated with the selective negative regulation of delayed type hypersensitivity (DTH) after the introduction of antigen into the eye. An accumulation of splenic NKT cells is absolutely required for the development of ACAID. Preliminary data show that MIP-2 is associated with NKT cell recruitment. We will use molecular, cellular and morphological techniques to identify and define the role of the chemokines in the tolerance inducing process. Aim One will define the chemokine profile by RNase Protection Assay and multi-color flow cytometry. The second aim will use classic chemotaxis assays to define the migratory response of NKT cells to ACAID associated chemokines, along with molecular techniques to confirm the expression of chemokine receptors on these cells. The third aim will explore the mechanisms of chemokine-NKT cell interaction during ACAID induction by reconstituting NKT cell knockout mice with NKT cells from chemokine receptor knockout mice. A local adoptive transfer assay will measure if regulator T cells were generated. Finally, the fourth aim will explore the hypothesis that the cells recruited to the spleen for the induction of ACAID must necessarily form interactive cell clusters. After identifying such clusters and cells within, we will modulate chemokines and potential adhesion molecules and evaluate the outcome by quality and quantity of clusters. NKT cell defects and/or deficiency is associated with a variety of autoimmune disorders in both mice and humans (lupus, type 1 diabetes, systemic scleroderma). Thus, the mechanisms of NKT cell mediated induction of T regulatory cells might function in the maintenance of self tolerance in a variety of organs and tissues in addition to immune privileged sites such as the eye. The novel postulates about chemokines, innate cells and peripheral tolerance presented in this proposal, represent a heretofore totally unexplored area of research.

Website: http://crisp.cit.nih.gov/crisp/Crisp_Query.Generate_Screen

- **Project Title: CLINICAL CENTER**

Principal Investigator & Institution: Wofsy, David; Professor; University of California San Francisco 500 Parnassus Ave San Francisco, Ca 941222747

Timing: Fiscal Year 2003; Project Start 01-JUL-2003; Project End 30-JUN-2008

Summary: The University of California, San Francisco (UCSF) conducts clinical trials in a wide range of autoimmune diseases. This proposal focuses on three of these diseases (SLE, MS, and IDDM), and presents detailed descriptions of two potential clinical trials that demonstrate our interests and our ability to develop collaborative multicenter clinical trials for patients with autoimmune diseases. The two proposed clinical trials are: Protocol 1: Treatment of lupus nephritis with CTLA4Ig, a fusion protein that inhibits T cell costimulation via the CD28 pathway. This trial represents the culmination of a comprehensive bench-to-bedside research program conducted at UCSF by the PI of the Clinical Center and the PI of Project 2 in this application. The proposed trial will determine: (i) whether CTLA4Ig augments the benefit of cyclophosphamide (CTX) therapy in patients with lupus nephritis; (ii) whether CTLA4Ig can minimize the duration of therapy with CTX; (iii) whether combined therapy with CTX and CTLA4Ig can eliminate the need for maintenance therapy (induce 'tolerance'); and (iv) whether CTLA4Ig is better tolerated/safer than CTX. Protocol 2: Treatment with atorvastatin to prevent progression to MS after a clinically isolated first attack of CNS demyelination. This trial also represents a true bench-to-bedside collaboration among basic and clinical scientists involved in this application. It arose from studies by Dr. Scott Zamvil at UCSF, demonstrating that 3-hydroxy-3-methylglutaryl coenzyme A (HMG-CoA) reductase inhibitors ('statins') can prevent or reverse paralysis in murine models for MS. The proposed trial will determine whether atorvastatin can prevent progression to MS in patients at high risk for the developing the disease. Although it is not represented in this application by a detailed protocol, the Diabetes program at UCSF also has a very strong clinical trials component. The short-term goal of our clinical trials program in diabetes is to extend recent studies of anti-CD3 therapy to determine the potential of this approach to treat early IDDM and/or to prevent IDDM in people at high risk for the disease. We also are conducting trials to examine new strategies to facilitate islet transplantation. In addition to our studies in SLE, MS, and IDDM, investigators affiliated with our Center are currently conducting clinical trials in numerous other autoimmune diseases, including rheumatoid arthritis, ankylosing spondylitis, psoriatic arthritis, Sjogren syndrome, **scleroderma,** and Wegener's granulomatosis. This breadth of interests and experience at UCSF provides evidence of our ability to contribute across a broad range of potential ACE trials.

Website: http://crisp.cit.nih.gov/crisp/Crisp_Query.Generate_Screen

- **Project Title: CLONING AND FUNCTIONAL STUDIES OF PLATELET RECEPTOR FOR TYPES I AND III COLLAGEN**

Principal Investigator & Institution: Chiang, Thomas M.; University of Tennessee Health Sci Ctr Memphis, Tn 38163

Timing: Fiscal Year 2002

Summary: (provided by applicant): Ongoing microvascular injury is a hallmark of systemic sclerosis (SSc). The injury is associated with microthrombi formation secondary to platelet aggregation. One of the initial events in hemostasis is the interaction of platelets with the underlying collagen in damaged vessels. The specific mechanism of collagen induced platelet aggregation and its role in pathological thrombosis are not well understood. Recently, nitric oxide (NO) has also been reported to be involved in the collagen-platelet interactive process. The role of NO in cellular signaling has become one of the most rapidly growing areas in biology. In many instances NO mediates its biological effects including platelets. We propose 1) to define the structural features of the CIR and CIIIR that are essential for binding to CI and CIII, 2) to develop synthetic oligopeptides patterned after deduced CIR and CIIIR protein amino acid sequences that inhibit binding of CI and CIII to normal platelets and determine their effect on the binding of SSc platelets to CI and CIII. The results obtained in specific aim 1) will provide clues as to what size and amino acid sequence are most effective in blocking platelet interaction with CI and CIII, 3) to determine the functional significance of the recombinant protein and its signal transduction pathway, 4) to explore whether nitrosylation of specific platelet protein(s) occurs on tyrosine residues upon collagen platelet interaction of SSc patients and whether nitrosylation contributes stimulatory or inhibitory effects on platelet function in SSc patients and 5) to extend our assessment of the content of NOS in red blood cells of SSc patients. Binding assays will be used to determine the direct interaction of both [32PO4]-labeled rCIR and CIIIR and [125I]-labeled peptides to immobilized collagen on microtiter wells. Western blot with anti-nitrotyrsine will be used to detect platelet protein nitrusylation. The activity of NOS will be assayed with the conversion of [3H]-arginine to [3H]-citrulline. Functional studies will be performed by inhibiting both types I and III collagen-induced platelet aggregation and release reaction, by binding assay, protein phosphorylation, and flow experiments. We hope to understand more about the structure and functional significance of the platelet CIR and CIIIR. The defined reactive site(s) of CIR and CIIIR will aid in the design of active peptide(s), which could be used to modulate collagen-platelet interaction. These results will be important in understanding collagen-platelet interaction and may pave the way for the intervention of pathological thrombi formation in SSc.

Website: http://crisp.cit.nih.gov/crisp/Crisp_Query.Generate_Screen

- **Project Title: CORE--METHODOLOGY**

Principal Investigator & Institution: Tiley, Barbara C.; Medical University of South Carolina 171 Ashley Ave Charleston, Sc 29425

Timing: Fiscal Year 2003; Project Start 01-JAN-2003; Project End 31-DEC-2007

Summary: The overall objective of the Methodology Core is to provide rigorous methodological and biostatistical support to the MCRC. As specific aims the Core will provide: (1) data management; (2) statistical collaboration; (3) data and safety monitoring and (4) teaching regarding clinical research methodology.

Website: http://crisp.cit.nih.gov/crisp/Crisp_Query.Generate_Screen

- **Project Title: CORE--MOLECULAR RESOURCES LABORATORY**

Principal Investigator & Institution: Raghow, Rajendra; Professor; University of Tennessee Health Sci Ctr Memphis, Tn 38163

Timing: Fiscal Year 2002

Summary: (provided by applicant): We propose to set up a Molecular Resources Core Laboratory (MRCL) to fully support the methodologic requirements of the **scleroderma** SCOR. Thus, we envision MRCL as an efficient and economical facility equipped with specialized instruments and expertise to generate key reagents, and to continue to engage in developing state of the art techniques to facilitate the specific aims of the various sub-components of the **scleroderma** SCOR. The MRCL will be responsible for the purification, characterization and quality control of types I and III collagen and production and purification of cyanogen bromide sub-fragments of type I and III collagen. The Core will help design recombinant DNA vectors that are optimally suited to produce large amounts of wild type and site-specifically mutated 90-kDa receptor used for types I and III collagen binding on platelets. Furthermore, the MRCL personnel will collaborate with the leaders of the individual sub-projects of **scleroderma** SCOR to carry out the nucleic acid manipulations needed to quantify expression of multiple gene families. Finally, the MRCL will develop expression vectors that may be employed to produce dominant negative proteins (e.g., Smads) or antisense oligoribonucleotides in various types of mesenchymal cells. Thus, MRCL is proposed not only as a centralized resource for specialized biological reagents and equipment, but housed with a staff who will keep abreast of the newer experimental approaches of cell and molecular biology, deemed to be instrumental in successfully accomplishing the mission of the **scleroderma** SCOR.

Website: http://crisp.cit.nih.gov/crisp/Crisp_Query.Generate_Screen

- **Project Title: CORE--PATIENT RESOURCE**

Principal Investigator & Institution: Smith, Edwin A.; Medical University of South Carolina 171 Ashley Ave Charleston, Sc 29425

Timing: Fiscal Year 2003; Project Start 01-JAN-2003; Project End 31-DEC-2007

Summary: The Patient Resource Core will serve each project within the MCRC for Rheumatic Diseases in African-Americans, as well as other MCRC investigators interested in the study of **scleroderma** (SSc) and systemic lupus erythematosus (SLE). The overall objective of the Patient Resource Core is to serve MCRC investigators as a resource of patients and biological samples, upon which ongoing and future clinical research will be conducted. As specific aims the Core will: (1) facilitate the recruitment and retention of African-American patients with SSc and SLE for proposed and future clinical research projects under the umbrella of the MCRC; (2) provide MCRC investigators a source of clinically well characterized SSc and SLE patients for the performance of clinical research; and (3) serve as a repository of biological specimens (blood cells and serum, dermal and lung fibroblasts, urine and renal tissue, bronehoalveolar lavage fluid and cells) for research conducted by MCRC investigators. The availability of clinical data and biological samples for a large population of understudied African-American patients with SSc and SLE is a unique feature of this Core.

Website: http://crisp.cit.nih.gov/crisp/Crisp_Query.Generate_Screen

- **Project Title: CORE--TISSUE CULTURE LABORATORY**

  Principal Investigator & Institution: Milewicz, Dianne; University of Texas Hlth Sci Ctr Houston Box 20036 Houston, Tx 77225

  Timing: Fiscal Year 2002

  Summary: The Tissue Culture Core will prepare, store and process RNA, protein and DNA from cultured dermal fibroblasts (and keratinocytes) from patients with **scleroderma** and controls for the studies proposed in Projects 1 and 3. Epstein-Barr virus (EBV) transformed lymphoblastoid cell lines from the Choctaw SSC cases, relatives and controls also are stored here and are regrown/processed for genomic DNA as needed. This core guarantees a perpetual source of DNA (and RNA and proteins from fibroblasts) from these well characterized study patients.

  Website: http://crisp.cit.nih.gov/crisp/Crisp_Query.Generate_Screen

- **Project Title: CTGF STIMULATION OF COLLAGEN PRODUCTION IN SCLERODERMA**

  Principal Investigator & Institution: Rosenbloom, Joel; Professor; Anatomy and Cell Biology; University of Pennsylvania 3451 Walnut Street Philadelphia, Pa 19104

  Timing: Fiscal Year 2002; Project Start 20-SEP-2002; Project End 31-AUG-2004

  Summary: One of the cardinal manifestations of **Scleroderma** or **Systemic Sclerosis** (SSc) is excessive production of connective tissue matrix which impairs function in the skin and multiple internal organs. While the pathogenic mechanisms underlying this disease are complex and incompletely understood, it is likely that many of the harmful aspects with respect to connective tissue are mediated by the manifold effects of TGF-beta acting as a final common pathway. Strong evidence suggests that many of the effects of TGF-beta on fibroblast extracellular matrix may be mediated by connective tissue growth factor (CTGF) Our preliminary data demonstrate that CTGF expression by cultured SSC and normal fibroblasts is greatly stimulated by TGF-beta1 aqnd we have confirmed the presence of excess CTGF in the dermis of SSc patients by immunolocalization. We pose the following hypotheses: (1) TGF-beta stimulation of CTGF expression requires the activity of prenylated protein(s) and protein kinase C (PKC) in addition to the Smads. (2) CTGF is a major mediator of the fibroproliferative response, exerting its activity through binding to integrin cell surface receptor(s). (3) Alteration in the regulation of CTGF expression and/or its activity is a significant feature of the pathogenic fibrotic response found in SSc. In order to test these hypotheses, we propose the following aims: (1) To identify and characterize the molecular mechanisms whereby TGF-beta stimulates expression of CTGF in normal and SSC fibroblasts. (2) To define the signaling pathways whereby CTGF increases expression of collagen in normal and SSC fibroblasts. (3) To identify and characterize CTGF cis- responsive elements in the promoter of the COLIA1 gene and their cognate transacting factors. Identification of the mechanisms of action of CTGF and the pathways regulating its expression are of considerable importance, since CTGF may play a key role in the pathogenesis of SSC and blocking its abnormal production may ameliorate the most harmful features of the fibrotic response.

  Website: http://crisp.cit.nih.gov/crisp/Crisp_Query.Generate_Screen

- **Project Title: CUTANEOUS BIOLOGY OF NITRIC OXIDE**

  Principal Investigator & Institution: Lerner, Ethan A.; Associate Professor; Massachusetts General Hospital 55 Fruit St Boston, Ma 02114

Timing: Fiscal Year 2002; Project Start 30-SEP-1998; Project End 31-AUG-2004

Summary: It is proposed that nitric oxide (NO) is a critical messenger and effector molecule in skin physiology and homeostasis and that altered levels of NO in the skin cause disease. The goal of the proposal is to define the role of NO in skin with an emphasis towards determining the functional effects of this gas. Human, but not murine, keratinocytes have been demonstrated to have the capacity to express inducible form of nitric oxide synthase (iNOS) and produce NO. This critical difference between mice and men may explain why mice do not develop cutaneous eruptions analogous to those found in humans. Transgenic mice in which NOS is targeted to the skin mimic are shown here to develop phenotype found in human conditions. In conventional mice, iNOS is expressed in Langerhans cells (LC). NO is also produced by the LC-like cell line XS-52. NO produced in LC may affect LC function and, as NO is freely diffusible across cell membranes, it has the capacity to affect adjacent cells in the epidermis. Toxic effects of NO on melanocytes and keratinocytes suggest that NO may be an effector molecules in a number of skin conditions, including post-inflammatory hypo-pigmentation, vitiligo, graft versus host disease (GVH), **scleroderma** and the often fatal process, toxic epidermal necrolysis (TEN). In the proposed studies, purified LC will be evaluated for the production of iNOS using RT-PCR and measurement of NO using the Griess reaction and the conversion of radioactive L-arginine to citrulline. The effects of selected cytokines in the regulation of NOS will be examined. The effects of NO on XS-52 cells themselves will be studied. The mechanism of NO- induced killing of melanocytes and keratinocytes will be examined in co- culture experiments with XS-52 cells and via incubation with NO donors. Transgenic mice in which NOS expression is targeted to the epidermis have been produced, phenotypically develop white hair and histopathologically, **scleroderma**. These animals will be characterized further. Mice expressing NOS under the control of an inducible promoter will be generated. The transgenic mice will be tested as models for disorders of pigmentation, antigen presentation, **scleroderma,** TEN and GVH. These results have the potential to lead to novel therapeutic strategies for the treatment of human disease.

Website: http://crisp.cit.nih.gov/crisp/Crisp_Query.Generate_Screen

- **Project Title: CYTOKINE REGULATION OF RA SYNOVIOCYTE PHENOTYPE**

Principal Investigator & Institution: Ivashkiv, Lionel B.; Associate Professor; Hospital for Special Surgery 535 E 70Th St New York, Ny 10021

Timing: Fiscal Year 2002; Project Start 27-SEP-1999; Project End 31-AUG-2004

Summary: Certain pro-inflammatory cytokines, especially IL-1 and TNFalpha, are expressed in the majority of patients with RA and play an important role in pathogenesis. Important targets for pro-inflammatory cytokines are synovial fibroblasts, which proliferate, assume an invasive morphology, and invade and degrade cartilage. One striking characteristic of RA synovitis is the consistently high expression of immunosuppressive and anti-inflammatory cytokines, such as IL10 and TGF-beta, and of members of the IL-6 family of cytokines. Although IL-6-related cytokines have often been considered pro-inflammatory, more recent results suggest that they (and the downstream transcription factor Stat3) have anti-inflammatory actions on synovial fibroblasts and possibly macrophages. One major school of thought holds that the balance between pro- and anti-inflammatory factors determines the progression of disease, and that defects in the de-activation phase of inflammation play a critical role in the pathogenesis of RA. One important issue is why abundant expression of anti-inflammatory cytokines does not lead to resolution of inflammation in RA? We have explored the possibility that the anti-inflammatory actions of IL-10 and IL-6-related cytokines may be blocked in RA synovium at the level of signal transduction. We have found that IL-1, TNFalpha, and H2O2 suppress IL-6 and IL-10 activation of Stat3 DNA-binding and tyrosine phosphorylation by a mechanism that appears dependent on mitogen-activated protein kinases (MAPKs). Inhibition of Stat3 correlated with inhibition of expression of IL-6-inducible genes that have an anti-inflammatory function. We hypothesize that inhibition of IL-6 and IL-10 signaling and Stat3 activity by inflammatory factors that are present during synovitis contributes to pathogenesis by blocking de-activation of synovial inflammation. We propose to delineate the mechanisms underlying crosstalk between inflammatory/MAPK and IL-6/IL-10 Jak-STAT signaling pathways in synovial fibroblasts, and to investigate the functional consequences of this crosstalk in the context of RA pathogenesis. Greater understanding of mechanisms that block anti-inflammatory cytokine action will be helpful in designing novel therapeutic approaches to shift the balance of cytokine activity to limit inflammation and progression of disease. Our specific aims are to: (1) Identify the molecular mechanism by which the inflammatory cytokines IL-1 and TNFalpha, and ROIs, inhibit activation of Stat3 by IL-6-related cytokines and IL-10 in RA synovial fibroblasts. (2) Determine which MAPKs play an important role in inhibition of IL-6 and IL-10 signaling in RA synovial fibroblasts. (3) Characterize the functional consequences of modulation of IL-6 and IL-10 signal transduction by inflammatory factors on synovial fibroblast phenotype.

Website: http://crisp.cit.nih.gov/crisp/Crisp_Query.Generate_Screen

- **Project Title: DIFFERENTIAL GENE EXPRESSION IN SCLERODERMA FIBROBLASTS**

Principal Investigator & Institution: Korn, Joseph H.; Professor of Medicine in Rheumatology; Medicine; Boston University Medical Campus 715 Albany St, 560 Boston, Ma 02118

Timing: Fiscal Year 2002; Project Start 01-SEP-2000; Project End 30-JUN-2004

Summary: The underlying basis of **systemic sclerosis, scleroderma,** is unknown. Cultured dermal fibroblasts from **scleroderma** patients overexpress extracellular matrix components, thus retaining a feature of **scleroderma** skin in the culture model. We used differential display and hybridization to large arrays of expressed sequence tags to compare gene expression in **scleroderma** and healthy fibroblasts. Our recently published data show that protease nexin 1, a protein that regulates matrix metabolism, is expressed in **scleroderma** skin but not in skin from healthy individuals. Because protease nexin 1 is known to inhibit the activation of collagenase, and because we have shown that protease nexin 1 induces collagen transcription, we created transgenic mice containing the human protease nexin 1 cDNA in a cytomegalovirus transcription unit. Part of the current proposal is to examine these mice as a potential model of fibrotic disease. We recently found another gene with more dramatic differential expression. Hybridization to large arrays of expressed sequence tags demonstrated that heat shock protein 90 (hsp90) is overexpressed in **scleroderma** fibroblasts. Northern analysis showed that hsp90 is highly expressed in **scleroderma** fibroblasts and not detected in healthy fibroblasts. Overexpression in healthy cells or heat shock itself caused a significant increase in endogenous collagen message. Overexpression of hsp90 also causes a 3.6-fold reduction in collagenase promoter activity (MMP1). Furthermore, a specific inhibitor of hsp90, geldanamycin, obliterates TGFbeta-induced collagen transcription. Hsp90 is known as a molecular chaperone. The chaperone activity of hsp90 is essential to the normal function of the hormone receptor. TGFbeta activates a receptor system, which in turn causes phosphorylation of a cytoplasmic protein called

Smad. Phosphorylation of Smad causes its transport to the nucleus where it binds to a specific transcriptional regulatory sequence. Our recent novel finding is that hsp90 is a component of the Smad signaling complex. The second aim of this proposal is therefore to more firmly understand the overexpression of hsp90 in **scleroderma** skin. The final aim in this proposal is to define the nature of the interactions between Smad, hsp90 and related proteins in the Smad signaling complex and thus to understand how hsp90 functions in regarding TGF-beta signaling.

Website: http://crisp.cit.nih.gov/crisp/Crisp_Query.Generate_Screen

- **Project Title: EPIDEMIOLOGIC CLINICAL GENETIC FEATURES OF SYSTEMIC SCLEROSIS IN TWINS**

Principal Investigator & Institution: Wright, Timothy M.; Director; University of Pittsburgh at Pittsburgh 350 Thackeray Hall Pittsburgh, Pa 15260

Timing: Fiscal Year 2002

Summary: Systemic sclerosis (SSc) or **scleroderma** is an autoimmune connective tissue disease of unknown etiology. Twins provide a unique opportunity to assess the role of inherited vs. acquired genetic/environmental factors in disease development and provide the ideal controls for examining changes in gene expression at the tissue level. The aims of the proposed study are: (1) examination of a cohort of twins with SSc to determine concordance for disease; (2) confirmed pairs of twins with SSc (monozygotic and dizygotic, concordant and discordant) will be further analyzed by a detailed physical and laboratory examination (including cytogenetic analysis on peripheral blood and dermal fibroblasts, analysis of differential gene expression in dermal fibroblasts).

Website: http://crisp.cit.nih.gov/crisp/Crisp_Query.Generate_Screen

- **Project Title: FIBROBLAST CD 90 EXPRESSION IN FIBROGENIC SKIN DISORDERS**

Principal Investigator & Institution: Hagood, James S.; Associate Professor; Pediatrics; University of Alabama at Birmingham Uab Station Birmingham, Al 35294

Timing: Fiscal Year 2002; Project Start 01-AUG-2000; Project End 31-JUL-2003

Summary: (Taken from the application): Following skin injury, fibroblasts enter the wound, proliferate, and produce and reorganize connective tissue, restoring strength and function to the wounded site. If this process is disordered or excessive, fibrotic scarring results. Keloids and hypertrophic scars are painful and disfiguring examples. In **scleroderma,** fibrotic scarring forms in skin and other organs without prior injury, causing deformity, debilitation, and in some cases, death. The long-term goal to which the proposed research is directed is to understand how excessive fibrosis occurs and to develop new ways to prevent or treat it. Fibroblasts isolated from fibrotic tissues have many distinctive features, but it remains unclear how they acquire these features and whether all fibroblasts are equally involved. Prior investigations have defined heterogeneous features of normal rodent fibroblast subsets based on whether they express the cell surface marker Thy-1. However, to date Thy-1 expression in fibrotic states has not been explored, nor has there been correlation of expression of CD90, the human Thy-1 equivalent, with human 'fibroblast heterogeneity. We hypothesize that absence of Thy-1CD90 on the fibroblast surface correlates with a phenotype predisposed to participate in fibrotic responses, and that examination of fibrogenic lesions in human skin will demonstrate a higher proportion of fibroblasts lacking CD90 compared to normal skin. Thus, the aims of the project are: 1) to characterize fibroblast CD90 expression in hypertrophic scars. keloids, and scleroderma-affected skin in comparison to normal skin and normal scars, by immunostaining of tissue sections and cultured fibroblasts; 2) to characterize expression of type I collagen and connective tissue growth factor in sorted CD90 (-/+) and Thy-l (-/+) fibroblast populations: and to define the profile of differential gene expression in CD90 and Thv-l(-/+) subpopulations. Establishing the role of fibroblast Thy-1/CD90 expression in human fibrogenic skin diseases is likely to unlock mechanisms of fibroblast activation and lead to more effective treatments for fibrotic disorders in skin and other tissues.

Website: http://crisp.cit.nih.gov/crisp/Crisp_Query.Generate_Screen

- **Project Title: FINE SPECIFICITY OF SCLERODERMA AUTOANTIBODIES**

  Principal Investigator & Institution: James, Judith A.; Associate Professor; Oklahoma Medical Research Foundation Oklahoma City, Ok 73104

  Timing: Fiscal Year 2002; Project Start 26-SEP-2001; Project End 31-MAY-2006

  Summary: (provided by applicant): **Systemic sclerosis** (scleroderma) is a disfiguring, multi-system disease of unknown etiology, which is characterized by a broad spectrum of disease manifestations with varying organ involvement. Raynaud's phenomenon, the dysregulated vascular contraction of the terminal arteries of the circulatory system, is present in almost every case. Vascular insufficiency in these patients is associated with a vasculopathy causing tissue ischemia, which is directly linked to progressive fibrosis of specific target organs, such as the skin, lung, heart, gastrointestinal tract, and kidney. Although the underlying pathophysiology of this disorder remains an enigma, the presence of anti-nuclear antibodies in **scleroderma** patients is nearly universal. Targets of these autoantibodies include topoisomerase 1 (Scl-70), nuclear ribonucleoproteins (nRNP), centromere, PM-Scl, and Ku. Anti-topoisomerase-1 (topo-1) autoantibodies are quite specific for **scleroderma.** and are present in precipitating levels in 20-40% of patients. Anti-topo 1 is associated with diffuse skin thickening, lung involvement, and the development of lung, colon, and brain cancer. **Scleroderma** patients with anti-nRNP autoantibodies may have a more cutaneous form of the disease and universally suffer from Raynaud's phenomenon. Over the past decade we have extensively characterized the immunochemistry of lupus autoantigens. These previous studies provide the technical background for this proposal. Epitope mapping experiments of the lupus spliceosomal autoantigens have led to a peptide induced model of lupus autoimmunity. These studies have identified a potential etiological trigger and pathogenic mechanisms. We will now apply these well-honed techniques, as well as a similar scientific strategy, to analyze the humoral fine specificity of the anti-nRNP and anti-topoisomerase autoantibodies found in **scleroderma.** Preliminary data suggest a dramatic difference in the anti-nRNP response of SLE patients and **scleroderma** patients with nRNP autoantibodies. This project seeks to identify the common humoral epitopes of nRNP and topoisomerase-1 in **scleroderma** and primary Raynaud's, to describe the development of these humoral autoimmune responses over time (and with therapy), to establish potential etiological triggers of these rheumatic diseases, and to understand the role of these specific autoantibodies in **scleroderma,** disease pathogenesis.

  Website: http://crisp.cit.nih.gov/crisp/Crisp_Query.Generate_Screen

- **Project Title: GENETIC & PROTEIN STUDIES OF FIBRILLIN 1 IN SCLERODERMA**

  Principal Investigator & Institution: Tan, Filemon K.; Assistant Professor; University of Texas Hlth Sci Ctr Houston Box 20036 Houston, Tx 77225

  Timing: Fiscal Year 2002; Project Start 01-MAR-2002; Project End 28-FEB-2003

Summary: This abstract is not available.

Website: http://crisp.cit.nih.gov/crisp/Crisp_Query.Generate_Screen

- **Project Title: GENETIC ASPECTS OF PULMONARY HYPERTENSION**

Principal Investigator & Institution: Morse, Jane H.; Associate Professor of Medicine; Medicine; Columbia University Health Sciences New York, Ny 10032

Timing: Fiscal Year 2004; Project Start 23-AUG-1999; Project End 30-NOV-2007

Summary: (provided by applicant): The pathogenesis of primary pulmonary arterial hypertension (PAH) is unknown. The main goal of this project continues to be the identification of genes that cause PAH and how these genes contribute to the pathophysiology of the disease and its clinical subsets. The familial form of primary pulmonary hypertension (FPPH), inherited as an autosomal dominant disease with incomplete penetrance, was known to have a gene, PPH1 located on chromosome 2q32,33. After narrowing this large locus, our studies found mutations of bone morphogenetic protein receptor 2 (BMPR2) caused disease in 9 of 21 FPPH families. Others found BMPR2 mutations in 26% of sporadic PPH. BMPR2 mutations were also found 9% of fenfluramine appetite-associated PAH whereas no mutations were found in PAH patients with HIV-infection or with scleroderma spectrum of disease. BMPR2 mutations remain to be determined in large PAH cohorts of children and adults with anatomically large congenital pulmonary to systemic communications and with sporadic PPH. Our clinical resources include 100 FPPH families and 5 hereditary hemorrhagic telangiectasia (HHT1) families, four have mutations in activin-like receptor 1 (ALK-1), another gene associated with PPH. The identification of BMPR2 gene, a member of the TGF-B superfamly has focused the BMP/TGF-B signaling pathway for new explorations into the pathogenesis of PPH. Our newer aims will investigate the mechanism by which BMPR2 mutations cause disease, identify genetic mutations that cause disease in the 50% of FPPH cases that do not contain mutations in the exons of BMPR2, and identify DNA variations that alter the penetrance of BMPR2 mutations. We are most interested in the long C-terminal tail of BMPR2, which is unique in the TGF-B superfamily. Hopefully, these aims and the large available clinical material should provide pathophysiological information on the functional relevance of BMPR2 mutations, provide an in vitro method of BMPR2 evaluation, and provide the identification of additional risk factors and genes required for disease penetrance. Longitudinal follow of the FPPH and sporadic cases and of the HHT families should give information on the natural history of disease. The results could also define further avenues for therapeutic interventions and potentially provide in vitro models for drug testing.

Website: http://crisp.cit.nih.gov/crisp/Crisp_Query.Generate_Screen

- **Project Title: GENETIC DEFECT OF FIBRILLIN AND SCLERODERMA**

Principal Investigator & Institution: Bona, Constantin A.; Professor; Mount Sinai School of Medicine of Cuny New York, Ny 10029

Timing: Fiscal Year 2002

Summary: Tight skin (TSK) is an autosomal dominant mutation in mice characterized by excessive accumulation of type I and III collagens and glycosaminoglycans in the skin and various internal organs. The TSK mouse represents an animal model for human scleroderma because it has similar involvement of the skin and is associated with autoimmune phenomena. Recently, the TSK syndrome has been linked to a partial duplication of fibrillin-1 gene predicted to encode a 418kD polypeptide containing 948 amino acids in addition to 312kD normal protein. However, there is no formal demonstration that TSK mutation is similar to fibrillin-1 (Fbn-1) mutation. Fibrillins are constitutes of microfibrils. The production of microfibrils is increased and their structure is altered in **scleroderma** and TSK mouse. Ongoing studies carried out in the laboratory showed a high incidence of anti Fbn-1 autoantibodies in TSK/+ mice and in Choctaw Indian tribe compared to normal mice or healthy Choctaw individuals. The specific aims of the proposal are: 1. To study whether Tg mice expressing duplicated Fbn-1 gene exhibit the TSK syndrome and whether the fibroblasts express a stable fibrogenic phenotype and to determine whether injection of naked DNA expressing mutated Fbn-1 gene causes local sclerosis. 2. The preparation of characterization of Fbn-1 or elastin specific T cell clones and to study their effects on the production of extracellular matrix proteins by fibroblasts. 3. To study the presence of anti-Fbn-1 autoantibodies in Ssc and other kindred connective tissue diseases.

Website: http://crisp.cit.nih.gov/crisp/Crisp_Query.Generate_Screen

- **Project Title: GENETIC VS ENVIRONMENT IN SCLERODERMA OUTCOMES STUDY**

Principal Investigator & Institution: Reveille, John D.; Professor; University of Texas Hlth Sci Ctr Houston Box 20036 Houston, Tx 77225

Timing: Fiscal Year 2002; Project Start 01-SEP-2002; Project End 31-AUG-2003

Summary: The hypothesis to be tested in this proposal is that **systemic sclerosis** (SSC) is a more aggressive disease in non-Caucasians who manifest a higher occurrence of critical organ involvement and a worse prognosis, and that reasons for this may include both genetic factor factors as well as sociodemographic or behavioral determinants. To ascertain this we have established a multi-ethic cohort of 175 patients with SSC of relatively recent onset (<five years) deemed the GENISOS cohort (Genetics versus Environment In **Scleroderma** Outcome Study) which are following at regular intervals. Our specific aims are: 1) To continue followup of the GENISOS cohort of Caucasians, Hispanics and African Americans with SSc of five years of less duration at the University of Texas Health Science Center at Houston, the University of Texas Medical Branch at Galveston and the University of Texas Health Science Center at San Antonio in order to follow their course and outcome at regular intervals for a period of five to seven years and to enroll 80 new cases at the three centers, focusing especially on African American patients. 2) To determine the HLA class II genotypes (HLA-DRB1, DQA1, DQB1 and DPB1 alleles) as well as disease-associated alleles of other candidate genes found to be associated with SSc in ongoing studies in our Division and elsewhere (e.g. fibrillin, SPARC, and others). 3) To determine the sociodemographic parameters (income, education, insurance status) and behavioral features (illness behavior, health care utilization and attitudes, compliance) of these patients. 4) To determine pertinent clinical and laboratory parameters, including disease manifestations (e.g. extent of organ system involvement and co- morbidities), laboratory features (CBC, urinalysis, serum creatinine, serial pulmonary function tests, high resolution CT(HRCT), chest Xray and selected SSc-associated autoantibodies (anti-centromere antibodies (ACA), anti-topoisomerase I (anti-topo I), anti-fibrillin (anti-fib, etc) whose expression has been shown to e associated with specific clinical features of SSc as well as with certain HLA class II alleles. 5) To follow disease progression to outcomes manifested by: a) the development of end-stage pulmonary fibrosis (manifested by a forced vital capacity of 3.0 mg/dl not drug related; c) **scleroderma** heart disease, defined as either congestive heart failure (defined as a left ventricular ejection fraction of <40%) or malignant arrhythmias requiring therapy; d) functional disability (determined by the SF36 and the mHAQ); e) skin score; f) cumulative disease damage (as measured by the Disease Severity Scale proposed by Medsger et al (1) or death. 6) To examine how gene expression (of fibroblasts from involved and uninvolved skin and from peripheral blood leukocytes) at one point early in disease course predict disease progression (using the outcomes stated above). 7) To examine the relative contributions and interactions of genetic, demographic, socioeconomic, cultural, family history and initial and followup clinical and laboratory features on the course and outcome of early SSc through time dependent statistical analytic approaches including proportional hazard Cox-regression models and longitudinal analysis methods. By elucidating the sociodemographic, behavioral and genetic contributions to morbidity and mortality in SSC, interventions would be possible that could improve the course and outcome of this disease.

Website: http://crisp.cit.nih.gov/crisp/Crisp_Query.Generate_Screen

- **Project Title: IMMUNE MECHANISMS THAT LEAD TO IRREVERSIBLE SCLERODERMA**

Principal Investigator & Institution: Gilliam, Anita C.; Associate Professor of Dermatology; Dermatology; Case Western Reserve University 10900 Euclid Ave Cleveland, Oh 44106

Timing: Fiscal Year 2004; Project Start 01-FEB-2004; Project End 31-JAN-2009

Summary: (provided by applicant): **Scleroderma** is a chronic autoimmune disease characterized by fibrosis of organs and skin, due to upregulated synthesis of collagen by fibroblasts. There is no effective treatment for **scleroderma** to date. We are using murine sclerodermatous graft versus host disease (Scl GVHD) to model early **scleroderma**, which may be more amenable to therapy. In this model, we can generate measurable (up to 40% thicker) skin thickening within 21-28 days post bone marrow transplantation in mice with Scl GVHD. We and others have shown that in **scleroderma** and in early inflammatory Scl GVHD, the chemokine macrophage chemotactic protein-1 (MCP-1), an infiltrating monocyte/macrophage cell population and the cytokine transforming growth factor-beta TGF-beta are major players. We have also prevented murine Scl GVHD with early administration of a specific inhibitor of TGF-beta, latency-associated peptide (LAP) in vivo. In later fibrosing disease, inflammation subsides, and the fibroblasts are thought to have a permanently altered phenotype of unregulated collagen synthesis. The triggers for the switch from early reversible inflammatory disease and later noninflammatory fibrotic disease are not known. We hypothesize that the unique cutaneous environment in early inflammatory fibrosis involves cross talk between immune cells and fibroblasts. Critical fibroblast signals are required for immune cells to home to skin and become activated, and critical immune signals are required to produce an irreversible fibroblast phenotype. We plan to examine the cross talk between immune cells and fibroblasts in the following studies that are focused on cutaneous dendritic cells as initiators of the immune response, monocyte/macrophages and MCP-1. Aim 1: Immune cell studies. A. When can LAP no longer prevent or reverse skin fibrosis? This will establish "reversible" versus " irreversible" disease clinically. B. What are the effects of interventions stimulating (Fit3 ligand) or inhibiting (CTLA41g) dendritic cells, which are essential to initiate an immune response? C. What are the effects of monocyte/ macrophage interventions? Can we still generate Scl GVHD with macrophage-depleted bone marrow or by depleting macrophages in vivo after BMT? Can we generate Scl GVHD in MCP-1 knockout mice? Aim II. Fibroblast studies. A. Do cutaneous fibroblasts secrete immunomodulatory molecules (particularly MCP-1) in early inflammatory Scl GVHD? Can we inhibit fibroblast MCP-1 with interference RNA (RNAi) and block activation of immune cells and an altered fibroblast phenotype in vitro? B. What immunologic triggers are related to the excessive and persistent secretion of collagen by fibroblasts? Is SMAD dysregulation a critical event? Do clones of cells resistant to apoptosis explain the irreversible fibroblast phenotype? Are increased numbers of myofibroblasts generated in Scl GVHD that signal the onset of irreversible fibrosis? We are one of the few laboratories using this valuable model for **scleroderma.** We have the expertise in cutaneous immunobiology, and in dendritic cell and monocyte/macrophage biology. We are ideally suited to carry out this project to examine the cross talk between immune cells and fibroblasts in fibrosing disease, an entirely new and exciting area of research in **scleroderma** research. Developing more effective diagnostic tools and immunomodulatory therapies for early **scleroderma** is the ultimate goal of this research.

Website: http://crisp.cit.nih.gov/crisp/Crisp_Query.Generate_Screen

- **Project Title: IMMUNE RECOGNITION OF MODIFIED ANTIGEN IN SCLERODERMA**

Principal Investigator & Institution: Hoffman, Robert W.; Director; Internal Medicine; University of Missouri Columbia 310 Jesse Hall Columbia, Mo 65211

Timing: Fiscal Year 2002; Project Start 21-SEP-2001; Project End 31-MAY-2004

Summary: (provided by applicant): Small nuclear ribonucleoproteins (snRNP) are prominent self antigens targeted in **scleroderma** and other autoimmune conditions. The overall goal of this proposal is to characterize the role of antibodies directed against snRNP in the pathogenesis of **scleroderma.** In recent work, we have shown that patients who recognize the oxidative modified form of 70k have scleroderma-spectrum clinical characteristics. Furthermore, we have demonstrated that the lupus-associated apoptotic form of 70k is antigenically distinct from intact 70k. We hypothesize that oxidative modified 70k exposes previously cryptic epitopes, driving the development of scleroderma-associated anti-70k immune response. This proposal will seek to test this hypothesis and define the antigenetically distinct epitopes of oxidative 70k recognized by human anti-snRNP antibodies. The four Specific Aims of this proposal are: 1) identify antibodies that specifically bind at high affinity to oxidative 70k but not to native or apoptotic 70k from scleroderma-spectrum disease patient sera; 2) define the structural modification of 70k produced by metal-catalyzed oxidation that are sufficient to induce exposure of oxidative-specific 70k epitopes; 3) map oxidative-specific 70k antibody epitopes; 4) generate monoclonal anti-oxidative 70k antibodies from phage display expression libraries. To accomplish Aim 1, we will examine at least 40 sera known to have anti-70k antibodies from our large well-characterized cohort of patients using oxidative 70k and immunoblotting. Specificity will be determined in blocking studies using molar excess of either intact, apoptotic 70k or oxidative modified 70k pre-incubated prior to immunoblotting. We anticipate that we will be able to define a panel of patients with oxidative-specific antibodies. In Aim 2, we will use expression cloning and site-directed mutagenesis to define the products of 70k produced by metal-catalyzed oxidation. We anticipate that we will be able to define the sites of 70k that preferentially express oxidative-specific epitopes. In Aim 3, we will use truncation and point mutation of the 70k fusion protein, along with synthetic polypeptides and oxidative-specific 70k antibodies, to define the linear B cell epitopes on oxidative-modified 70k. We predict that these experiments will serve to define the B cell epitope on oxidative-modified 70k and anticipate that this will reside in p94-194 region of 70k. Finally, in Aim 4, we will use phage Fab expression libraries to identify antibodies that specifically bind at high affinity to oxidative 70k. We anticipate that these experiments will determine whether heavy and light chain gene usage patterns are similar between libraries generated from different patients. These Fab may then serve as valuable reagents for a series of future experiments derived directly from the work proposed.

Website: http://crisp.cit.nih.gov/crisp/Crisp_Query.Generate_Screen

- **Project Title: IMMUNOTOXICOLOGY OF A HEAVY METAL**

Principal Investigator & Institution: Pollard, Kenneth Michael.; Associate Professor; Scripps Research Institute Tpc7 La Jolla, Ca 92037

Timing: Fiscal Year 2002; Project Start 01-AUG-1996; Project End 31-MAR-2005

Summary: (Applicant's Abstract): Exposure to toxins and chemicals can produce aberrant immune reactions that may include autoimmunity. The observation that eludes explanation is the restriction of the autoantibody response to a single, or a limited number of intracellular antigens the specificity of which appears dependent in part upon the toxin or chemical involved. We have shown that the heavy metal mercury induces a genetically restricted autoantibody response in mice that targets the nucleolar protein fibrillarin. Mercury-induced cell death results in modification of the molecular properties of fibrillarin, however mercury-modified fibrillarin is a poor antigen for HgCl2-induced antifibrillarin autoantibodies. These observations suggest that mercury-modified fibrillarin might be a source of (cryptic) T cell determinants. Immunization studies with bacterial recombinant fibrillarin, modified by mercury, where not successful in eliciting the same spectrum of antifibrillarin antibodies as HgC12-treatment. Alternative antigen sources appear more promising, including fragments of fibrillarin produced following cell death associated proteolysis, and eukaryotic cellular material resulting from HgCl2-induced cell death. The investigators propose to continue to examine the immunogenicity of fibrillarin by using eukaryotic expression systems to determine if the nature of the antigen is a limiting factor in autoantibody production. This will be achieved by examination of the fine specificity of anti-fibrillarin antibodies produced by immunization, or HgCl2-treatment. Additional studies will examine the fine specificity of fibrillarin specific T cells, to determine if cryptic epitopes are important in the autoantibody response and whether immunization elicits cryptic epitope specific T cells. The importance of T cell specificity in the anti-fibrillarin autoantibody response will be determined by examining the ability of antigen specific T cells to drive B cells to produce antibody. Analysis of the interaction between fibrillarin, mercury and cells of the lymphoid system may lead to insights into how an imunotoxin renders self-antigen immunogenic.

Website: http://crisp.cit.nih.gov/crisp/Crisp_Query.Generate_Screen

- **Project Title: IMPACT OF GENETIC, SOCIODEMOGRAPHIC & BEHAVIORAL FACTORS IN SYSTEMIC SCLEROSIS**

Principal Investigator & Institution: Fischbach, Michael; University of Texas Hlth Sci Ctr San Ant 7703 Floyd Curl Dr San Antonio, Tx 78229

Timing: Fiscal Year 2002

Summary: Systemic sclerosis (SS) is an uncommon disease of uncertain etiology in which both genetic and environmental causes are postulated to play a role. However it is hypothesized that the disease is more aggressive in non-Caucasians who manifest a higher occurrence of organ involvement and a worse prognosis. The reasons for this may include genetic factors or organic or behavioral factors. At the three Texas medical centers, cohorts of Caucasians, African American, and Hispanics will be studied from early onset. The study will determine the HLA class II genotypes by DNA oligotyping and disease-associated alleles of other candidate genes found to be associated with SS;

determine the sociodemographic parameters and behavioral features of the patients; determine pertinent clinical and laboratory parameters including disease manifestations; follow disease progression to outcomes; and examine the relative contributions and interactions of genetic, demographic, socioeconommic, cultural, familial, and initial clinical and laboratory features on the course and outcome of the disease.

Website: http://crisp.cit.nih.gov/crisp/Crisp_Query.Generate_Screen

- **Project Title: INHIBITION OF COLLAGEN SYNTHESIS BY RNA INTERFERENCE**

Principal Investigator & Institution: Yoon, Kyonggeun; Associate Professor; Dermatology/Cutaneous Biology; Thomas Jefferson University Office of Research Administration Philadelphia, Pa 191075587

Timing: Fiscal Year 2002; Project Start 23-SEP-2002; Project End 31-MAY-2004

Summary: (provided by applicant): The pathological hallmark of **scleroderma** is progressive fibrosis of the skin and various internal organs caused by a deposition of excessive amount of collagen as a result of elevated production of newly synthesized collagen. To develop molecular approaches applicable for treatment of fibrotic diseases, we propose to inhibit the type I collagen synthesis using a novel strategy of gene silencing by RNA interference (RNAi). Although a double-stranded RNA (dsRNA) has specifically silenced its cognate gene in many organisms, its application to mammalian cells has been difficult due to the interferon response. With the recent discovery of small interfering RNA (siRNA), various forms of small dsRNA are now emerging as a novel class of therapeutics, which cause degradation of the target mRNA in a sequence-specific manner, thus suppressing gene expression in mammalian cells. In preliminary studies, we have shown that siRNA for the COL1A1 caused over 50% of inhibition in the Type I collagen synthesis in fibroblasts. This inhibition was specific since unrelated siRNA did not cause any decrease in the collagen synthesis. We will further evaluate several different forms of dsRNA with various lengths and sequences for their efficacy and specificity in the collagen gene silencing. Inhibition of collagen synthesis will be quantitated at mRNA and protein levels for both a1(I) and a2(I) polypeptides of the type I collagen. Once the most effective form of dsRNA is identified, we will evaluate its in vivo efficacy. RNAi gene silencing in mammalian cells is expected to be transient and to inhibit only a de novo synthesis of protein. Thus, we will utilize a skin wound-healing model that showed a transient but dramatic increase in the type I collagen synthesis. Skin is also an ideal organ for testing and developing such novel strategy, because it is accessible to administer therapeutics locally and to monitor the treated and control sites simultaneously. Several in vivo delivery methods will be developed and wounds will analyzed by molecular and histological methods. The amount of collagen in the wound area will be quantitated at mRNA and protein levels. The importance of such feasibility testing is that information gained from the skin can be extended to the treatment of **scleroderma,** a frequently fatal systemic disorder affecting not only skin, but also lungs, kidneys, and other internal organs, for which no effective treatment is available.

Website: http://crisp.cit.nih.gov/crisp/Crisp_Query.Generate_Screen

- **Project Title: INHIBITION OF COLLAGENASE STIMULATION IN SCLERODERMA**

Principal Investigator & Institution: Hasty, Karen A.; Associate Professor; University of Tennessee Health Sci Ctr Memphis, Tn 38163

Timing: Fiscal Year 2002

Summary: (provided by applicant): Our preliminary data that collagenase (MMP-1) expression in **scleroderma** (SSc) fibroblasts is inhibited even after stimulation with TNFalpha, IL-1 Beta and PMA is extremely relevant for the accumulation of collagen in this disease. Both rnRNA and protein are reduced in stimulated cells and that these phenomena are seen in the, lesion but not the non-lesion fibroblasts. We will focus on the phenotype of the **scleroderma** fibroblast in relation to the level and degree of collagenase inhibition with regard to transcriptional or translational control in SSc fibroblasts stimulated with TNF-alpha or PMA as compared to collagenase induction in normal fibroblasts, Our study of transcriptional regulation of MMP- 1 levels will investigate the level and function of AP- 1 complexes as these represent the predominant intersection of the signaling pathways of the different stimuli. We will quantitate the amount and activity of different Fos and Jun family members which have been identified in these complexes in extracts of basal and stimulated SSc and normal fibroblasts and determine their ability to bind to the two AP-1 sequences which are active in the MMP-1 promoter. We will also examine levels of the many other genes known to affect collagenase expression using DNA microarray analyses of mRNA from stimulated and unstimulated cultures of SSc and normal fibroblasts. Finally, we will address the relevancy of the observation that icIRAP is elevated in Sscby using a retroviral vector to transfect antisense for icIRAP into SSc cells. The cells will then be stimulated with TNF and PMA to determine if collagenase responsiveness is recovered (or possibly exaggerated). The mRNA for collagenase and the collagenase protein synthesized will be correlated with the amounts of icIRAP protein. Modeling of observed effects in SSc collagenase pathways will be done using normal fibroblasts transfected with retrovirus containing cDNA for icIRAP or stimulated with peptide fragments of icIRAP. The experiments should provide information for the control of collagenase expression in this disease as well as to provide information for the association of icIRAP with collagenase inhibition.

Website: http://crisp.cit.nih.gov/crisp/Crisp_Query.Generate_Screen

- **Project Title: INHIBITION OF EFFECTOR CELLS IN SCLERODERMATOUS GVHD**

Principal Investigator & Institution: Zhang, Yan; Dermatology; Case Western Reserve University 10900 Euclid Ave Cleveland, Oh 44106

Timing: Fiscal Year 2002; Project Start 01-JUN-2002

Summary: We are using murine sclerodermatous graft versus host disease (Scl GVHD) to model human **scleroderma,** an autoimmune disease of unknown etiology. In our animal model, BALB/c mice (H-2d) develop skin thickening rather than classic GVHD when transplanted across minor histocompatibility loci with bone marrow and spleen cells from B10.D2 (H-2d) mice. Based on data from the literature and our published studies, we hypothesize that TGF-beta1 producing monocyte/macrophages are the crucial effector cells in Scl GVHD, where increased TGF-beta1 leads to upregulation of proalpha1(I)collagen by fibroblasts in early disease. To test this hypothesis, we propose in Aim I to characterize cells infiltrating skin of animals with Scl GVHD in several ways: (1) by FISH analysis to determine if they are male donor or female recipient cells, (2) by immunostaining and multiparameter flow cytometry analysis with specific antibodies to monocyte/macrophages and NK cell markers to determine the predominant cell in skin, and (3) by RT/PCR analysis of sorted cells to determine which cell type is making TGF-beta, and which isoform of TGF-beta predominates (beta1, beta2, beta3). In Aim II, we will test the hypothesis by depleting or inhibiting homing to skin of monocytes and other immune cells using several strategies. The final readout is ability to prevent and reverse skin thickening. This animal model provides the unique opportunity to study monocyte/macrophage biology, basic immunology in an autoimmune fibrosing disorder, and to develop novel therapies for **scleroderma** and Scl GVHD.

Website: http://crisp.cit.nih.gov/crisp/Crisp_Query.Generate_Screen

- **Project Title:** MAPPING SCLERODERMA SUSCEPTIBILITY GENES IN THE CHOCTAW

Principal Investigator & Institution: Arnett, Frank C.; Chairperson; University of Texas Hlth Sci Ctr Houston Box 20036 Houston, Tx 77225

Timing: Fiscal Year 2002

Summary: Scleroderma or **systemic sclerosis** (SSc) is a multi-system disease with high morbidity and mortality whose etiology and pathogenesis are unknown. The pathological picture in SSc includes widespread cutaneous and visceral fibrosis, obliterative small vessel disease, and autoimmune phenomena. Increasingly, evidence is being accumulated that SSC is a complex and heterologous in which several (or many) genes interact, perhaps also with environmental factors. Identification of these genes using conventional family-based genome wide scans is made difficult by the rarity of SSc and its infrequency of familial recurrence. In this project, however, a relatively isolated and inbred human population has been identified (Choctaw Native Americans) in which SSc occurs with high frequency and displays clinical homogeneity. Having genealogically traced the origins of the affected Choctaw to common founders, microsatellite and single nucleotide polymorphism (SNP) mapping strategies in candidate gene regions are being used to identify genes relevant to SSC in this population (with extension to other ethnic groups in Project 3). Evidence is presented that fibrillin-1 (FBN1), SPARC (or osteonectin) and the MHC are genetically associated with SSC, while a large number of other candidate genes have been excluded. A genome-wide scan in the in the Choctaw using over 400 microsatellite markers and LD mapping strategies to confirm and identify candidate regions for genetic fine mapping is currently being conducted. In addition, cDNA microarrays are being used to examine gene expression in SSC fibroblasts is currently being conducted. In addition, cDNA microarrays are being used to examine gene expression in SSC fibroblasts, so as to better understand molecular pathogenesis and identify relevant genes. Thus, the overall aims of the project remain the same, namely the justification of genes predisposing to SSC susceptibility and expression. Specific aims are as follows: 1) to perform genetic fine mapping of candidate genes/regions using SNPs at high density (300 kb) with genetic analysis performed using LD mapping and case-control methods; 2) genes identified in #1 will then be tested using SNPs and SNP haplotypes in the Project 3 SSc cohort (GENISOS) of unrelated, ethnically-defined but diverse, and clinically well-characterized SSc cases, as well ethnically-matched normal controls, to determine their impact on disease susceptibility and/.or clinical and/or serological expression, and outcomes; 3) to define and compare gene expression profiles using cDNA microarrays in SSc dermal fibroblasts and other tissue (muscle, peripheral blood mononuclear cells) vs their normal counterpart tissues, especially in the context of known biochemical pathways; and, 4) explore whether SSC serum factors, especially specific autoantibodies, can induce SSC-like gene expression changes (seen in microarrays) in normal fibroblasts and endothelial cells, the likely primary target tissues resulting in the **scleroderma** phenotype. The relatively inbred and isolated Choctaw population with its extraordinary high prevalence of SSc, the well-characterized GENISOS cohort and the application of newer gene technology (SNPs and arrays) combine to afford a unique opportunity to discover genes relevant to SSC.

Website: http://crisp.cit.nih.gov/crisp/Crisp_Query.Generate_Screen

- **Project Title: MECHANISMS OF ALTERED VASOREACTIVITY IN SCLERODERMA**

Principal Investigator & Institution: Flavahan, Nicholas A.; Professor of Medicine & Physiology; Internal Medicine; Ohio State University 1960 Kenny Road Columbus, Oh 43210

Timing: Fiscal Year 2002; Project Start 01-SEP-1998; Project End 30-JUN-2004

Summary: Scleroderma (SSc) is a disease of unknown etiology associated with high mortality and morbidity. An early feature of SSc is reversible vasospasm occurring in peripheral, myocardial, renal and pulmonary circulations - Raynaud's phenomenon is present in 95 percent of cases. Small arteries/arterioles subsequently develop concentric intimal thickening and adventitial fibrosis. In preliminary studies, small dermal arteries (100-300 mu diameter) were isolated from skin biopsies of SSc patients and from age/sex-matched controls and mounted in a microperfusion system. Vascular smooth muscle of SSc arteries (clinically-uninvolved skin) demonstrated a dramatic and selective increase (300-fold) in contractile reactivity to stimulation of alpha2-adenoceptors (alpha2-ARs). Endothelial function, as assessed by NO- mediated, endothelium-dependent relaxation to acetylcholine or bradykinin, was normal. In SSc arteries from involved skin, endothelium-dependent response to bradykinin was impaired suggesting the presence of endothelial dysfunction. The hypothesis of this proposal is that an early feature of SSc is an increased reactivity of microvascular smooth muscle alpha2-ARs. This causes inappropriate and exaggerated vasoconstriction in response to physiologic stimuli (e.g. nerve stimulation, cold). The resulting cycles of ischemia and reperfusion, characteristic of SSc, leads to dysfunction of microvascular endothelial cells, promoting vascular lesion development and the extravascular complications of the disease process. To test this hypothesis, experiments will be performed on isolated dermal arteries from subjects with SSc or primary Raynaud's disease, and from age/sex matched controls. Pharmacological, biochemical and molecular techniques will be used to address 3 specific aims: 1) to determine the mechanisms(s) underlying increased responsiveness to alpha-AR stimulation in SSc, 2) to determine whether the neural regulation of SSc microvascular contraction is dysfunctional, and 3) to analyze endothelial function, and the mechanisms underlying development of endothelial dysfunction in SSc. These studies should increase our understanding of the SSc disease process and may provide a scientific basis for therapeutic intervention.

Website: http://crisp.cit.nih.gov/crisp/Crisp_Query.Generate_Screen

- **Project Title: MECHANISMS OF AUTOANTIBODY PRODUCTION IN SLE**

Principal Investigator & Institution: Reeves, Westley H.; Professor; Medicine; University of Florida Gainesville, Fl 32611

Timing: Fiscal Year 2002; Project Start 01-AUG-1991; Project End 28-FEB-2006

Summary: There is no text on file for this abstract.

Website: http://crisp.cit.nih.gov/crisp/Crisp_Query.Generate_Screen

- **Project Title: MECHANISMS OF CHRONIC GVHD INITIATION AND PATHOGENESIS**

Principal Investigator & Institution: Shlomchik, Mark J.; Associate Professor; Laboratory Medicine; Yale University 47 College Street, Suite 203 New Haven, Ct 065208047

Timing: Fiscal Year 2002; Project Start 01-MAR-2001; Project End 28-FEB-2005

Summary: (Applicant's Abstract) Allogeneic stem cell transplantation (alloSCT) is a potentially curative therapy for hematologic malignancies and inherited hematopoietic stem cell disorders. Graft vs. host disease (GVHD) is a major cause of morbidity and mortality in alloSCT. Strategies to reduce GVHD are limited because they can adversely affect graft vs. tumor stem cell engraftment, and immune reconstitution. Thus, a better understanding of GVHD is needed. GVHD has two manifestations, acute and chronic. Acute GVHD (aGVHD) is relatively well studied and treated. By comparison, chronic GVHD (cGVHD) is less well understood. Nonetheless, cGVHD is becoming an increasing problem due to longer survival of recipients, better therapy of aGVHD, the use of peripheral blood stem cells (PBSC), treatment of older patients with nonmyeloablative alloSCT, and delayed leukocyte infusions (DLI). Murine models of aGVHD involving lethal irradiation, and crossing only minor histocompatibility Ags (MiHAs) as in the most common human transplant situation, have been invaluable. However, the same has not generally been true of cGVHD. The most commonly used models are parent into Fl transplants (P to F1) and use huge doses of donor spleen cells and little or no host irradiation and no donor bone marrow. All of these are substantial deviations from the common human transplant situations. The applicant's long term goal is to understand the mechanisms of initiation and pathogenesis of cGVHD. To this end, he has further explored the lethal irradiation, MHC-matched B1O.D2 to BALB that was originally reported to have features resembling cGVHD or **scleroderma.** This model, little worked on over the last 10 yrs., may be the only known realistic model of cGVHD, although it is unclear why a chronic rather than acute syndrome ensues. One clue may be that unlike most aGVHD situations, CD4 cells rather than CD8 cells play a dominant role. Thus, the B10.D2 to BALB/c model is also an excellent one for understanding the role of CD4 cells in cGVHD. In this application the applicant plans to use this model to test key hypotheses about the initiation, maintenance and pathogenesis of cGVHD. He proposes to: 1) Determine the mechanism of antigen presentation for initiation and host tissue recognition and destruction; 2) Test the hypothesis that cGVHD is a Th2 cytokine dominated alloimmune response; 3) Test the hypothesis that host factors including genetic background and residual host T cells modulate cGVHD.

Website: http://crisp.cit.nih.gov/crisp/Crisp_Query.Generate_Screen

Project Title: MEDIATORS OF FIBROSIS IN SCLERODERMA SKIN AND LUNG

Principal Investigator & Institution: Feghali, Carol A.; Medicine; University of Pittsburgh at Pittsburgh 350 Thackeray Hall Pittsburgh, Pa 15260

Timing: Fiscal Year 2003; Project Start 30-SEP-2003; Project End 31-MAY-2007

Summary: (provided by applicant): **Systemic sclerosis** (SSc) is a connective tissue disease of unknown etiology that affects mostly women and is associated with significant morbidity and mortality. No effective therapies or cures for SSc are yet available. One of the hallmarks of SSc is overproduction of extracellular matrix components such as collagen and fibronectin by fibroblasts in the skin and internal organs. We have made the novel observation of a 20-fold increase in the expression of insulin-like growth factor binding protein 5 (IGFBP-5) in fibroblasts from the clinically affected skin of SSc patients. IGFBP-5, as well as IGFBP-3, are produced by fibroblasts and modulate the actions of IGF-I, including fibroblast activation and overproduction of collagen. We hypothesize that the IGFBP/IGF-I axis contributes to the development and perpetuation of skin and lung fibrosis in SSc. Our studies will use two unique sample sets available to us--fibroblasts and tissues from monozygotic (MZ) and dizygotic (DZ) twins discordant for SSc and from lungs of SSc patients undergoing lung transplant surgery and unused donor lungs-and target two organs affected by SSc--skin and lung. These samples constitute a unique and valuable resource. Our aims are 1) to determine the regulation of IGFBP-3 and IGFBP-5 in vitro and in vivo in skin an lung tissues of SSc patients and twin and non-twin controls; 2) to determine the function of IGFBPs on skin and lung fibroblasts and identify key molecules downstream of IGFBPs; 3) to determine the mechanism of IGFBP-mediated effects on fibroblasts, including whether the effect of IGFBPs is IGF-I-dependent or - independent, the identification of IGFBP binding partners, and the effect of suppressing IGFBP expression on the fibrotic phenotype. Our combined approach using lung and skin fibroblasts and tissues will allow us to identify the systemic mechanisms that underlie the skin and lung phenotype in SSc, while the use of samples from twins discordant for SSc will allow us to determine the importance of the inherited genetic background in the development of the 'scleroderma' phenotype. Our results will provide important insights into mechanisms of overproduction of extracellular matrix components by fibroblasts and thus the pathogenesis of fibrosis. Identifying key steps in the cascade of events culminating in fibrosis will facilitate the development of novel targeted therapies for **scleroderma** and for other fibrotic conditions.

Website: http://crisp.cit.nih.gov/crisp/Crisp_Query.Generate_Screen

- **Project Title: MENTORED PATIENT-ORIENTED RESEARCH CAREER DEVELOPMENT AW**

Principal Investigator & Institution: Robbins, Ivan M.; Medicine; Vanderbilt University 3319 West End Ave. Nashville, Tn 372036917

Timing: Fiscal Year 2002; Project Start 01-JUL-2000; Project End 30-JUN-2005

Summary: (Adapted from the applicant's abstract): PPH is a disease of high morbidity and mortality occurring predominately in young adult women. The etiology of this illness remains unknown, but increased production of thromboxane A(2) [TxA(2)] and decreased synthesis of prostacyclin [prostaglandin I] provide clues to the pathogenesis. Over the past decade, intravenous epoprostenol, the synthetic analogue of prostacyclin, has emerged as the most effective treatment of PPH. However, tolerance to the effects of epoprostenol occurs in the majority of patients necessitating progressive dose escalation to maintain efficacy. Furthermore, only 70% of patients benefit from treatment. Preliminary data derived from clinical studies of patients with PPH demonstrate that epoprostenol increases circulating levels of angiotensin II (AII), a potent vasoconstrictor and smooth muscle mitogen, which can stimulate production of both plasminogen activator inhibitor 1 (PAI- 1), a procoagulant protein, and vascular endothelial growth factor (VEGF), permeability and angiogenic growth factor. This proposal will explore two hypotheses: 1) activation of the renin- angiotensin system (RAS) during chronic administration of epoprostenol is the cause of increasing dose requirements; 2) direct and indirect effects of RAS activation and persistent TxA(2) production limit the clinical efficacy of epoprostenol. To evaluate these hypotheses, the applicant will: a) delineate the relationship between epoprostenol-induced RAS activation and compare biochemical changes with hemodynamic data obtained during right heart catheterization; b) delineate clinical data obtained from measurement of distance walked in six minutes, and structural changes obtained by wedge angiography of pulmonary circulation; and c) determine, in a collaborative study with other medical centers, whether concomitant treatment with and angiotensin converting enzyme inhibitor will improve the clinical efficacy of epoprostenol and prevent the need for chronic dose escalation. These studies will advance our knowledge of the mechanism of action of epoprostenol and pulmonary hypertension.

Website: http://crisp.cit.nih.gov/crisp/Crisp_Query.Generate_Screen

- **Project Title:** MODULATION OF AUTOREACTIVE B CELL REPERTOIRE IN SCLERODERMA BY IVIG

  Principal Investigator & Institution: Vazquez-Abad, Dolores; University of Connecticut Sch of Med/Dnt Bb20, Mc 2806 Farmington, Ct 060302806

  Timing: Fiscal Year 2002

  Summary: This abstract is not available.

  Website: http://crisp.cit.nih.gov/crisp/Crisp_Query.Generate_Screen

- **Project Title:** NEUROHORMONAL ACTIVATION IN PULMONARY HYPERTENSION

  Principal Investigator & Institution: Kawut, Steven; Medicine; Columbia University Health Sciences New York, Ny 10032

  Timing: Fiscal Year 2002; Project Start 01-SEP-2001; Project End 31-AUG-2006

  Summary: Candidate's Plans/Training: The candidate plans a career as an independent clinical investigator focusing on patient-oriented research related to pulmonary vascular disease. Training will include formal epidemiological course work in clinical research and closely mentored completion of the research protocol. Environment: The Center for Clinical Epidemiology and Biostatistics (CCEB) will provide formal coursework and structured mentoring. The CCEB, Pulmonary Vascular Disease Program, and General Clinical Research Center at the University of Pennsylvania Medical Center will provide research support. Research: Primary pulmonary hypertension (idiopathic) and secondary pulmonary hypertension (associated with portal hypertension, anorectic use, HIV, **scleroderma**, and other collagen vascular diseases) cause substantial morbidity and mortality. Although there are available therapies and interventions, they may be costly and risky in themselves. In addition, targeting therapy at the mechanism of morbidity and mortality and distinguishing highrisk patients have been suboptimal. There is evidence that certain vasoactive substances may play an important role in the disease process of pulmonary arterial hypertension. Studies have documented elevated levels of endothelin, natriuretic peptides, and norepinephine in patients with this disease. It is well known that these neurohormones play important mechanistic and predictive roles in left-sided heart failure. Similarly, there is much potential for these neurohormone levels in determining 1) the mechanism of disease and 2) the prognosis in pulmonary arterial hypertension. We propose an investigation of patients with pulmonary arterial hypertension to examine whether levels of these biomarkers at baseline and at six month follow-up are associated with right-sided heart failure and cardiovascular death. We will formulate prediction rules using neurohormone levels and clinical variables to improve prognostication and management in this disease.

  Website: http://crisp.cit.nih.gov/crisp/Crisp_Query.Generate_Screen

- **Project Title:** NIAMS CLINICAL RESEARCH CENTER FOR RHEUMATOID DISEASE

  Principal Investigator & Institution: Silver, Richard M.; Professer; Medicine; Medical University of South Carolina 171 Ashley Ave Charleston, Sc 29425

  Timing: Fiscal Year 2003; Project Start 15-APR-2003; Project End 31-MAR-2008

  Summary: (provided by applicant): The Medical University of South Carolina will establish a Multidisciplinary Clinical Research Center (MCRC) for the Study of

Rheumatic Diseases in African-Americans. This MCRC will focus on **scleroderma** (SSc) and systemic lupus erythematosus (SLE), two rheumatic diseases that disproportionately affect the African-American community. Outstanding leadership in three key areas - Rheumatology, Biometry/Epidemiology, and Health Services Research - provides a framework for successful design and implementation of meaningful clinical research in this understudied population of patients. Three projects and three supporting cores are proposed. Project A is designed to study the interactions between TGF-beta and sphingolipid signaling pathways in SSc and normal fibroblasts. The proposed studies will elucidate this heretofore-unknown interaction to shed light on the mechanism whereby TGF-beta signaling is integrated with other cellular signaling pathways leading to fibrosis. Project B addresses an important understudied area, namely psychosocial aspects of female adolescents with SLE, the majority of whom are African-American. MCRC investigators will assess the associations between adaptational processes and adjustment and health-related quality of life, and will conduct an interventional trial designed to enhance adjustment and quality of life for these patients. Project C will address the important issue of divergent racial trends in morbidity from lupus nephritis. Mortality has increased for African-American lupus patients while remaining stable in Caucasian lupus patients, and this divergence cannot be accounted for by differences in socioeconomic status alone. Utilizing the unique resources of the Carolina Lupus Study and the sea island Gullah population, MCRC investigators will address genetic and environmental influences on the development and progression of lupus nephritis. Each of these projects, as well as future pilot projects to be developed by the MCRC, will be served by two Cores: (1) a Methodology Core will provide rigorous methodological and biostatistical support; and (2) a Patient Resource Core will assure MCRC investigators access to a population of African-American patients who are clinically well characterized and from whom biological samples are obtained and stored. This MCRC will facilitate the translation of basic research into the clinical arena, support much needed behavioral research, and conduct epidemiology and health services research on rheumatic diseases affecting minorities and women disproportionately, thus exemplifying the "cross-cutting" nature of research proposed in NIAMS's strategic plan.

Website: http://crisp.cit.nih.gov/crisp/Crisp_Query.Generate_Screen

- **Project Title: NIAMS MULTIDICIPLINARY CLINICAL RESEARCH CENTER IN CINC***

Principal Investigator & Institution: Glass, David N.; Professor of Pediatrics and Director; Children's Hospital Med Ctr (Cincinnati) 3333 Burnet Ave Cincinnati, Oh 45229

Timing: Fiscal Year 2002; Project Start 01-SEP-2001; Project End 30-JUN-2006

Summary: OF THE OVERALL PROGRAM: (Taken from the application) This proposal from the Children's Hospital Medical Center in Cincinnati has the goal of impacting a clinical practice as it is applied to the most common rheumatic diseases of childhood. This proposal also represents in part the competing renewal for the Centers existing P60 MAMDC and is complimentary to the P30 Cincinnati Rheumatic Diseases Core Center submitted earlier this year. It is estimated that 140,000-200,000 children within the United States have rheumatic disease, many, but not all, of which are autoimmune. The major diseases are juvenile rheumatoid arthritis, systemic lupus erythematosus, **scleroderma** and juvenile dermatomyositis. Of increasing impact are illnesses with regional and generalized musculoskeletal pain syndromes of which fibromyalgia is particularly common and appears to be increasing in frequency and can present a major management problem. The five components of the Center are: A methods core interacting with all projects; A trial of etanercept in juvenile dermatomyositis; A study of psychological status in juvenile onset fibromyalgia; An imaging study using quantitative T2 mapping JRA; Methotrexate pharmacogenomics in JRA. In addition, there is an administrative unit which will exercise operational control and administrative oversight of all the projects through an executive committee, two Advisory Boards and a Community-Based Board of Directors. The short- and long-term goals are to improve the health of children with these conditions and to better ensure a smooth transition from childhood and adolescence through to young adulthood for the child with a chronic rheumatic disease.

Website: http://crisp.cit.nih.gov/crisp/Crisp_Query.Generate_Screen

- **Project Title: NUCLEAR PATHWAY FOR MESSENGER RNA DEGRADATION IN YEAST**

Principal Investigator & Institution: Butler, James S.; Associate Professor; Microbiology and Immunology; University of Rochester Orpa - Rc Box 270140 Rochester, Ny 14627

Timing: Fiscal Year 2002; Project Start 01-AUG-1999; Project End 31-JUL-2004

Summary: The biogenesis of mature eukaryotic RNA molecules requires posttranscriptional processing reactions that produce stable and functional mRNAs, rRNAs, snRNAs and tRNAs. Each of these RNA processing reactions provide targets for the regulation of gene expression, and thereby help to guide the proliferation and development of cells. Research into these RNA processing pathways has revealed steps within each that are used to regulate the rates of mature RNA production, yet little is known about how these RNA processing pathways are co-regulated to produce balanced levels of mature RNAs in response to changes in the cell's intracellular and extracellular environment. This proposal focuses on the roles of nuclear proteins implicated in the regulation of poly (A)+ mRNA and rRNA levels in S. cerevisiae. The yeast protein Rrp6p is a nuclear riboexonuclease homologous to an autoantigen produced in patients suffering from Polymyositis **Scleroderma** Overlap Syndrome (PM-Sc1), as well as to the Werner's and Bloom's syndrome proteins implicated in premature aging. Mutations in Rrp6p cause defects in rRNA processing and ribosome biogenesis. Rrp6p also plays a role in a nuclear mRNA degradation pathway, since loss of its function stabilizes an intermediate in the mRNA polyadenylation pathway. The experiments proposed here seek to determine the biochemical mechanism and physiological function of Rrp6p. The relationship of Rrp6p to other proteins will be determined using affinity purification and genetic techniques. Other proteins, whose connection to Rrp6p stems from our studies, include core components of an RNA processing complex called exosome, a subunit of RNA polymerase III and a riboexonuclease implicated in rRNA processing and mRNA nucleocytoplasmic transport. Rrp6p will be studied as a pure protein and complexed with its interacting partners. These studies will be carried out to determine which domains of Rrp6p are required for its ability to bind and hydrolyze RNAs, as well as which domains are required to interact with other proteins. The substrate specificity of Rrp6p will also be analyzed to determine what features of its RNA substrates are required for recognition by the enzyme and what features of the enzyme and its substrates are necessary for its ability to distinguish between mRNAs and rRNAs. These studies will illuminate the enzymatic properties of Rrp6p, as well as its role in nuclear mRNA degradation and rRNA processing. Moreover, the results of these experiments should provide basic knowledge regarding the functions of the PM-Sc1 autoantigens and the Bloom's and

Werner's syndrome proteins, thereby contributing to an understanding of the processes leading to autoimmune disease and aging.

Website: http://crisp.cit.nih.gov/crisp/Crisp_Query.Generate_Screen

- **Project Title: ORAL CYCLOPHOSPHAMIDE VS ORAL PLACEBO IN SSC ALVEOLITIS**

Principal Investigator & Institution: Read, Charles; Medicine; Georgetown University Washington, Dc 20057

Timing: Fiscal Year 2002; Project Start 10-AUG-1999; Project End 30-JUN-2004

Summary: In **Systemic Sclerosis** (SSc), interstitial pulmonary fibrosis is frequent (80%) and is now the leading cause of death. The mortality rate of patients with a forced vital capacity (FVC) 2.0% eosinophils in BAL fluid. Secondarily, we will assess the impact of CYC on quality of life (SF36), functional activity (SSc Health Assessment Questionnaire), dyspnea (Mahler Transition Dyspnea Index) and diffusing capacity for carbon monoxide (DLCO) in these patients. Patients will be recruited for study during the first 3 years (from 6 mos. to 2 yrs, 9 mos) of the 5-year project period. Randomized participants will be treated with study drug for 1 year and followed at 3-month intervals for 2 years. Overall study coordination and data collection, management and analysis will be centralized at UCLA. Proven methods for analyzing time-oriented data employed by the investigators in previous controlled studies of **scleroderma** will be used to evaluate whether oral CYC (1-2 mg/kg/day) is better than placebo a) in improving or preventing worsening of FVC (the primary outcome variable) and b) in improving or preventing worsening of quality of life, functional ability, breathlessness and DLCO (secondary outcome variables).

Website: http://crisp.cit.nih.gov/crisp/Crisp_Query.Generate_Screen

- **Project Title: PATHOGENESIS OF MARFAN SYNDROME AND RELATED DISORDERS**

Principal Investigator & Institution: Sakai, Lynn Y.; Associate Professor; Biochem and Molecular Biology; Oregon Health & Science University Portland, or 972393098

Timing: Fiscal Year 2002; Project Start 01-MAR-2001; Project End 28-FEB-2005

Summary: (from applicant's abstract): Mutations in FBN1 result in the pleiotropic cardiovascular, skeletal, and ocular phenotypic features of the Marfan syndrome as well as in several of the individual phenotypic features of the Marfan syndrome in isolation, such a isolated aortic aneurysm, isolated ectopia lentis, and isolated tall statures. Mutations have also been found in Shprintzen-Goldberg syndrome and the MASS phenotype, and FBN1 has been implicated in Weill-Marchesani syndrome, pseudoexfoliation of the lens, and **scleroderma**. More than 200 different mutations in FBNI have bee identified. Mutations in FBN2 have been identified in individuals with congenital contractural arachnodactyly, disorder affecting skeletal but usually not ocular or cardiovascular tissues. With the notable exception of the mutations causing "neonatal" Marfan syndrome, efforts correlate genotype with phenotype been unsuccessful. In this application, two potential mechanisms by which mutations in fibrillins may result in disease are proposed. In the first case, mutant fibrillin molecules would create weak spots in all microfibrils; over time, microfibrils, which are normally very long, would be fragmented into short microfibrillar pieces, precipitating a cascade of events leading to the development of disease. A second possible mechanism is based on the hypothesis that some mutations in fibrillins will inhibit assembly of microfibrils. In this case, most of the microfibrils will be short, and severe early onset disease is predicted. Specific aims are proposed to test these mechanisms of disease pathogenesis. In the first specific aim, novel "coculture assay" will be utilized to precisely define domains in fibrillins required for assembly of microfibrils. In this assay, effects of epitope-mapped monoclonal antibodies will be monitored, and cells transfected with both wildtype and mutant constructs will be tested. In the second specific aim, in order to test whether the results obtained in the first specific aim hold within the context of full-length fibrillin, fibrillin constructs containing selected mutation will be overexpressed in cells which assemble overexpressed wildtype fibrillin into fibrils. In addition, selected mutant constructs will be tested for protease susceptibility in comparison to analogous wildtype constructs.

Website: http://crisp.cit.nih.gov/crisp/Crisp_Query.Generate_Screen

- **Project Title: PATHOPHYSIOLOGY OF CUTANEOUS VASCULAR LESIONS**

Principal Investigator & Institution: Arbiser, Jack L.; Assistant Professor; Dermatology; Emory University 1784 North Decatur Road Atlanta, Ga 30322

Timing: Fiscal Year 2002; Project Start 15-SEP-1998; Project End 31-AUG-2004

Summary: This Career Development Award Proposal focuses on the pathogenesis of cutaneous vascular lesions. Hemangiomas are the most common cutaneous vascular lesions of childhood, and are present in 10 percent of infants at 1 year of age. These hemangiomas may grow to large size, resulting in compression of vital structures, high output cardiac failure, and coagulopathy. The coagulopathy phenomenon is known as the Kasabach- Merritt syndrome. Treatment of large hemangiomas requires lengthy treatment with steroids or alpha interferon, and surgery. A significant number of these hemangiomas do not respond to treatment, resulting in death. Little is known of the pathophysiology of these lesions, but preliminary evidence points to an imbalance of angiogenesis stimulators and inhibitors. We have developed a murine model of proliferative vascular lesions through the sequential introduction of SV40 large T antigen and H-ras into endothelial cells. This model recapitulates clinical and histologic features of both nonproliferative and proliferative hemangiomas. I wish to study the signal transduction pathways involved in upregulation of angiogenesis stimulators and downregulation of angiogenesis inhibitors. In addition, I have found that transformed endothelial cells express both VEGF and its receptor, flk-1, suggesting a possible autocrine loop. Finally, the novel angiogenesis inhibitor endostatin has been isolated from a spontaneous hemangioendothelioma cell line. Its mechanism of action is unknown. I hope to learn the signal transduction pathways through which endostatin mediates angiogenesis inhibition. Interruption of angiogenic autocrine loops and targeting of signal transduction pathways activated in proliferative vascular lesions may provide novel therapies for hemangiomas. The Folkman laboratory has extensive experience in the isolation and characterization of angiogenesis stimulators and inhibitors. In order to become an independent investigator in angiogenesis, proficiency in these techniques is necessary. The opportunity to carry out the studies outlined in this proposal and receive formal training in cell biology, protein purification and characterization, and surgical procedures will afford the applicant the training which is required toward the establishment of his career as an independent physician-scientist.

Website: http://crisp.cit.nih.gov/crisp/Crisp_Query.Generate_Screen

- **Project Title: PERSISTENT FETAL CELLS IN THE IMMUNOPATHOGENESIS OF SSC**

Principal Investigator & Institution: Artlett, Carol M.; Medicine; Thomas Jefferson University Office of Research Administration Philadelphia, Pa 191075587

Timing: Fiscal Year 2002; Project Start 15-AUG-1998; Project End 30-JUN-2003

Summary: (Adapted from the applicant's abstract) - SSc is a disease of unknown origin with the highest incidence occurring in females predominantly after child-bearing years. Recent research has revealed that fetal cells can survive in the maternal circulation for many years. Graft-versus-Host Disease (GVDH) has many similar clinical features to SSc although no evidence for GVHD in SSc has been identified. This investigator has identified by PCR and fluorescence in-situ hybridization (FISH) the presence of Y chromosome nucleated cells in 58% of skin biopsies from active lesions in patients with SSc and 46% of peripheral blood tested of female SSc patients. The investigato hypothesizes that these cells have become activated and have established a GVHD-like response in some female SSc patients. The investigator proposes in the current studies to identify and characterize the fetal cells in frozen and paraffin-embedded section of affected lung, skin, and kidneys in patient with early disease by a combination of magnetic cell sorting, immunophenotyping, and FISH. In addition, she proposes to examine the pattern of cytokine expression of the fetal cells in histologic sections and to isolate, clone, and expand Y chromosome nucleated cells from active lesions. She will also investigate whether expanded lymphocytes from the active lesion can induce Type I collagen mRNA in normal fibroblasts. The studies proposed in this application will identify and functionally characterize the Y chromosome positive cells found in the active lesion of SSc women. Obviously, the aims of this proposal cannot address the pathogenesis of SSc occurring in males, or in woman who have not had recognized pregnancies or male offspring.

Website: http://crisp.cit.nih.gov/crisp/Crisp_Query.Generate_Screen

- **Project Title: PHOSPHORYLATION OF LUPUS AUTOANTIGENS IN APOPTOSIS**

Principal Investigator & Institution: Utz, Paul J.; Medicine; Stanford University Stanford, Ca 94305

Timing: Fiscal Year 2002; Project Start 01-APR-1998; Project End 31-MAY-2003

Summary: The broad, long-term objective of this proposal is to characterize a recently identified serine kinase activity that is responsible for phosphorylating seven autoantigens during apoptosis. Recent studies have demonstrated that some autoantigens undergo posttranslational modifications such as proteolytic cleavage and phosphorylation during apoptosis, and it is hypothesized that these and other modifications allow these proteins to bypass or overcome normal mechanisms of tolerance, contributing to the production of autoantibodies. Kinase cascades play critical roles in important cellular functions such as cell cycle regulation and receptor-mediated signalling, and protein phosphorylation has been directly implicated in the regulation of apoptosis. There are two specific aims of this proposal: i.) To identify autoantigens that are phosphorylated during apoptosis using combined biochemical and antibody affinity purification techniques; and ii.) To characterize and identify the kinase that phosphorylates the substrates identified in the first specific aim. In the later years of the proposal, cDNAs encoding the kinase will be expressed in mammalian cells, and the effects of the kinase on programmed cell death pathways using several complementary assays will be addressed. Once achieved, this system will be utilized to screen known serine kinase inhibitors for their ability to block autoantigen phosphorylation, with the long- term goal to better understand the mechanisms underlying autoantibody production. The results of this proposal may prove useful in drug screening and rational drug design for treatment of diseases including SLE, Sjogren's disease and **scleroderma**. This award will be instrumental in preparing the candidate for a career as a clinician-scientist in the field of autoimmune disease. The proposal includes attendance at several basic science courses directly related to the field, and acquisition of expertise in several new techniques including molecular cloning, library screening, biochemical purification, and protein expression. Dr. Anderson and members of an Advisory Committee will provide hands-on training in performance of the techniques and interpretation of the results. The commitment of Dr. Anderson and the Division to the applicant's development as a fully independent investigator, together with the rich intellectual environment provided by Harvard Medical School and Brigham and Women's Hospital, make this an ideal environment in which to complete this proposal.

Website: http://crisp.cit.nih.gov/crisp/Crisp_Query.Generate_Screen

- **Project Title: PILOT INVESTIGATION OF THE SAFETY AND EFFICACY OF THALIDOMIDE IN SCLERODERMA**

Principal Investigator & Institution: Oliver, Stephen J.; Rockefeller University New York, Ny 100216399

Timing: Fiscal Year 2002

Summary: Scleroderma is a connective tissue disease of unknown etiology characterized by excessive fibrosis of the skin and visceral organs. **Scleroderma** patients have not responded to traditional immunosuppressive and anti-inflammatory regimens, and the majority of these patients experience progressive disease with marked morbidity and mortality. Chronic graft versus host disease that occurs in bone marrow transplant patients shares many characteristics with **scleroderma.** In addition, recent reports have suggested that maternal-fetal exchange of cells across placental membranes and persistent microchimerism may contribute to **scleroderma** pathogenesis. The drug thalidomide, previously known for its teratogenic effects in the early 1960's, has since been found to have anti-inflammatory and immune-modulating effects in a number of immune mediated diseases, including graft-versus-host disease. Furthermore, preliminary studies suggest that the conventional treatment of graft-versus-host disease, cyclosporin A, may be effective in treating **scleroderma.** Thalidomide use has not been reported in **scleroderma** patients. This pilot study will obtain preliminary data on the safety and tolerability of thalidomide in **scleroderma** patients by establishing baseline clinical and serological profiles of patients and then follow those parameters during daily exposure to thalidomide over an initial dose escalation course over 12 weeks, with continued maintenance therapy for up to one year.

Website: http://crisp.cit.nih.gov/crisp/Crisp_Query.Generate_Screen

- **Project Title: PKC SIGNALING IN THROMBIN-ACTIVATED LUNG FIBROBLASTS**

Principal Investigator & Institution: Bogatkevich, Galina S.; Medicine; Medical University of South Carolina 171 Ashley Ave Charleston, Sc 29425

Timing: Fiscal Year 2002; Project Start 20-MAY-2002

Summary: (provided by applicant):Scleroderma (systemic sclerosis, SSc) is an autoimmune, connective tissue disease characterized by microvascular injury and fibrosis, affecting 250,000 people (mostly women) in the USA. A leading cause of death in **scleroderma** patients is pulmonary dysfunction as a result of progressive interstitial lung fibrosis. It is postulated that activated fibroblasts (myofibroblasts) are involved in the pathogenesis of lung fibrosis. One mediator of lung fibroblast activation is thrombin, a multifunctional serine protease and G-protein coupled receptor ligand, which is generated immediately at sites of vascular injury. Recently we observed that exposure of normal cultured human lung fibroblasts to thrombin induces the myofibroblast phenotype. This change to an SSc phenotype occurs via protein kinase C epsilon (PKC-e) signal transduction. These observations open an interesting avenue in the investigation of the pathogenesis of SSc. Our overlying hypothesis is that thrombin triggers distinct PKC signaling mechanisms in normal and SSc lung fibroblasts. Specificity of the responses mediated in these two cell types can be explained by interaction of PKC with specific anchoring proteins. Better understanding of the mechanisms of these interactions may provide a useful target for novel therapeutic interventions in **scleroderma** lung disease, for which no proven, effective therapy exists.

Website: http://crisp.cit.nih.gov/crisp/Crisp_Query.Generate_Screen

- **Project Title: PKCEPSILON-RELATED PROTEINS IN LUNG FIBROSIS**

Principal Investigator & Institution: Hoffman, Stanley R.; Associate Professor of Medicine and Cell; Medicine; Medical University of South Carolina 171 Ashley Ave Charleston, Sc 29425

Timing: Fiscal Year 2003; Project Start 01-SEP-2003; Project End 31-AUG-2007

Summary: (provided by applicant): This RFA asks investigators to identify novel targets that play a role in fibrogenesis, then to validate that altering the expression or function of targets does indeed inhibit pulmonary fibrosis. We already have identified a set of interconnected novel targets and have partially validated one target. Our central target is the e isoform of protein kinase C (PKC-epsilon). Cells cultured from the fibrotic lung tissue of **scleroderma** patients have altered PKC-epsilon signaling. The extracellular matrix protein tenascin is overexpressed in **scleroderma** lung fibroblasts due to altered PKC-epsilon signaling. Altered PKC-epsilon signaling is also revealed by the facts that: 1) Curcumin, from the Indian spice turmeric, inhibits collagen expression in **scleroderma** lung fibroblasts then causes the cells to undergo apoptosis while normal lung fibroblasts are unaffected by curcumin; and 2) **Scleroderma** lung fibroblasts can be made curcumin-resistant by PKC-epsilon overexpression while PKC-epsilon depletion makes normal cells sensitive to curcumin. Moreover, three "binding partners" for PKC-epsilon (calponin, caveolin- 1, and RACK2) have altered levels of expression and subcellular localizations in **scleroderma** lung fibroblasts. The overexpression of tenascin and calponin in vivo has been confirmed in sections of lung tissue from **scleroderma** patients. Based on these observations, we will test the hypothesis that altering the expression or function of PKC-epsilon, of tenascin, or of binding partners for PKC-epsilon will inhibit pulmonary fibrosis. Experiments will be performed using: 1) Cultured lung fibroblasts from **scleroderma** patients and matched normal subjects and 2) Mice in which lung fibrosis in induced using bleomycin. Specifically we will: 1) Optimize the delivery of potential treatments via lentivirus into the lungs of mice. 2) Perturb PKC-epsilon expression and function using curcumin, using virus that enhance or inhibit PKC-epsilon expression, and using a peptide that blocks PKC-epsilon translocation and function. These experiments will include a determination of why **scleroderma** fibroblasts are particularly sensitive to curcumin. 3) Perturb the expression of PKC-epsilon binding partners using virus. 4) Inhibit tenascin expression using virus and test the idea that tenascin is a downstream mediator of the effects observed when PKC-epsilon expression is manipulated. The effects of these perturbations will be read out in terms of collagen expression and curcumin-induced apoptosis in cell cultures and in terms of survival, lung tissue morphology, and collagen levels in bleomycin-treated mice. These approaches will allow us to validate the role in lung fibrosis of the several target proteins that we have already identified.

Website: http://crisp.cit.nih.gov/crisp/Crisp_Query.Generate_Screen

- **Project Title: PREGNANCY, MICROCHIMERISM AND AUTOIMMUNE DISEASE**

Principal Investigator & Institution: Nelson, J Lee.; Professor; Fred Hutchinson Cancer Research Center Box 19024, 1100 Fairview Ave N Seattle, Wa 98109

Timing: Fiscal Year 2002; Project Start 01-JUL-1997; Project End 31-MAY-2006

Summary: In the prior grant period we investigated the hypothesis that persistent fetal microchimerism contributes to the pathogenesis of autoimmune disease. In studies of women with **systemic sclerosis** (SSc) we found that parous women had significantly greater levels of persistent fetal microchimerism compared to healthy parous controls. Fetal microchimerism was not uncommon, however, among healthy women. Fetal microchimerism was detected in immune competent peripheral blood cellular subsets in women with SSc and also in healthy women. The simple presence of persistent fetal cells is therefore not necessarily detrimental to the host. However, the hypothesis we proposed to test is that non-host cells contribute to autoimmune disease in the context of particular HLA alleles and HLA-relationships of host and donor cells. We found a nine-fold increased risk of SSc in women who had previously given birth to a child who was compatible for HLA-DRB1. Because cell traffic is bi-directional during pregnancy, and maternal cells can also persist in her progeny, women are uniquely potential recipients of microchimerism across generations. We found that HLA-DRB1 compatibility of the patient's mother from the perspective of her child was also associated with increased risk of SSc. T lymphocytes are implicated in the pathogenesis of SSc. Persistent fetal microchimerism among T lymphocytes was associated with specific HLA alleles of the mother and even more so of her child. Because significant findings were consistently greatest for the DRB1 locus, results point to the DRbeta1 molecule, and/or peptides derived from DRbeta1 as important to the interaction of host and non-host cells. The first aim of the current proposal is to define the role of HLA-relationships over three generations in risk of SSc in parous women. The second aim will evaluate familial HLA-relationships and HLA alleles in nulligravid women, children, and men who can also develop SSc. Specific Aim 3 studies will exploit Real-Time PCR techniques to quantitatively assess fetal microchimerism in the peripheral blood of parous women. Specific Aim 4 will quantitatively determine fetal microchimerism in immunologically active cellular subsets. Cell surface expression of candidate molecules that could interfere with maternal immune recognition will also be tested. Studies of Specific Aim 5 will provide a functional context from which to correlate results of prior aims. Artificial antigen presenting cells will be made and a T cell capture assay used to investigate T cells that respond to disease associated HLA-DR molecules/peptides. Women are disproportionately affected by autoimmune diseases. The current studies are designed to examine a long-term immunologic consequence of pregnancy. If, within the context of HLA-DRB1 compatible relationships and particular HLA alleles, persistent fetal microchimerism contributes to the pathogenesis of SSc, new therapies could be developed for this difficult disease.

Website: http://crisp.cit.nih.gov/crisp/Crisp_Query.Generate_Screen

- **Project Title: PSYCHOSOCIAL INTERVENTIONS FOR SCLERODERMA**

Principal Investigator & Institution: Haythornthwaite, Jennifer A.; Associate Professor; Psychiatry and Behavioral Scis; Johns Hopkins University 3400 N Charles St Baltimore, Md 21218

Timing: Fiscal Year 2002; Project Start 01-AUG-2000; Project End 31-JUL-2004

Summary: (adapted from investigator's abstract): **Systemic sclerosis** (scleroderma: SSc) is a rare, disfiguring connective tissue disease characterized by inflammation vascular injury, and fibrosis. Despite the significant physical disability, pain, disfigurement, negative prognosis, and lack of a cure associated with SSc, no psychosocial interventions have been developed and tested to guide these individuals in managing the daily challenges of living with a chronic illness and improving the quality of their lives. The proposed research will examine the efficacy of two psychological interventions designed to target important areas of daily living: pain, depression, and distress about disfigurement (Specific Aim #1). Individual differences in treatment outcome will be examined by determining whether clinical depression predicts the effects of professionally guide self-help materials (Specific Aim #2). Since psychological interventions requiring a trained professional can be costly and are often not available to the majority of patients, professional involvement in the proposed interventions will be minimal. Two hundred and one patients with **systemic sclerosis** who report symptoms of pain, depression, or distress about disfigurement will be recruited and randomized to one of three interventions: individual cognitive-behavioral therapy, self-help cognitive-behavioral intervention facilitated by a Psychologist, or a disease/health education intervention. Measures of pain, functioning, distress about disfigurement, and mood will be collected at baseline and following the 8-week intervention period by an individual blind to intervention assignment. Both the cognitive-behavioral self-help materials and the educational materials (8 written chapters and audiotapes) will be designed for home use but will be supplemented by individual sessions (2) and telephone contacts (2) with the professional. Patients will be followed for one year after completing the active intervention phase (Specific Aim #3). It is hypothesized that the therapist administered CB intervention and the self-help CB intervention will result in greater declines in pain, depression, and distress about disfigurement both at the end of the active intervention and at one year follow-up as compared to the disease/health educational intervention. Depression is expected to reduce the efficacy of the CB self-help intervention. These findings will increase our understanding of the quality of life of individuals with **scleroderma** and determine whether self-help interventions can be used effectively to manage pain, depression, and distress about disfigurement.

Website: http://crisp.cit.nih.gov/crisp/Crisp_Query.Generate_Screen

- **Project Title: REGULATION OF COLLAGEN GENE EXPRESSION BY TGF BETA**

Principal Investigator & Institution: Varga, John M.; Professor of Medicine; Medicine; University of Illinois at Chicago 1737 West Polk Street Chicago, Il 60612

Timing: Fiscal Year 2002; Project Start 01-DEC-1993; Project End 30-NOV-2003

Summary: The uncontrolled tissue accumulation of Type I collagen characteristic of **scleroderma** is attributed to increased transcription of the collagen genes in **scleroderma** fibroblasts. TGF-Beta, a potent inducer of collagen synthesis, is strongly implicated in the development of pathological fibrosis in **scleroderma**. Other cytokines such as interferon-gamma antagonize the effects of TGF-Beta, and are likely to be important for prevention of scarring. Little is known about the intracellular signaling pathways involved in the physiologic regulation of collagen synthesis by cytokines, and the cis-acting elements of the collagen genes that are targets for these pathways. This information is of crucial importance for gaining a better understanding of the pathogenesis of fibrosis. We have shown that TGF-Beta stimulates transcription of the alpha1 (I) collagen gene (COL1A1) in fibroblasts. During the previous period of funding, we have identified cis-acting elements and their cognate transcription factors that play roles in regulating basal COL1A1 transcription. Our long-term goal is to understand the cellular mechanisms for modulation of collagen transcription in response to stimulatory and inhibitory extracellular signals, and to delineate alterations in the intracellular signaling pathways that result in constitutive up-regulation of the expression of collagen genes in **scleroderma.** In Specific Aim 1, we will ask which regions of the human COL1A1 promoter (and first intron) are responsive to TGF-Beta in fibroblasts, and what trans-acting proteins bind to these elements? We will confirm the functional role of TGF-Beta response elements in vivo by gene transfer in mice. In Specific Aim 2, we will examine the role of a novel family of intracellular signaling proteins in activation of collagen transcription by TGF-Beta in vitro. By gain- of-function and loss-of-function experiments, we will ask which Smad proteins are involved, and whether the Smads function as DNA-binding transcription factors in fibroblasts. We will ask if the Smads are molecular targets for antagonistic regulation by cytokines with opposing effects on collagen transcription. In Specific Aim 3, we will ask whether aberrant or deregulated Smad signaling underlies the constitutive up-regulation of collagen transcription in **scleroderma** fibroblasts. These studies should better define the signaling mechanisms that are important in regulating collagen transcription in normal and fibrotic fibroblasts. The results will facilitate the design of interventions to selectively inhibit this process.

Website: http://crisp.cit.nih.gov/crisp/Crisp_Query.Generate_Screen

- **Project Title: REGULATION OF FIBROGENESIS BY THE DIETARY FLAVONOIDS**

Principal Investigator & Institution: Ricupero, Dennis A.; Medicine; Boston University Medical Campus 715 Albany St, 560 Boston, Ma 02118

Timing: Fiscal Year 2002; Project Start 15-SEP-2001; Project End 31-AUG-2004

Summary: (provided by applicant) Excess deposition of type I collagen is characteristic of a number of fibrotic disorders including idiopathic pulmonary fibrosis, asthma, and **scleroderma.** Many fibrotic diseases have features of chronic inflammation. Reactive oxygen species (ROS) are abundant in inflammatory events, although the roles of ROS are not completely understood. TGF-Beta (TGF-B), considered to be the major pro-fibrotic effector, stimulates hydrogen peroxide (H_2O_2) production in myofibroblasts. The data presented here demonstrate, for the first time, that in myofibroblasts, H_2O_2 stimulates an increase in alpha1(I) collagen mRNA. Apigenin, a common dietary flavonoid with anti-inflammatory and anti-oxidant properties, blocks the TGF-B-stimulated increase of alpha1(I) collagen mRNA and the TGF-stimulated production of H_2O_2. The mechanism by which apigenin blocks the TGF-B-stimulated production of H_2O_2 remains unclear. Steady-state levels of alpha1(I) collagen mRNA are regulated by the rate of transcription of the alpha1(I) collagen gene and by the stability of the message. The investigators previously reported that inhibition of phosphatidylinositol 3-kinase (PI3K) decreased the stability of alpha1(I) collagen mRNA. They found that apigenin blocked the TGF-B-stimulated transcription of the alpha1(I)collagen gene and reduced the stability of the message. Most importantly, they found that in transgenic mice expressing the chloramphenicol acetyl transferase (CAT) reporter construct driven by the alpha1(I)collagen promoter, topically-applied apigenin blocked the CAT activity of skin samples. Thus, it appears that apigenin is a potent downregulator of alpha1(I) collagen expression both in vitro and in vivo. This proposal will (Aim 1) test the hypothesis that an apigenin-rich diet will attenuate the development of fibrosis and (Aim 2) identify the apigenin-sensitive mechanism by which TGF-B stimulates production of H_2O_2 and test the hypothesis that alpha1(I) collagen mRNA stability is modulated through PI3K activity.

Website: http://crisp.cit.nih.gov/crisp/Crisp_Query.Generate_Screen

- **Project Title: RELAXIN IN SYSTEMIC SCLEROSIS W/ DIFFUSE SCLERODERMA**

Principal Investigator & Institution: Medsger, Thomas A.; Professor; University of Pittsburgh at Pittsburgh 350 Thackeray Hall Pittsburgh, Pa 15260

Timing: Fiscal Year 2002

Summary: A multicenter, randomized, double blind Phase II/III study of the safety, efficacy and dose response of recombinant human relaxin (25 mcg or 10 mcg/kg/day) vs. placebo is proposed in patients with **systemic sclerosis** with diffuse **scleroderma** of less than five years duration. The drug will be administered by continuous subcutaneous infusion for 24 weeks. Endpoints will include mesurement of skin thickness and other laboratory tests. The objectives of this study are to replicate the efficacy of relaxin at 25ug/kg/day for 24 weeks in SSc patients with diffuse **scleroderma** and to support effectiveness of the 25ug/kg/day therapy using a panel of additional variables. Another objective is to evaluate the efficacy and safety of a 10 ug/kg/day dose of relaxin and to continue evaluation of the safety of relaxin.

Website: http://crisp.cit.nih.gov/crisp/Crisp_Query.Generate_Screen

- **Project Title: ROLE OF T CELLS IN LUNG DISEASE IN SYSTEMIC SCLEROSIS**

Principal Investigator & Institution: White, Barbara; Professor of Medicine; Medicine; University of Maryland Balt Prof School Baltimore, Md 21201

Timing: Fiscal Year 2003; Project Start 01-JUN-1995; Project End 30-JUN-2007

Summary: (provided by applicant): Pulmonary fibrosis is a major cause of death in **scleroderma.** Progressive pulmonary fibrosis in **scleroderma** is part of a mature, stable pathologic network that is ongoing in the lungs of certain patients, rather than the end of a unidirectional cascade. This pathology includes multiple components, linked in multiple ways. Preliminary work suggests that CD8+ T cells may be an essential component in this pathologic network. The hypothesis of this work is that T cells are essential to progressive pulmonary fibrosis in **scleroderma**, causing lung fibrosis through production of pro-fibrotic cytokines and growth factors as well as stimulation of TGF-betaa production and activation, alternative activation of macrophages and lung inflammation. The strategy is to delete T cells and monitor changes in profibrotic pathways in vivo, as well as clinical benefit on lung function. These experiments will include in-depth analyses of the effects of T cells on profibrotic pathways, assessed at the level of gene expression, protein expression and signal transduction. The expected outcome is that depletion of T cells will reduce T cell production of IL-4 and other profibrotic growth factors and reduce production and activation of TGF-beta. It will reduce alternative activation of alveolar macrophages and lung inflammation. These changes will be accompanied by arrest of pulmonary fibrosis. In this application, patients will receive alefacept therapy for 12 months, with bronchoalveolar lavage done at time 0, 6, and 12 months. Alefacept is a humanized LFA-3/IgG1 fusion protein that depletes CD2+ cells, which are largely T cells, through apoptosis, without T cell activation. The specific aims are given: 1) Show that alefacept therapy depletes T cells in the lungs of **scleroderma** patients and that T cell depletion stabilizes lung fibrosis; 2) Show that two major profibrotic pathways - IL-4 production and signaling and TGF-beta production, activation and signaling - are T cell-dependent processes in **scleroderma** lung disease; and 3) Show that alternative activation of macrophages and lung inflammation are T cell-dependent processes in **scleroderma** lung disease. The new information that is gained will advance knowledge of T-cell dependent mechanisms of pulmonary fibrosis in **scleroderma.**

Website: http://crisp.cit.nih.gov/crisp/Crisp_Query.Generate_Screen

- **Project Title: SCLERODERMA LUNG STUDY**

Principal Investigator & Institution: Tashkin, Donald P.; Professor of Medicine; Medicine; University of California Los Angeles 10920 Wilshire Blvd., Suite 1200 Los Angeles, Ca 90024

Timing: Fiscal Year 2002; Project Start 10-AUG-1999; Project End 30-JUN-2004

Summary: In **Systemic Sclerosis** (SSc), interstitial pulmonary fibrosis is frequent (80%) and is now the leading cause of death. The mortality rate of patients with a forced vital capacity (FVC) 2.0% eosinophils in BAL fluid. Secondarily, we will assess the impact of CYC on quality of life (SF36), functional activity (SSc Health Assessment Questionnaire), dyspnea (Mahler Transition Dyspnea Index) and diffusing capacity for carbon monoxide (DLCO) in these patients. Patients will be recruited for study during the first 3 years (from 6 mos. to 2 yrs, 9 mos) of the 5-year project period. Randomized participants will be treated with study drug for 1 year and followed at 3-month intervals for 2 years. Overall study coordination and data collection, management and analysis will be centralized at UCLA. Proven methods for analyzing time-oriented data employed by the investigators in previous controlled studies of **scleroderma** will be used to evaluate whether oral CYC (1-2 mg/kg/day) is better than placebo a) in improving or preventing worsening of FVC (the primary outcome variable) and b) in improving or preventing worsening of quality of life, functional ability, breathlessness and DLCO (secondary outcome variables).

Website: http://crisp.cit.nih.gov/crisp/Crisp_Query.Generate_Screen

- **Project Title: SCOR ON THE PATHOGENESIS OF SCLERODERMA**

Principal Investigator & Institution: Postlethwaite, Arnold E.; Professor; Medicine; University of Tennessee Health Sci Ctr Memphis, Tn 38163

Timing: Fiscal Year 2002; Project Start 24-AUG-2001; Project End 31-JUL-2006

Summary: (provided by applicant): We propose the establishment of a SCOR on the Pathogenesis of **Scleroderma** (SSc) at the University of Tennessee, Memphis. This application brings together a diverse and highly talented group of biomedical scientific investigators with a remarkable history of scientific collaborations and accomplishments in research related to SSc whose attention has now been focused on selected aspects of the biology of the collagenous matrix in SSc which are 1) collagen-induced outgrowth of fibroblast-like cells from cultures of SSc peripheral blood mononuclear cells (PBMC), 2) refractoriness of matrix metalloproteinase (MMP)-1 in SSc lesional fibroblasts to upregulation by cytokines, and 3) collagen-induced platelet aggregation. Project #1 will characterize mechanisms by which type I collagen (CI) induces the outgrowth of FLC from PBMC, a potentially extremely important mechanism by which collagen-producing fibroblasts populate tissues and organs involved in fibrogenesis of SSc. Project #2 addresses the pervasive problem of an inherent resistance of MMP-1 upregulation in lesional SSc fibroblasts by cytokines such as IL-1, TNFalpha, and bFGF. This dysregulation of MMP-1 likely contributes to fibrosis in SSc by leading to decreased removal of collagen in sites where it is being produced. Project #3 will clone and perform functional studies on platelet CI and CIII receptors (R) and will develop blocking peptides that may prove therapeutically useful in halting excessive CI and CIII induced platelet aggregation in SSc patients. An Administrative Core and Molecular Resources Core Laboratory will support the three projects of the SCOR, providing administrative oversight and necessary assistance to each SCOR project. This SCOR will provide a vehicle through which a highly synergistic multidisciplinary approach can be focused on SSc. The spirit of cooperation and collaboration that has been the hallmark over the years of the members of the UT-VAMC Connective Tissue Research Group combined with the commitment of the University of Tennessee, Memphis to this SCOR will assure a successful and expeditious attaining of its goal.

Website: http://crisp.cit.nih.gov/crisp/Crisp_Query.Generate_Screen

- **Project Title: SELF-AND FOREIGN-LIPIDS PRESENTED BY CD1 IN SCLERODERMA**

Principal Investigator & Institution: Vincent, Michael S.; Brigham and Women's Hospital 75 Francis Street Boston, Ma 02115

Timing: Fiscal Year 2002; Project Start 28-SEP-2001; Project End 31-MAY-2004

Summary: (provided by applicant): The CD1 family of proteins serves as a molecular system for the presentation of the universe of lipid antigens to T cells. The five human CD1 isoforms include two groups:. Group I CD1 consists of the CD1a, b, and c molecules expressed on dendritic cells and found in humans and all other mammals except mice. Group 2 is represented by CD1d and found in all animals including mice. The physiologic function of CD1d is emerging and evidence exists supporting a role in host defense, immune tolerance, tumor immunity, and autoimmune disease such as systemic lupus, **systemic sclerosis,** and type I diabetes. In contrast, the group I CD1a, b, and c molecules are thought to provide for recognition of foreign microbial lipids. This proposal considers an alternative function of CD1a, b, and c, namely, presentation of self-lipids and the capacity to provoke immunoregulatory T cell functions bearing relationship to those proposed for the CDld-restricted T cell population. A large panel of cloned, autoreactive group 1 CD1-restricted T cells has been derived, which shares features of T cells restricted by CD1d. These clones secrete abundant cytokines in diverse patterns, are efficient cytolytic T cells, and express NK cell markers. Quantification of CD1 self-reactive cells ex vivo by ELISPOT indicates that this population is substantial. Surprisingly, a synthetic lipid spermicide, nonoxynol-9, was found to be a much more potent agonist than the self-lipid for one T cell clone. This suggested the hypothesis that self-lipid reactive CD1-restricted regulatory T cells might be influenced by exogenous lipids. Specifically, the illness in the epidemic "toxic oil syndrome" that occurred in Spain in 1981 was highly correlated with a contaminant closely matching the classic CD1 antigen general structure. Approximately 20% of patients with this syndrome went on to develop a chronic disease closely resembling **scleroderma.** Preliminary studies suggest that the toxic oil contaminants can promote T cell cytokine production in the presence of CD1-expressing immature dendritic cells. The long-term objectives of the proposed work are to structurally characterize foreign and self-lipid CD1 antigens, measure CD1 -restricted T cell responses in patients with **scleroderma** in comparison to healthy individuals, and identify therapeutic targets for amelioration of this disease by modulation of the immune system with candidate hydrophobic antigens. Just as previous work has focused on the role of CD1 a, b, and c in host defense against microbes, it is now possible, here, to begin to unravel the molecular basis for T cells autoreactive to self-lipids presented by CD1 a, b, and c.

Website: http://crisp.cit.nih.gov/crisp/Crisp_Query.Generate_Screen

- **Project Title: SPHINGOSINE KINASE IN SYSTEMIC SCLEROSIS (SCLERODERMA)**

Principal Investigator & Institution: Trojanowska, Maria; Professor; Medical University of South Carolina 171 Ashley Ave Charleston, Sc 29425

Timing: Fiscal Year 2003; Project Start 01-JAN-2003; Project End 31-DEC-2007

Summary: Our long term objective is to understand the regulation of extracellular matrix (ECM) production by human fibroblasts and its dysregulation in fibrotic diseases such as **scleroderma** (systemic sclerosis, SSc). Organ fibrosis, a main pathologic manifestation of SSc, is the result of excessive deposition of ECM. Numerous studies have established a central role for transforming growth factor-beta (TGF-beta) in the fibrogenic process occurring in various organs and diseases including SSc. Rapid progress made in the past several years has led to the identification and characterization of the several key components of the TGF-beta signaling pathway. However, it is still not fully understood how TGF-beta signaling is integrated with other cellular signaling pathways to achieve diverse tissue-specific responses. Furthermore, the nature of the specific alterations of TGF-beta signaling that contribute to the fibrogenic process in SSc is not yet clear. We have made a novel observation that in human fibroblasts TGF-beta regulates levels and activities of the enzymes involved in regulation of lipid metabolism. Specifically, TGF-beta upregulates the levels and activity of the sphingosine kinase (SPHK) and down regulates activity of the sphingosine phosphate phosphatase (S1Pase). Furthermore, our preliminary data using ectopically expressed SPHK suggest that SPHK inhibits TGF-beta stimulation of collagen production. Significantly, basal and TGF-beta-induced activity of SPHK is lower in SSc skin and lung fibroblasts. Based on these observations we hypothesize that in normal fibroblasts TGF-beta activates SPHK and induces the levels of sphingosine 1-phosphate (S1P), which in turn provides a counter regulatory signal (negative autofeedback loop) affecting duration and/or intensity of TGF-beta stimulation of collagen production, and that this signaling pathway is defective in SSc fibroblasts. We propose three specific aims to test these hypotheses and to start unraveling the molecular mechanisms of the cross-talk between sphingolipids and the TGF-beta. In Specific Aim 1 we will determine whether the sphingolipid pathway is dysregulated in SSc fibroblasts by examining the levels and activities of the key lipid enzymes and determining the intracellular concentrations of ceramide, sphingosine, and sphingosine 1-phosphate (S1P) in SSc and healthy dermal fibroblasts at the basal level and after TGF-beta stimulation. In Specific Aim 2 we will determine the mechanism by which the SPHK/S1P pathway regulates ECM production in response to TGF-beta signaling. in Specific Aim 3 we will determine the role of sphingosine phosphate phosphatase (S1Pase) and sphingosine phosphate lyasc (S1P lyase), two important enzymes involved in regulation of the cellular levels of S1P, in TGF-beta signaling and collagen metabolism in SSc and healthy fibroblasts.

Website: http://crisp.cit.nih.gov/crisp/Crisp_Query.Generate_Screen

- **Project Title: STUDIES IN SCLERODERMA AND CYSTIC FIBROSIS OSTEOPOROSIS**

Principal Investigator & Institution: Merkel, Peter A.; Assistant Professor; Medicine; Boston University Medical Campus 715 Albany St, 560 Boston, Ma 02118

Timing: Fiscal Year 2002; Project Start 18-JUL-2001; Project End 30-JUN-2006

Summary: (provided by applicant): To provide support for research projects in the field of rheumatology that will form the basis of a structured mentoring program for young investigators pursuing careers in patient-oriented clinical research. This application has two major specific research aims: 1) Develop new outcome measures for skin assessment in **scleroderma** for use in clinical trials and 2) Determine the prevalence and progression of osteoporosis in patients with cystic fibrosis (CF). Both projects will have direct relevance to furthering the health of the populations under study. Clinical research in **scleroderma,** including therapeutic trials, is greatly hampered by a lack of reliable and precise outcome measurements of disease activity. Skin thickening and fibrosis are major causes of morbidity and dysfunction for patients with **scleroderma.** The great success in extending the life expectancy of patients with CF gained in the last 20 years has resulted in patients now experiencing diseases as adults not formerly encountered in this population. Among these diseases is osteoporosis. Patients with CF appear to be at high risk for osteoporosis due to nutritional, pharmacologic, and genetic factors but the pathophysiology and extent of the problem is not known. Patients with **scleroderma** will be followed prospectively and evaluated for skin disease activity by skin scoring, durometer readings (thickness), light-based technologies, skin biopsies, self-assessments, and functional status instruments. These data will be analyzed to determine a core set of outcome measures for **scleroderma.** and validated by an expert panel of national researchers in this disease. An observational cohort of patients with CF will be studied. Baseline and 2-year measurements of bone density, nutritional status, and biochemical markers of bone turnover will performed. A comprehensive program for training new clinical investigators by the principal investigator is proposed. This program includes trainees taking an active and integral role in the research studies described. Additionally, trainees will be enrolled in formal coursework in biostatistics, epidemiology, and clinical research techniques leading to a master degree. A unique seminar and a series of support services at the host institution will further complement the training program.

Website: http://crisp.cit.nih.gov/crisp/Crisp_Query.Generate_Screen

- **Project Title: STUDIES OF COLLAGEN GENE REGULATION IN TWO MURINE MODELS**

Principal Investigator & Institution: Clark, Stephen H.; Associate Professor; Medicine; University of Connecticut Sch of Med/Dnt Bb20, Mc 2806 Farmington, Ct 060302806

Timing: Fiscal Year 2002; Project Start 26-SEP-2001; Project End 31-MAY-2006

Summary: (provided by applicant): This proposal will utilize two mouse mutations that are models for **scleroderma,** tight skin (Tsk) and tight skin 2 (Tsk2). Both mutations display excessive accumulation of collagen and other extracellular matrix components in the skin, a hallmark feature of the human disease. The long range of objective of the proposed research is to utilize these two mutations combined with several lines of transgenic mice as experimental tools to dissect molecular mechanisms of disease pathogenesis. Specific experiments are proposed for the identification of genes involved in the regulation of extracellular matrix synthesis in dermal fibroblasts. Two experimental strategies are planned and are encompassed in three specific aims. Specific aim 1 focuses on identifying cis-acting elements in the type I collagen gene required for the increased production of Col1al mRNA in mutant dermal fibroblasts. Defining "fibrotic" specific elements will provide a basis for the identification of the transacting factors that interact with these DNA segments to increase Collagen gene expression. These elements will be defined by studying the expression of Col1al CAT reporter transgenes bearing various segments of the 5' promoter region as well as specific deletions of the first intron. The expression of each transgene will be evaluated in skin samples isolated from Tsk, Tsk2 and normal mice. Also, transgene expression will be measured in dermal fibroblasts cultured from skin explants isolated from these mice. To generate experimental mice, Tsk and Tsk2 mutant mice will be crossed with transgenic mice bearing the various collagen transgene constructs. A potential role of the Col1al first intron in the upregulation of transcription of the Col1al gene has been shown with the Tsk and Tsk2 mutations (our preliminary data) as well as in **scleroderma** dermal fibroblasts. In specific aim 2 the role of the Col1al first intron in regulating transcription of the Col1al gene and the development of the Tsk and Tsk2 fibrotic skin phenotype will be determined. For these experiments a targeted deletion in the Col1a1 first intron will be employed. This experimental model has a unique feature permitting the determination of the levels of Col1a1 mRNA produced by the deleted and normal allele in the same RNA preparation. Further this genetic system allows the monitoring of gene expression in the context of the endogenous gene. A second experimental direction involves identifying genes in dermal fibroblasts that are associated with elevated levels of collagen production employing micorarray analysis. The experimental plan outlined in specific aim 3 includes the development of reagents to isolate specific populations of dermal fibroblasts cultured from both mutant and normal animals based on their collagen gene expression. This will be accomplished by employing a collagen promoter GFP reporter transgene that has been documented to display elevated expression in dermal fibroblasts isolated from both Tsk and Tsk2 mutant mice. Flow cytometric analysis of dermal fibroblasts expressing this transgene will permit the isolation of cell populations based on their level of collagen expression. RNA's will be extracted from high collagen and low collagen producing cell populations. These RNA's will be utilized in a microarray analysis to identify genes differentially expressed in high collagen producing cells compared to low collagen producing cells and visa versa. It is anticipated that genes identified in this experimental paradigm will permit the dissection of molecular pathways that are involved with the onset of **scleroderma** and potentially lead to therapies to control extracellular matrix metabolism.

Website: http://crisp.cit.nih.gov/crisp/Crisp_Query.Generate_Screen

- **Project Title: STUDY OF PERSISTENT INFECTION IN SSC SKIN AND VESSELS**

Principal Investigator & Institution: Mayes, Maureen D.; Professor; Internal Medicine; University of Texas Hlth Sci Ctr Houston Box 20036 Houston, Tx 77225

Timing: Fiscal Year 2002; Project Start 26-SEP-2001; Project End 31-MAY-2004

Summary: (provided by applicant): The overall objective of this proposal is to study the possibility that in some **systemic sclerosis** patients, a persistent bacterial infection involving dermal microvascular endothelium or other cells that are resident in skin results in the obliterative microvasculopathy and/or the fibrosing features of this disease. As a first step in addressing this issue, we will test the following hypothesis: persistent bacterial infection of skin or microvasculature occurs more commonly in **systemic sclerosis** cases than in matched controls and participates in the disease process. Specific aims are: (1) to test skin biopsies from 60 systemic **scleroderma** patients and 30 matched normal controls for evidence of bacterial persistence by pan-bacterial and chlamydia-specific molecular screening; (2) to microdissect dermal vessels from these same cases and controls and test this tissue by panbacterial and chlamydia-specific molecular probes; (3) to prepare PBMC'S from these individuals and screen with these probes; and (4) depending on positive results, to perform immunohistochemistry studies for these organisms on skin biopsies/vessels from selected patients and appropriate controls. **Scleroderma** small vessel vasculopathy shares some key features with large vessel atherosclerosis, a condition also characterized by intimal proliferation and luminal narrowing among multiple other abnormalities. Inflammation may play an important role in the pathogenesis of atherosclerosis raising the possibility of infectious agents as mediators in this process. There are several examples of infection resulting in chronic inflammatory autoimmune diseases including Lyme disease (Borrelia burgdorferii), and reactive arthritis (ReA), an inflammatory joint disease associated with prior infection by a number of specific bacterial pathogens, including Chlamydia trachomatis and various species of the Genera Salmonella, Yersinia, Campylobacter, and others. This research team is comprised of individuals with expertise in clinical

scleroderma, the vascular abnormalities of primary and secondary Raynaud's disease, and autoimmunity related to persistent bacterial infections with relevant pathogens. If positive results are obtained in at least a subset of **scleroderma** cases, intervention trials could be devised with therapy targeted to specific organisms.

Website: http://crisp.cit.nih.gov/crisp/Crisp_Query.Generate_Screen

- **Project Title: STUDY OF T CELL CHARACTERISTICS AND ADHESION MOLECULES**

Principal Investigator & Institution: Bergasa, Nora V.; Columbia University Health Sciences New York, Ny 10032

Timing: Fiscal Year 2003; Project Start 01-SEP-2003; Project End 31-AUG-2008

Summary: Primary biliary cirrhosis (PBC) is chronic liver disease of unknown etiology. Histologically, PBC is characterized by a progressive immunologically mediated inflammation known as chronic nonsuppurative destructive cholangitis (CNSDC) that leads to bile duct destruction, ductopenia and biliary cirrhosis. At present there is no cure for PBC. The most common symptoms associated with PBC are fatigue and pruritus. More than 90% of patients with PBC are women. The average age of diagnosis is about 50 years. Asymptomatic patients have a four-fold increase in mortality when compared to the U.S.A. population matched for age and the median survival from the onset of symptoms is 7.5 to 9 years. PBC is considered a model autoimmune disease; it is associated with hypergammaglobulinemia, autoantibodies, defects of immune regulation, and an increased incidence of other autoimmune conditions (thyroiditis, Sjogren's syndrome, scleroderma). The liver injury is characterized by a rich inflammatory infiltrate composed of CD4+ and CD8+ cells, cytokines, adhesion molecules and other immunologic mediators. The consequence of CNSDC is biliary cirrhosis and liver failure. The only treatment approved to treat PBC is ursodeoxycholic acid (UDCA), which appears to delay the time to liver transplantation but does not cure for the disease. Thus, the need for the provision of effective and safe treatments for PBC is clear. Patients with PBC may benefit from treatment with an appropriate immunosuppressive drug. Mycophenolate mofetil meets the criteria of a superior immunosuppressive agent. In this proposal we are going to explore immune mediators of PBC including T cells and adhesion molecules in patients with PBC and the effect of treatment with MMF in combination with UDCA on these factors in patients who are participants in a clinical trial.

Website: http://crisp.cit.nih.gov/crisp/Crisp_Query.Generate_Screen

- **Project Title: SYSTEMIC SCLEROSIS--SOCIODEMOGRAPHIC, BEHAVIORAL, AND IMMUNOGENETIC FACTOR**

Principal Investigator & Institution: Mcnearney, Terry; University of Texas Medical Br Galveston 301 University Blvd Galveston, Tx 77555

Timing: Fiscal Year 2002

Summary: Systemic Sclerosis (SSc) is a autoimmune disease that affects 1:17,000 persons. Patients with this disease can experience problems with arthritis, muscles, swallowing, the stomach and intestines, the kidney and the heart. The disease can be painful and debilitating and can lead to premature death. There is no cure for **Scleroderma** and treatment is usually aimed at treating the symptoms. The clinical course and organ involvement in **Scleroderma** can be variable, so what is a complication in one patient may not occur in another. The objective of the current study is to study environmental, behavioral, cultural, genetic and laboratory factors in a cohort of **Scleroderma** patients, in order to identify trends, and risk factors for serious complications of the disease. These factors will be studied in Caucasian, Black and Hispanic populations who have been diagnosed less than five years. It will be important to identify patients at high risk for developing serious complications of **Scleroderma** so that treatment can be modified to impact on their disease.

Website: http://crisp.cit.nih.gov/crisp/Crisp_Query.Generate_Screen

- **Project Title: T CELLS IN THE PATHOGENESIS OF SYSTEMIC SCLEROSIS**

Principal Investigator & Institution: Platsoucas, Chris D.; Professor and Chairman; Microbiology and Immunology; Temple University 406 Usb, 083-45 Philadelphia, Pa 19122

Timing: Fiscal Year 2002; Project Start 21-SEP-2001; Project End 31-MAY-2006

Summary: (provided by applicant): **Systemic Sclerosis** (SSc) is a chronic disease characterized by extensive fibrosis, microvascular fibrointimal proliferation and autoantibody production. T cells and monocytes infiltrate early skin lesions of patients with SSc. We have demonstrated that skin-biopsies in five of five patients with SSc contain oligoclonal populations of T cells. Hemopoeitic fetal cells have been identified in women with SSc who had previously been pregnant. Activation of these fetal T cells in the mother results in clinical disease designated as maternal SSc, which resembles GVHD. Microchimerism of maternal cells has been identified in women who have not been previously pregnant or in men. Activation of these maternal T cells results in offspring SSc. The hypothesis to be tested in this RO1 application is: (a) whether T-cells infiltrating skin-biopsies from patients with maternal SSc are of fetal origin and whether their recognize alloantigens of maternal origin, by the direct or the indirect antigen recognition pathways; (b) whether T-cells infiltrating skin-biopsies from patients with offspring SSc are of maternal origin and whether their recognize alloantigens of offspring origin, by the direct or the indirect antigen recognition pathways. Our specific aims are: 1. To determine whether fresh (not expanded in culture) T cells infiltrating skin-biopsies from patients with maternal SSc or offspring SSc contain substantial proportions of monoclonal T cells. To determine whether these clonally expanded T cells are of fetal origin in maternal SSc or of maternal origin in offspring SSc. 2. To identify the antigens recognized by T cells employing the clonally expanded alpha- and beta-chain TCR transcripts in maternal SSc or offspring SSc skin-biopsies. a. To express the clonally expanded in SSc skin-biopsies TCR transcripts into ap TCR-negative J.RT3T3.5 Jurkat cells by transfection, or into normal CTL by infection with retroviral vectors. b. To determine whether these transduced or transfected T cells with the clonally expanded TCR, recognize alloantigen by the direct or the indirect recognition pathway. 3. To develop by limiting dilution T-cell clones specific for alloantigens or for putative SSc antigens (CMV and DNA topoisomerase I) from the same SSc patients studied in specific aim #1. a. To determine whether these T-cell clones are of fetal origin in maternal SSc or maternal origin in offspring SSc. To determine whether they recognize alloantigen. b. To characterize these T-cell clones phenotypically and functionally and to determine whether they recognize: (i) alloantigens; by the direct or the indirect recognition pathway; (ii) the putative SSc antigen(s) listed above. To determine whether these T-cell clones exhibit suppressor activity to allospecific responses or to CTL activity. c. To compare the TCR sequences utilized by these antigen-specific T-cell clones to those of fresh (not expanded in culture) SSc infiltrating T cells from the same patients, in order to determine whether clonal. populations of these fresh infiltrating T cells have the same antigenic specificities to those of antigen-specific T-cell clones. d. To identify Thl, Th2, suppressor, anergic and CTL T-cell clones from those developed above, on the basis of expression patterns of their genes, using DNA array technology.

Website: http://crisp.cit.nih.gov/crisp/Crisp_Query.Generate_Screen

- **Project Title: TBI, CYCLOPHOSPHAMIDE, GLOBULIN & STEM CELL RESCUE IN SYSTEMIC SCLEROSIS**

Principal Investigator & Institution: Mcdonagh, Kevin T.; Associate Professor of Internal Medicine; University of Michigan at Ann Arbor 3003 South State, Room 1040 Ann Arbor, Mi 481091274

Timing: Fiscal Year 2002

Summary: This abstract is not available.

Website: http://crisp.cit.nih.gov/crisp/Crisp_Query.Generate_Screen

- **Project Title: TGF BETA ACTIVATION IN PULMONARY DISEASE**

Principal Investigator & Institution: Munger, John; New York University School of Medicine 550 1St Ave New York, Ny 10016

Timing: Fiscal Year 2002

Summary: This abstract is not available.

Website: http://crisp.cit.nih.gov/crisp/Crisp_Query.Generate_Screen

- **Project Title: THE MOLECULAR BASIS FOR ENDOTHELIAL DYSFUNCTION IN SSC**

Principal Investigator & Institution: Kahaleh, Bashar Bashar.; Medicine; Medical College of Ohio at Toledo Research & Grants Admin. Toledo, Oh 436145804

Timing: Fiscal Year 2002; Project Start 21-SEP-2001; Project End 31-MAY-2004

Summary: Scleroderma (SSc) is an autoimmune disease of unknown etiology characterized by endothelial cell injury and tissue fibrosis. Considerable body of evidence indicates that the vascular disease in SSc precedes, and may well be, a driving force behind enhanced biosynthetic activity of fibroblasts. To better understand the molecular events, which operate in the pathogenesis of SSc, we have undertaken an investigation of gene expression in microvascular endothelial (MVEC) cells isolated from involved and uninvolved skin of patients with diffuse **systemic sclerosis.** Preliminary data indicate that MVEC derived from unaffected and affected skin of SSc patients exhibit qualitatively similar aberrations in the constitutive expression of certain pathogenically relevant genes when compared with MVEC of sex- and age-matched normal volunteers. The main goal for the current proposal is to explore the basis for the development of the aberrant EC phenotype in SSc. Understanding disease related process that leads to endothelial dysfunction may provide insights into pathogenic processes associated with **scleroderma** and may help in the design of future therapeutic intervention. The three specific aims for the proposal are: 1. To study SSc MVEC gene expression phenotype under different experimental conditions, particularly under mechanical shear stress forces, to examine the persistence of the phenotype. 2. To investigate the possibility that SSc MVEC phenotype may result from an, in vivo. DNA methylation, and that cytotoxic T cells may play a role in this process. 3. To explore the possibility that SSc MVEC phenotype results from, in vivo, selection through clonal expansion of a heterogeneous population of EC. Involvement of the vascular endothelial cells is a major event in the pathogenesis of **scleroderma.** Our longterm goal is to precisely define the mechanisms leading to endothelial dysfunction and to investigate potential therapy that may help in preventing or modifying the vascular abnormalities.

Website: http://crisp.cit.nih.gov/crisp/Crisp_Query.Generate_Screen

- **Project Title: TRANSGENIC ANIMAL MODELS FOR FIBROTIC DISEASE**

Principal Investigator & Institution: De Crombrugghe, Benoit; Professor and Chair; University of Texas Hlth Sci Ctr Houston Box 20036 Houston, Tx 77225

Timing: Fiscal Year 2002

Summary: The overall objective of this application is to establish new mouse models of fibrotic diseases. To achieve this objective we propose two approaches, one is to disrupt in fibroblasts of transgene mice the TGF- beta signalling pathway, the other is to alter the balance between metalloproteinases and their tissue inhibitors in the extracellular matrix of fibroblasts. Our application is anchored on our previous identification and characterization of a promoter/enhancer in the mouse gene for the proalpha2 chain of mous4e type I collagen (Co11alpha2) that has the ability to direct expression of reporter genes specifically to fibroblasts of transgene mice. To avoid undesirable effects during embryonic development we use a dual system. This system, based on Cre mediated recombination, allows to switch-on the DNAs that we propose to activate in fibroblasts at a specific time after birth. The system used throughout this proposal is based on a Cre recombinase, developed by others, which becomes activated only after administration of Tamoxifen. In this proposal, expression of the DNA for this recombinase is directed by the Co11alpha2 promoter/enhancer which restricts its expression to fibroblastic cells. The genes that we propose to express in fibroblasts postnatally are cloned downstream of the potent and ubiquitously active ROSA26 promoter. Interposed between this promoter and the DNAs that we propose to express we placed a transcription stop cassette, flanked by two Lox P sites, which are substrates for Cre recombinase. Thus expression of the DNAs is only possible after Cre-mediated removal of the STOP cassette. Hence in this dual system, Tamoxifen controls expression of these DNAs which is restricted to fibroblasts because Cre is only expressed in fibroblasts. We hypothesize that the expression of DNA for a constitutively active TGF-beta1 receptor in fibroblasts as well as the over-expression of TIMP1, in fibroblasts will produce fibrotic phenotypes. To attempt to correct the postulated fibrotic phenotype caused by expression of the constitutively active TGF-beta type I receptor, we propose to over- expression in fibroblasts a DNA for a dominant-negative Smad3. In each case of the phenotype of transgene mice and that of their fibroblasts in culture will be extensively characterized with the use of specific molecular markers and gene expression arrays. The results of such gene profiling of fibroblasts from fibrotic animals will also be compared to those performed with fibroblasts of **scleroderma** patients performed by Dr. Frank Arnett.

Website: http://crisp.cit.nih.gov/crisp/Crisp_Query.Generate_Screen

- **Project Title: TSK-2: A NEW ANIMAL MODEL FOR SCLERODERMA**

Principal Investigator & Institution: Christner, Paul J.; Research Associate Professor; Medicine; Thomas Jefferson University Office of Research Administration Philadelphia, Pa 191075587

Timing: Fiscal Year 2002; Project Start 09-JAN-1995; Project End 31-MAR-2005

Summary: Systemic sclerosis (SSc) is a serious disease of unknown cause, characterized by excessive accumulation of collagen and other connective tissue components in the skin and internal organs. An animal model to study the molecular mechanisms of SSc would be extremely useful. We have recently initiated studies of such a model, the Tight

Skin 2 or the Tsk2 mouse. During the previous period of funding we have conclusively demonstrated that Tsk2 is a different mutation than Tsk1; we have located the mutation on the proximal arm of chromosome I; and we have narrowed the interval in which the mutation lies from over 50 cM to 2.1 cM. We have shown that the Tsk2 mouse displays marked thickening of the dermis and excessive accumulation of dermal collagen. We found that collagen protein synthesis and type I, III, V and VI collagen mRNA levels were markedly elevated in either Tsk2 mouse skin or dermal fibroblasts. The elevated expression of type I and III collagen genes was due to increased transcription of the corresponding genes. These results demonstrated that the Tsk2 mutant mouse displays connective tissue abnormalities, which resemble those present in the skin of both SSc patients and Tsk1 mice. The discovery of an additional Tsk mutation will allow us to pursue a second avenue of approach to understanding the mechanisms controlling collagen gene expression at the molecular level and should greatly increase our chances of eventually finding an effective treatment for SSc. The overall goal of this renewal application is to identify the Tsk2 gene. To accomplish this goal we will pursue the following specific aims: (1) To further narrow the region on chromosome 1 on which Tsk2 is known to reside by;continuing to type and map the N2 offspring from the intersubspecific backcross of [(Mus castaneus x C57BL/6-+/Tsk2)F1 x Mus castaneus] mice; (2) to continue to identify screen candidate genes which are known to reside in or near the region of interest; (3) to establish YAC and BAC contigs encompassing Tsk2 and establish refined proxinal and distal boundaries with recombinant markers; (4) to identify coding regions within the contigs by means of identifying CpG islands, exon trapping and cDNA selecton; and (5) to screen and identify the novel gene sequences. These studies will allow us to identify and clone Tsk2 and to characterize the mutation as a prelude to understanding its function. It is expected that the knowledge gained from these studies will be of direct relevance to the understanding of the pathogenesis of the excessive collagen deposition characteristic of Ssc and will provide a more rational approach to develop possible modes of therapy for this incurable and devastating disease.

Website: http://crisp.cit.nih.gov/crisp/Crisp_Query.Generate_Screen

- **Project Title: TYPE I BOVINE COLLAGEN THERAPY OF SYSTEMIC SCLERODERMA**

Principal Investigator & Institution: Mckown, Kevin M.; University of Tennessee Health Sci Ctr Memphis, Tn 38163

Timing: Fiscal Year 2003

Summary: This abstract is not available.

Website: http://crisp.cit.nih.gov/crisp/Crisp_Query.Generate_Screen

- **Project Title: UV-INDUCED COLLAGEN REDUCTION: TREATING SKIN SCLERODERMA**

Principal Investigator & Institution: Kang, Sewon; Associate Professor; Dermatology; University of Michigan at Ann Arbor 3003 South State, Room 1040 Ann Arbor, Mi 481091274

Timing: Fiscal Year 2002; Project Start 26-SEP-2001; Project End 30-JUN-2006

Summary: (provided by applicant): **Scleroderma** is a progressive, potentially life-threatening disease of the connective tissue that can cause hardening of the skin, and damage to lungs, heart, kidney, and gastrointestinal tract, The disease may also affect blood vessels, muscles and joints. **Scleroderma** typically strikes between ages 25 and 55, and women are four times more likely than men to be stricken. An estimated 300,000 persons in the United States have **scleroderma.** The exact causes of **scleroderma** are unknown, however, the hallmark of the disease process is over-production of collagen. Currently, there is no safe and effective therapy for the disease. Acute exposure to relatively low and safe doses of ultraviolet (UV) irradiation has been shown to reduce skin collagen. This reduction occurs through two simultaneous mechanisms; 1) induction of matrix metalloproteinases (MMP) that degrade skin collagen, and 2) inhibit of new procollagen synthesis. UV irradiation is composed of electromagnetic energy with wavelengths between 290-400nm, and the ability of UV to reduce skin collagen is wavelength-dependent. Short wavelengths-dependent between 290-320nm (referred to as UVB) and long wavelengths between 360-400mn (referred to as UVA1) are most effective. In light-colored people, acute exposure to UVB can cause sun turn, and chronic exposure over many years can cause skin cancer. However, the risks of sunburn and cancer from UVA1 are at least one thousand fold less than from UVB exposure. Therefore, UVA1 phototherapy holds great potential for treatment of cutaneous **scleroderma** in light-colored persons. In dark-colored people, the ability of UV A1 to reduce skin collagen is largely attenuated by skin pigment, likely making this form of phototherapy ineffective. However, for dark-colored people the risk of sunburn and skin cancer from UVB exposure is substantially less than for light-colored people. Therefore, UVB phototherapy for cutaneous **scleroderma** in dark-colored persons holds great promise. The broad, long-term objectives of this application are to optimize, evaluate, and investigate the molecular basis of UV phototherapy for the treatment of cutaneous **scleroderma.** The hypothesis that UV irradiation reduces cutaneous fibrosis of **scleroderma** by inducing MMPS and simultaneously inhibiting procollagen synthesis, and that efficacy of treatment is dependent on patients' skin pigmentation in combination with the UV wavelength used for treatment will be tested. This application contains five specific aims. Specific aims 1-3 focus on optimization of phototherapy conditions based on measurements of collagen reduction. Specific aim 1 will determine the UVA1 dose-, time- and skin color-dependence for induction of a) MMPs, b) tissue inhibitors of MMPs (TIMPS), c) collagen degradation, and d) inhibition of procollagen synthesis in light-pigmented human skin in vivo. Specific aim 2 will determine the broadband (290-320 nm) and narrowband UVB (311-313nm) dose- and time-dependence for reduction of collagen (as described for specific aim 1) in dark-pigmented human skin in vivo. Specific aim 3 will determine the kinetics and magnitude of UVA1-induced tanning, and the impact of this tanning on subsequent UV dose dependence for reduction of collagen (as described for specific aim 1) in lightly-pigmented human skin in vivo. Specific aims 4-5 focus on phototherapy clinical trials for treatment of **scleroderma.** Specific aim 4 will determine, based on information obtained from Specific Aims 1-3, whether a) an optimized regimen of UVA1 irradiation improves cutaneous **scleroderma** in light-pigmented patients, and b) an optimized regimen of UVB, improves cutaneous **scleroderma** in dark-pigmented patients. Specific Aim 5 will determine whether clinical improvement in **scleroderma** with UV phototherapy correlates with MMP induction, collagen degradation, inhibition of procollagen synthesis, levels of profibrotic (TGF-b, CTGF, IL-4, IL-6) and antifibrotic (TNF-a, IFN-g) cytokines, and infiltrating immune cells.

Website: http://crisp.cit.nih.gov/crisp/Crisp_Query.Generate_Screen

- **Project Title: VASCULOPATHY, APOPTOSIS AND AUTOIMMUNITY**

  Principal Investigator & Institution: Ahearn, Joseph M.; Associate Professor; Medicine; University of Pittsburgh at Pittsburgh 350 Thackeray Hall Pittsburgh, Pa 15260

  Timing: Fiscal Year 2002; Project Start 27-SEP-1999; Project End 31-AUG-2004

Summary: This proposal is focused upon the molecular mechanism by which vasculopathy leads to fibrotic and autoimmune manifestations of **systemic sclerosis.** Autoantibodies generated by patients with **systemic sclerosis** are uniquely targeted to nucleolar proteins such as DNA topoisomerase I (topo-I). It has been demonstrated that topo-I is a substrate for protease(s) specific to the apoptotic process, resulting in novel cleavage fragments that may reveal cryptic epitopes to which the host has not previously been tolerized. It has also been recently demonstrated that several of the autoantigens targeted in diffuse **scleroderma** are uniquely susceptible to cleavage by metal-catalyzed oxidation reactions similar to what may occur during ischemia-reperfusion in the presence of appropriate metals. This process may also reveal immunocryptic epitopes and provides a molecular explanation for why certain proteins are uniquely targeted by the immune response in **systemic sclerosis.** However, it is well known that a cryptic epitope alone is not sufficient to generate autoreactivity, which also requires the participation of a molecular adjuvant, and uptake of the potential autoantigen by an antigen presenting cell (APC) with costimulatory capacity. The central hypothesis of this proposal is that chronic ischemia-reperfusion injury in patients with **systemic sclerosis** not only generates immunocryptic epitopes within nucleolar autoantigens of cutaneous origin, but it also generates complement ligands that provide the molecular adjuvant required to break immune tolerance. The specific aims of this proposal are to: 1) Determine the capacity of apoptotic blebs bearing complement ligands to modulate the cytokine expression and costimulatory capacity of antigen presenting cells, 2) characterize the immune responses to self antigen- containing apoptotic blebs, and 3) examine the role of complement ligand C3d during induction of autoreactive T and B cell responses to topo I in vitro. Although **systemic sclerosis** is the focus of this proposal, the data generated by these studies should provide insight into our understanding of vasculopathic and autoimmune processes in general.

Website: http://crisp.cit.nih.gov/crisp/Crisp_Query.Generate_Screen

- **Project Title: VITAMIN D METABOLITE, CALCITRIOL IN SCLERODERMA**

Principal Investigator & Institution: Lemire, Jacques; University of California San Diego 9500 Gilman Dr, Dept. 0934 La Jolla, Ca 92093

Timing: Fiscal Year 2002

Summary: This abstract is not available.

Website: http://crisp.cit.nih.gov/crisp/Crisp_Query.Generate_Screen

- **Project Title: ZINC THERAPY FOR SCLERODERMA--PHASE I STUDY**

Principal Investigator & Institution: Wigley, Frederick M.; Johns Hopkins University 3400 N Charles St Baltimore, Md 21218

Timing: Fiscal Year 2002

Summary: This abstract is not available.

Website: http://crisp.cit.nih.gov/crisp/Crisp_Query.Generate_Screen

E-Journals: PubMed Central[3]

PubMed Central (PMC) is a digital archive of life sciences journal literature developed and managed by the National Center for Biotechnology Information (NCBI) at the U.S. National Library of Medicine (NLM).[4] Access to this growing archive of e-journals is free and unrestricted.[5] To search, go to **http://www.ncbi.nlm.nih.gov/entrez/query.fcgi?db=Pmc**, and type "scleroderma" (or synonyms) into the search box. This search gives you access to full-text articles. The following is a sample of items found for scleroderma in the PubMed Central database:

- **Altered decorin expression of systemic sclerosis by UVA1 (340 --400 nm) phototherapy: Immunohistochemical analysis of 3 cases.** by Sawada H, Isogai Z, Morita A.; 2003;
  http://www.pubmedcentral.gov/articlerender.fcgi?tool=pmcentrez&artid=153525

- **Angiogenic and angiostatic factors in systemic sclerosis: increased levels of vascular endothelial growth factor are a feature of the earliest disease stages and are associated with the absence of fingertip ulcers.** by Distler O, del Rosso A, Giacomelli R, Cipriani P, Conforti ML, Guiducci S, Gay RE, Michel BA, Bruhlmann P, Muller-Ladner U, Gay S, Matucci-Cerinic M.; 2002;
  http://www.pubmedcentral.gov/articlerender.fcgi?tool=pmcentrez&artid=153841

- **Anti-Endothelial Cell Antibodies in Systemic Sclerosis.** by Renaudineau Y, Revelen R, Levy Y, Salojin K, Gilburg B, Shoenfeld Y, Youinou P.; 1999 Mar;
  http://www.pubmedcentral.gov/articlerender.fcgi?tool=pmcentrez&artid=95679

- **Autoantibodies from a Patient with Scleroderma CREST Recognized Kinetochores of the Higher Plant Haemanthus.** by Mole-Bajer J, Bajer AS, Zinkowski RP, Balczon RD, Brinkley BR.; 1990 May 1;
  http://www.pubmedcentral.gov/articlerender.fcgi?tool=pmcentrez&rendertype=abstract&artid=53949

- **Bilateral linear scleroderma "en coup de sabre" associated with facial atrophy and neurological complications.** by Gambichler T, Kreuter A, Hoffmann K, Bechara FG, Altmeyer P, Jansen T.; 2001;
  http://www.pubmedcentral.gov/articlerender.fcgi?tool=pmcentrez&artid=61032

- **Characterization of two scleroderma autoimmune antigens that copurify with human ribonuclease P.** by Eder PS, Kekuda R, Stolc V, Altman S.; 1997 Feb 18;
  http://www.pubmedcentral.gov/articlerender.fcgi?tool=pmcentrez&artid=19751

- **Deficient Smad7 expression: A putative molecular defect in scleroderma.** by Dong C, Zhu S, Wang T, Yoon W, Li Z, Alvarez RJ, ten Dijke P, White B, Wigley FM, Goldschmidt-Clermont PJ.; 2002 Mar 19;
  http://www.pubmedcentral.gov/articlerender.fcgi?tool=pmcentrez&artid=122622

- **Determination of an epitope of the diffuse systemic sclerosis marker antigen DNA topoisomerase I: sequence similarity with retroviral p30gag protein suggests a**

---

[3] Adapted from the National Library of Medicine: **http://www.pubmedcentral.nih.gov/about/intro.html**.

[4] With PubMed Central, NCBI is taking the lead in preservation and maintenance of open access to electronic literature, just as NLM has done for decades with printed biomedical literature. PubMed Central aims to become a world-class library of the digital age.

[5] The value of PubMed Central, in addition to its role as an archive, lies in the availability of data from diverse sources stored in a common format in a single repository. Many journals already have online publishing operations, and there is a growing tendency to publish material online only, to the exclusion of print.

possible cause for autoimmunity in systemic sclerosis. by Maul GG, Jimenez SA, Riggs E, Ziemnicka-Kotula D.; 1989 Nov;
http://www.pubmedcentral.gov/picrender.fcgi?tool=pmcentrez&action=stream&blobtype=pdf&artid=298308

- **Genetic epidemiology: Systemic sclerosis.** by Herrick AL, Worthington J.; 2002;
  http://www.pubmedcentral.gov/articlerender.fcgi?tool=pmcentrez&artid=128927

- **Histometric data obtained by in vivo confocal laser scanning microscopy in patients with systemic sclerosis.** by Sauermann K, Gambichler T, Jaspers S, Radenhausen M, Rapp S, Reich S, Altmeyer P, Clemann S, Teichmann S, Ennen J, Hoffmann K.; 2002;
  http://www.pubmedcentral.gov/articlerender.fcgi?tool=pmcentrez&artid=122067

- **Impaired Smad7-Smurf --mediated negative regulation of TGF-[beta] signaling in scleroderma fibroblasts.** by Asano Y, Ihn H, Yamane K, Kubo M, Tamaki K.; 2004 Jan 15;
  http://www.pubmedcentral.gov/articlerender.fcgi?tool=pmcentrez&artid=310747

- **Increased Levels of Alternatively Spliced Interleukin 4 (IL-4[delta]2) Transcripts in Peripheral Blood Mononuclear Cells from Patients with Systemic Sclerosis.** by Sakkas LI, Tourtellotte C, Berney S, Myers AR, Platsoucas CD.; 1999 Sep;
  http://www.pubmedcentral.gov/articlerender.fcgi?tool=pmcentrez&artid=95750

- **Interleukin 4 in Systemic Sclerosis: Not Just an Increase.** by Atamas SP, White B.; 1999 Sep;
  http://www.pubmedcentral.gov/articlerender.fcgi?tool=pmcentrez&artid=95749

- **Isolation and Characterization of cDNA Encoding the 80-kDa Subunit Protein of the Human Autoantigen Ku (p70/p80) Recognized by Autoantibodies from Patients with Scleroderma-Polymyositis Overlap Syndrome.** by Mimori T, Ohosone Y, Hama N, Suwa A, Akizuki M, Homma M, Griffith AJ, Hardin JA.; 1990 Mar 1;
  http://www.pubmedcentral.gov/articlerender.fcgi?tool=pmcentrez&rendertype=abstract&artid=53566

- **Rare Scleroderma Autoantibodies to the U11 Small Nuclear Ribonucleoprotein and to the Trimethylguanosine Cap of U Small Nuclear RNAs.** by Gilliam AC, Steitz JA.; 1993 Jul 15;
  http://www.pubmedcentral.gov/articlerender.fcgi?tool=pmcentrez&rendertype=abstract&artid=47016

- **Sixth International Workshop on Scleroderma Research, Oxford, UK, 30 July --2 August 2000.** by Wollheim FA, Denton CP, Abraham DJ.; 2001;
  http://www.pubmedcentral.gov/articlerender.fcgi?tool=pmcentrez&artid=128881

- **The human exosome: an autoantigenic complex of exoribonucleases in myositis and scleroderma.** by Brouwer R, Pruijn GJ, van Venrooij WJ.; 2001;
  http://www.pubmedcentral.gov/articlerender.fcgi?tool=pmcentrez&artid=128886

- **The inhibitory effects of camptothecin, a topoisomerase I inhibitor, on collagen synthesis in fibroblasts from patients with systemic sclerosis.** by Czuwara-Ladykowska J, Makiela B, Smith EA, Trojanowska M, Rudnicka L.; 2001;
  http://www.pubmedcentral.gov/articlerender.fcgi?tool=pmcentrez&artid=64844

- **Von Willebrand factor propeptide as a marker of disease activity in systemic sclerosis (scleroderma).** by Scheja A, Akesson A, Geborek P, Wildt M, Wollheim CB, Wollheim FA, Vischer UM.; 2001;
  http://www.pubmedcentral.gov/articlerender.fcgi?tool=pmcentrez&artid=30710

The National Library of Medicine: PubMed

One of the quickest and most comprehensive ways to find academic studies in both English and other languages is to use PubMed, maintained by the National Library of Medicine.[6] The advantage of PubMed over previously mentioned sources is that it covers a greater number of domestic and foreign references. It is also free to use. If the publisher has a Web site that offers full text of its journals, PubMed will provide links to that site, as well as to sites offering other related data. User registration, a subscription fee, or some other type of fee may be required to access the full text of articles in some journals.

To generate your own bibliography of studies dealing with scleroderma, simply go to the PubMed Web site at **http://www.ncbi.nlm.nih.gov/pubmed**. Type "scleroderma" (or synonyms) into the search box, and click "Go." The following is the type of output you can expect from PubMed for scleroderma (hyperlinks lead to article summaries):

- **A bioactive triterpenoid and vulpinic acid derivatives from the mushroom Scleroderma citrinum.**
  Author(s): Kanokmedhakul S, Kanokmedhakul K, Prajuabsuk T, Soytong K, Kongsaeree P, Suksamrarn A.
  Source: Planta Medica. 2003 June; 69(6): 568-71.
  http://www.ncbi.nlm.nih.gov:80/entrez/query.fcgi?cmd=Retrieve&db=PubMed&list_uids=12865983&dopt=Abstract

- **A case of linear scleroderma with muscle calcification.**
  Author(s): Jinnin M, Ihn H, Asano Y, Yamane K, Yazawa N, Tamaki K.
  Source: The British Journal of Dermatology. 2002 June; 146(6): 1084-6.
  http://www.ncbi.nlm.nih.gov:80/entrez/query.fcgi?cmd=Retrieve&db=PubMed&list_uids=12072084&dopt=Abstract

- **A cross-sectional comparison of three self-reported functional indices in scleroderma.**
  Author(s): Smyth AE, MacGregor AJ, Mukerjee D, Brough GM, Black CM, Denton CP.
  Source: Rheumatology (Oxford, England). 2003 June; 42(6): 732-8. Epub 2003 April 16.
  http://www.ncbi.nlm.nih.gov:80/entrez/query.fcgi?cmd=Retrieve&db=PubMed&list_uids=12730528&dopt=Abstract

- **A pediatric case of sclerodermatous chronic graft-versus-host disease.**
  Author(s): Terasaki K, Kanekura T, Setoyama M, Kanzaki T.
  Source: Pediatric Dermatology. 2003 July-August; 20(4): 327-31.
  http://www.ncbi.nlm.nih.gov:80/entrez/query.fcgi?cmd=Retrieve&db=PubMed&list_uids=12869155&dopt=Abstract

---

[6] PubMed was developed by the National Center for Biotechnology Information (NCBI) at the National Library of Medicine (NLM) at the National Institutes of Health (NIH). The PubMed database was developed in conjunction with publishers of biomedical literature as a search tool for accessing literature citations and linking to full-text journal articles at Web sites of participating publishers. Publishers that participate in PubMed supply NLM with their citations electronically prior to or at the time of publication.

- **A randomized, controlled trial of methotrexate versus placebo in early diffuse scleroderma.**
  Author(s): Pope JE, Bellamy N, Seibold JR, Baron M, Ellman M, Carette S, Smith CD, Chalmers IM, Hong P, O'Hanlon D, Kaminska E, Markland J, Sibley J, Catoggio L, Furst DE.
  Source: Arthritis and Rheumatism. 2001 June; 44(6): 1351-8.
  http://www.ncbi.nlm.nih.gov:80/entrez/query.fcgi?cmd=Retrieve&db=PubMed&list_uids=11407694&dopt=Abstract

- **A variant of acrokeratoelastoidosis in systemic scleroderma: report of 7 cases.**
  Author(s): Tajima S, Tanaka N, Ishibashi A, Suzuki K.
  Source: Journal of the American Academy of Dermatology. 2002 May; 46(5): 767-70.
  http://www.ncbi.nlm.nih.gov:80/entrez/query.fcgi?cmd=Retrieve&db=PubMed&list_uids=12004321&dopt=Abstract

- **Abnormal responses to endothelial agonists in Raynaud's phenomenon and scleroderma.**
  Author(s): Freedman RR, Girgis R, Mayes MD.
  Source: The Journal of Rheumatology. 2001 January; 28(1): 119-21.
  http://www.ncbi.nlm.nih.gov:80/entrez/query.fcgi?cmd=Retrieve&db=PubMed&list_uids=11196511&dopt=Abstract

- **Abnormalities in fibrillin 1-containing microfibrils in dermal fibroblast cultures from patients with systemic sclerosis (scleroderma).**
  Author(s): Wallis DD, Tan FK, Kielty CM, Kimball MD, Arnett FC, Milewicz DM.
  Source: Arthritis and Rheumatism. 2001 August; 44(8): 1855-64.
  http://www.ncbi.nlm.nih.gov:80/entrez/query.fcgi?cmd=Retrieve&db=PubMed&list_uids=11508439&dopt=Abstract

- **Achalasia in a patient with scleroderma false-positive ectopic thyroid scintigraphy.**
  Author(s): Peksoy I, Kiratli PO, Sari O, Erbas B.
  Source: Clinical Nuclear Medicine. 2000 November; 25(11): 931.
  http://www.ncbi.nlm.nih.gov:80/entrez/query.fcgi?cmd=Retrieve&db=PubMed&list_uids=11079600&dopt=Abstract

- **Acro-osteolysis in a patient with scleroderma.**
  Author(s): Zandman-Goddard G, Tal S.
  Source: Isr Med Assoc J. 2002 March; 4(3): 231. No Abstract Available.
  http://www.ncbi.nlm.nih.gov:80/entrez/query.fcgi?cmd=Retrieve&db=PubMed&list_uids=11908276&dopt=Abstract

- **Acute mechanical obstruction of the colon in scleroderma.**
  Author(s): Sayfan J, Becker A, Lev A.
  Source: Isr Med Assoc J. 2001 June; 3(6): 468-9. No Abstract Available.
  http://www.ncbi.nlm.nih.gov:80/entrez/query.fcgi?cmd=Retrieve&db=PubMed&list_uids=11433650&dopt=Abstract

- **Age and risk of pulmonary arterial hypertension in scleroderma.**
  Author(s): Schachna L, Wigley FM, Chang B, White B, Wise RA, Gelber AC.
  Source: Chest. 2003 December; 124(6): 2098-104.
  http://www.ncbi.nlm.nih.gov:80/entrez/query.fcgi?cmd=Retrieve&db=PubMed&list_uids=14665486&dopt=Abstract

- **Altered negative regulation of transforming growth factor beta signaling in scleroderma: potential involvement of SMURF2 in disease.**
  Author(s): Zuscik MJ, Rosier RN, Schwarz EM.
  Source: Arthritis and Rheumatism. 2003 July; 48(7): 1779-80. Review.
  http://www.ncbi.nlm.nih.gov:80/entrez/query.fcgi?cmd=Retrieve&db=PubMed&list_uids=12847669&dopt=Abstract

- **Animal models for scleroderma: an update.**
  Author(s): Zhang Y, Gilliam AC.
  Source: Curr Rheumatol Rep. 2002 April; 4(2): 150-62. Review.
  http://www.ncbi.nlm.nih.gov:80/entrez/query.fcgi?cmd=Retrieve&db=PubMed&list_uids=11890881&dopt=Abstract

- **Antibodies to Th/To ribonucleoprotein in patients with localized scleroderma.**
  Author(s): Yamane K, Ihn H, Kubo M, Kuwana M, Asano Y, Yazawa N, Tamaki K.
  Source: Rheumatology (Oxford, England). 2001 June; 40(6): 683-6.
  http://www.ncbi.nlm.nih.gov:80/entrez/query.fcgi?cmd=Retrieve&db=PubMed&list_uids=11426027&dopt=Abstract

- **Antibody-mediated gastrointestinal dysmotility in scleroderma.**
  Author(s): Goldblatt F, Gordon TP, Waterman SA.
  Source: Gastroenterology. 2002 October; 123(4): 1144-50. Erratum In: Gastroenterology 2002 December; 123(6): 2164.
  http://www.ncbi.nlm.nih.gov:80/entrez/query.fcgi?cmd=Retrieve&db=PubMed&list_uids=12360477&dopt=Abstract

- **Anti-Ku antibody-positive scleroderma-dermatomyositis overlap syndrome developing Graves' disease and immune thrombocytopenic purpura.**
  Author(s): Kamei N, Yamane K, Yamashita Y, Nakanishi S, Watanabe H, Fujikawa R, Hiyama K, Ishioka S, Mendoza C, Kohno N.
  Source: Intern Med. 2002 December; 41(12): 1199-203.
  http://www.ncbi.nlm.nih.gov:80/entrez/query.fcgi?cmd=Retrieve&db=PubMed&list_uids=12521216&dopt=Abstract

- **Antineutrophil cytoplasmic antibodies in scleroderma patients: first report of a case with anti-proteinase 3 antibodies and review of the literature.**
  Author(s): Caramaschi P, Biasi D, Tonolli E, Carletto A, Bambara LM.
  Source: Joint, Bone, Spine : Revue Du Rhumatisme. 2002 March; 69(2): 177-80.
  http://www.ncbi.nlm.nih.gov:80/entrez/query.fcgi?cmd=Retrieve&db=PubMed&list_uids=12027309&dopt=Abstract

- **Antiphospholipid antibody in localised scleroderma.**
  Author(s): Sato S, Fujimoto M, Hasegawa M, Takehara K.
  Source: Annals of the Rheumatic Diseases. 2003 August; 62(8): 771-4.
  http://www.ncbi.nlm.nih.gov:80/entrez/query.fcgi?cmd=Retrieve&db=PubMed&list_
  uids=12860735&dopt=Abstract

- **Anti-thymocyte globulin in scleroderma.**
  Author(s): Denman AM.
  Source: Rheumatology (Oxford, England). 2001 October; 40(10): 1192.
  http://www.ncbi.nlm.nih.gov:80/entrez/query.fcgi?cmd=Retrieve&db=PubMed&list_
  uids=11600753&dopt=Abstract

- **Antitopoisomerase I antibody in patients with systemic lupus erythematosus/sicca syndrome without a concomitant scleroderma: two case reports.**
  Author(s): Al Attia HM, D'Souza MS.
  Source: Clinical Rheumatology. 2003 February; 22(1): 70-2.
  http://www.ncbi.nlm.nih.gov:80/entrez/query.fcgi?cmd=Retrieve&db=PubMed&list_
  uids=12605324&dopt=Abstract

- **Anti-U3 snRNP antibodies in localised scleroderma.**
  Author(s): Yimane K, Ihn H, Kubo M, Asano Y, Yazawa N, Tamaki K.
  Source: Annals of the Rheumatic Diseases. 2001 December; 60(12): 1157-8.
  http://www.ncbi.nlm.nih.gov:80/entrez/query.fcgi?cmd=Retrieve&db=PubMed&list_
  uids=11760725&dopt=Abstract

- **Anti-U5 snRNP antibody as a possible serological marker for scleroderma-polymyositis overlap.**
  Author(s): Kubo M, Ihn H, Kuwana M, Asano Y, Tamaki T, Yamane K, Tamaki K.
  Source: Rheumatology (Oxford, England). 2002 May; 41(5): 531-4.
  http://www.ncbi.nlm.nih.gov:80/entrez/query.fcgi?cmd=Retrieve&db=PubMed&list_
  uids=12011376&dopt=Abstract

- **Association of 5'-untranslated region of the Fibrillin-1 gene with Japanese scleroderma.**
  Author(s): Kodera T, Tan FK, Sasaki T, Arnett FC, Bona CA.
  Source: Gene. 2002 September 4; 297(1-2): 61-7.
  http://www.ncbi.nlm.nih.gov:80/entrez/query.fcgi?cmd=Retrieve&db=PubMed&list_
  uids=12384286&dopt=Abstract

- **Association of novel polymorphisms with the expression of SPARC in normal fibroblasts and with susceptibility to scleroderma.**
  Author(s): Zhou X, Tan FK, Reveille JD, Wallis D, Milewicz DM, Ahn C, Wang A, Arnett FC.
  Source: Arthritis and Rheumatism. 2002 November; 46(11): 2990-9.
  http://www.ncbi.nlm.nih.gov:80/entrez/query.fcgi?cmd=Retrieve&db=PubMed&list_
  uids=12428242&dopt=Abstract

- **Autoantibodies against B23, a nucleolar phosphoprotein, occur in scleroderma and are associated with pulmonary hypertension.**
  Author(s): Ulanet DB, Wigley FM, Gelber AC, Rosen A.
  Source: Arthritis and Rheumatism. 2003 February 15; 49(1): 85-92.
  http://www.ncbi.nlm.nih.gov:80/entrez/query.fcgi?cmd=Retrieve&db=PubMed&list_uids=12579598&dopt=Abstract

- **Autoantibodies and clinical subsets: relevance to scleroderma.**
  Author(s): Maddison PJ.
  Source: Wiener Klinische Wochenschrift. 2000 August 25; 112(15-16): 684-6. Review.
  http://www.ncbi.nlm.nih.gov:80/entrez/query.fcgi?cmd=Retrieve&db=PubMed&list_uids=11020957&dopt=Abstract

- **Autoantibody detection in scleroderma patients. Diagnostic and analytical performances of a new coupled particle light scattering immunoassay.**
  Author(s): Bizzaro N, Bonelli F, Tonutti E, Villalta D, Tozzolis R.
  Source: Clin Exp Rheumatol. 2002 January-February; 20(1): 45-51.
  http://www.ncbi.nlm.nih.gov:80/entrez/query.fcgi?cmd=Retrieve&db=PubMed&list_uids=11892707&dopt=Abstract

- **Autoimmunity in scleroderma: the origin, pathogenetic role, and clinical significance of autoantibodies.**
  Author(s): Harris ML, Rosen A.
  Source: Current Opinion in Rheumatology. 2003 November; 15(6): 778-84. Review.
  http://www.ncbi.nlm.nih.gov:80/entrez/query.fcgi?cmd=Retrieve&db=PubMed&list_uids=14569210&dopt=Abstract

- **Autologous skin grafting in the treatment of severe scleroderma cutaneous ulcers: a case report.**
  Author(s): Giuggioli D, Sebastiani M, Cazzato M, Piaggesi A, Abatangelo G, Ferri C.
  Source: Rheumatology (Oxford, England). 2003 May; 42(5): 694-6.
  http://www.ncbi.nlm.nih.gov:80/entrez/query.fcgi?cmd=Retrieve&db=PubMed&list_uids=12709550&dopt=Abstract

- **Bilateral breast cancer associated with diffuse scleroderma.**
  Author(s): Pineda V, Salvador R, Soriano J.
  Source: Breast (Edinburgh, Scotland). 2003 June; 12(3): 217-9.
  http://www.ncbi.nlm.nih.gov:80/entrez/query.fcgi?cmd=Retrieve&db=PubMed&list_uids=14659331&dopt=Abstract

- **Bilateral cricoarytenoid joint ankylosis in scleroderma.**
  Author(s): Viner DD, Sabri A, Tucker HM.
  Source: Otolaryngology and Head and Neck Surgery. 2001 June; 124(6): 696-7.
  http://www.ncbi.nlm.nih.gov:80/entrez/query.fcgi?cmd=Retrieve&db=PubMed&list_uids=11391267&dopt=Abstract

- **Bilateral keratomalacia in a cachectic scleroderma patient.**
  Author(s): al-Husainy S, Deane J.
  Source: Eye (London, England). 1999 August; 13 (Pt 4): 586-8.
  http://www.ncbi.nlm.nih.gov:80/entrez/query.fcgi?cmd=Retrieve&db=PubMed&list_uids=10692938&dopt=Abstract

- **Bilateral linear scleroderma "en coup de sabre" associated with facial atrophy and neurological complications.**
  Author(s): Gambichler T, Kreuter A, Hoffmann K, Bechara FG, Altmeyer P, Jansen T.
  Source: Bmc Dermatology [electronic Resource]. 2001; 1(1): 9. Epub 2001 December 04.
  http://www.ncbi.nlm.nih.gov:80/entrez/query.fcgi?cmd=Retrieve&db=PubMed&list_uids=11741509&dopt=Abstract

- **Blockade of endogenous transforming growth factor beta signaling prevents up-regulated collagen synthesis in scleroderma fibroblasts: association with increased expression of transforming growth factor beta receptors.**
  Author(s): Ihn H, Yamane K, Kubo M, Tamaki K.
  Source: Arthritis and Rheumatism. 2001 February; 44(2): 474-80.
  http://www.ncbi.nlm.nih.gov:80/entrez/query.fcgi?cmd=Retrieve&db=PubMed&list_uids=11229480&dopt=Abstract

- **Body image dissatisfaction among women with scleroderma: extent and relationship to psychosocial function.**
  Author(s): Benrud-Larson LM, Heinberg LJ, Boling C, Reed J, White B, Wigley FM, Haythornthwaite JA.
  Source: Health Psychology : Official Journal of the Division of Health Psychology, American Psychological Association. 2003 March; 22(2): 130-9.
  http://www.ncbi.nlm.nih.gov:80/entrez/query.fcgi?cmd=Retrieve&db=PubMed&list_uids=12683733&dopt=Abstract

- **Brachial plexopathy associated with diffuse edematous scleroderma.**
  Author(s): Mouthon L, Halimi C, Dussaule Md JC, Cayre-Castel Md M, Guillevin L.
  Source: Annales De Medecine Interne. 2000 June; 151(4): 303-5.
  http://www.ncbi.nlm.nih.gov:80/entrez/query.fcgi?cmd=Retrieve&db=PubMed&list_uids=10922959&dopt=Abstract

- **Bullous lesions in scleroderma.**
  Author(s): Rencic A, Goyal S, Mofid M, Wigley F, Nousari HC.
  Source: International Journal of Dermatology. 2002 June; 41(6): 335-9. Review.
  http://www.ncbi.nlm.nih.gov:80/entrez/query.fcgi?cmd=Retrieve&db=PubMed&list_uids=12100687&dopt=Abstract

- **Bullous scleroderma-like changes in chronic graft-versus-host disease.**
  Author(s): Moreno JC, Valverde F, Martinez F, Velez A, Torres A, Fanego J, Ocana MS.
  Source: Journal of the European Academy of Dermatology and Venereology : Jeadv. 2003 March; 17(2): 200-3.
  http://www.ncbi.nlm.nih.gov:80/entrez/query.fcgi?cmd=Retrieve&db=PubMed&list_uids=12705752&dopt=Abstract

- **Calculated glomerular filtration rate is a useful screening tool to identify scleroderma patients with renal impairment.**
  Author(s): Kingdon EJ, Knight CJ, Dustan K, Irwin AG, Thomas M, Powis SH, Burns A, Hilson AJ, Black CM.
  Source: Rheumatology (Oxford, England). 2003 January; 42(1): 26-33.
  http://www.ncbi.nlm.nih.gov:80/entrez/query.fcgi?cmd=Retrieve&db=PubMed&list_uids=12509609&dopt=Abstract

- **Cardiac arrest after labetalol and metoclopramide administration in a patient with scleroderma.**
  Author(s): Tung A, Sweitzer B, Cutter T.
  Source: Anesthesia and Analgesia. 2002 December; 95(6): 1667-8, Table of Contents.
  http://www.ncbi.nlm.nih.gov:80/entrez/query.fcgi?cmd=Retrieve&db=PubMed&list_uids=12456435&dopt=Abstract

- **Carotid and femoral arterial wall mechanics in scleroderma.**
  Author(s): Cheng KS, Tiwari A, Boutin A, Denton CP, Black CM, Morris R, Hamilton G, Seifalian AM.
  Source: Rheumatology (Oxford, England). 2003 November; 42(11): 1299-305. Epub 2003 May 30.
  http://www.ncbi.nlm.nih.gov:80/entrez/query.fcgi?cmd=Retrieve&db=PubMed&list_uids=12777634&dopt=Abstract

- **Case 26-2001: scleroderma renal crisis and polymyositis.**
  Author(s): Lopez-Ovejero JA.
  Source: The New England Journal of Medicine. 2002 June 13; 346(24): 1916-8; Author Reply 1916-8.
  http://www.ncbi.nlm.nih.gov:80/entrez/query.fcgi?cmd=Retrieve&db=PubMed&list_uids=12066816&dopt=Abstract

- **Case 26-2001: scleroderma renal crisis and polymyositis.**
  Author(s): Aldington D.
  Source: The New England Journal of Medicine. 2002 June 13; 346(24): 1916-8; Author Reply 1916-8.
  http://www.ncbi.nlm.nih.gov:80/entrez/query.fcgi?cmd=Retrieve&db=PubMed&list_uids=12066815&dopt=Abstract

- **Case 26-2001: scleroderma renal crisis and polymyositis.**
  Author(s): Shapiro LS.
  Source: The New England Journal of Medicine. 2002 June 13; 346(24): 1916-8; Author Reply 1916-8.
  http://www.ncbi.nlm.nih.gov:80/entrez/query.fcgi?cmd=Retrieve&db=PubMed&list_uids=12066814&dopt=Abstract

- **Case 26-2001: scleroderma renal crisis and polymyositis.**
  Author(s): Selva O'Callaghan A, Labrador Horrillo M, Vilardell Tarres M.
  Source: The New England Journal of Medicine. 2002 June 13; 346(24): 1916-8; Author Reply 1916-8.
  http://www.ncbi.nlm.nih.gov:80/entrez/query.fcgi?cmd=Retrieve&db=PubMed&list_uids=12063382&dopt=Abstract

- **Catheter angiography and angioplasty in patients with scleroderma.**
  Author(s): Dick EA, Aviv R, Francis I, Hamilton G, Baker D, Black C, Platts A, Watkinson A.
  Source: The British Journal of Radiology. 2001 December; 74(888): 1091-6.
  http://www.ncbi.nlm.nih.gov:80/entrez/query.fcgi?cmd=Retrieve&db=PubMed&list_uids=11777765&dopt=Abstract

- **Childbearing and the risk of scleroderma: a population-based study in Sweden.**
  Author(s): Lambe M, Bjornadal L, Neregard P, Nyren O, Cooper GS.
  Source: American Journal of Epidemiology. 2004 January 15; 159(2): 162-6.
  http://www.ncbi.nlm.nih.gov:80/entrez/query.fcgi?cmd=Retrieve&db=PubMed&list_uids=14718218&dopt=Abstract

- **Chronic constipation--a lethal danger in patients with systemic scleroderma.**
  Author(s): Exadaktylos A, Papagrigoriadis S.
  Source: European Journal of Emergency Medicine : Official Journal of the European Society for Emergency Medicine. 2001 December; 8(4): 333-5.
  http://www.ncbi.nlm.nih.gov:80/entrez/query.fcgi?cmd=Retrieve&db=PubMed&list_uids=11785605&dopt=Abstract

- **Class II HLA associations with autoantibodies in scleroderma: a highly significant role for HLA-DP.**
  Author(s): Gilchrist FC, Bunn C, Foley PJ, Lympany PA, Black CM, Welsh KI, du Bois RM.
  Source: Genes and Immunity. 2001 April; 2(2): 76-81.
  http://www.ncbi.nlm.nih.gov:80/entrez/query.fcgi?cmd=Retrieve&db=PubMed&list_uids=11393660&dopt=Abstract

- **Clinical trials for pediatric scleroderma.**
  Author(s): Rosenkranz ME, Lehman TJ.
  Source: Curr Rheumatol Rep. 2002 December; 4(6): 449-51.
  http://www.ncbi.nlm.nih.gov:80/entrez/query.fcgi?cmd=Retrieve&db=PubMed&list_uids=12427357&dopt=Abstract

- **Clinical trials for the treatment of systemic sclerosis/scleroderma.**
  Author(s): Varga J, Ponor I.
  Source: Curr Rheumatol Rep. 1999 October; 1(1): 13-4. Review. No Abstract Available.
  http://www.ncbi.nlm.nih.gov:80/entrez/query.fcgi?cmd=Retrieve&db=PubMed&list_uids=11123008&dopt=Abstract

- **Clinical utility of telangiectasia of hands in scleroderma and other rheumatic disorders.**
  Author(s): Robert-Thomson PJ, Mould TL, Walker JG, Smith MD, Ahern MJ.
  Source: Asian Pac J Allergy Immunol. 2002 March; 20(1): 7-12.
  http://www.ncbi.nlm.nih.gov:80/entrez/query.fcgi?cmd=Retrieve&db=PubMed&list_uids=12125921&dopt=Abstract

- **Coexistent linear scleroderma and juvenile systemic lupus erythematosus.**
  Author(s): Majeed M, Al-Mayouf SM, Al-Sabban E, Bahabri S.
  Source: Pediatric Dermatology. 2000 November-December; 17(6): 456-9. Review.
  http://www.ncbi.nlm.nih.gov:80/entrez/query.fcgi?cmd=Retrieve&db=PubMed&list_
  uids=11123778&dopt=Abstract

- **Comparative biochemistry of human skin: glycosaminoglycans from different body sites in normal subjects and in patients with localized scleroderma.**
  Author(s): Passos CO, Werneck CC, Onofre GR, Pagani EA, Filgueira AL, Silva LC.
  Source: Journal of the European Academy of Dermatology and Venereology : Jeadv.
  2003 January; 17(1): 14-9.
  http://www.ncbi.nlm.nih.gov:80/entrez/query.fcgi?cmd=Retrieve&db=PubMed&list_
  uids=12602961&dopt=Abstract

- **Congenital fascial dystrophy, a new scleroderma-like genetic disease with limitation of joint mobility: comment on the clinical image presented by Di Rocco.**
  Author(s): Jablonska S.
  Source: Arthritis and Rheumatism. 2002 July; 46(7): 1978-80.
  http://www.ncbi.nlm.nih.gov:80/entrez/query.fcgi?cmd=Retrieve&db=PubMed&list_
  uids=12124894&dopt=Abstract

- **Constitutive connective tissue growth factor expression in scleroderma fibroblasts is dependent on Sp1.**
  Author(s): Holmes A, Abraham DJ, Chen Y, Denton C, Shi-wen X, Black CM, Leask A.
  Source: The Journal of Biological Chemistry. 2003 October 24; 278(43): 41728-33. Epub
  2003 July 29.
  http://www.ncbi.nlm.nih.gov:80/entrez/query.fcgi?cmd=Retrieve&db=PubMed&list_
  uids=12888575&dopt=Abstract

- **Continuous intravenous epoprostenol for pulmonary hypertension due to the scleroderma spectrum of disease. A randomized, controlled trial.**
  Author(s): Badesch DB, Tapson VF, McGoon MD, Brundage BH, Rubin LJ, Wigley FM, Rich S, Barst RJ, Barrett PS, Kral KM, Jobsis MM, Loyd JE, Murali S, Frost A, Girgis R, Bourge RC, Ralph DD, Elliott CG, Hill NS, Langleben D, Schilz RJ, McLaughlin VV, Robbins IM, Groves BM, Shapiro S, Medsger TA Jr.
  Source: Annals of Internal Medicine. 2000 March 21; 132(6): 425-34.
  http://www.ncbi.nlm.nih.gov:80/entrez/query.fcgi?cmd=Retrieve&db=PubMed&list_
  uids=10733441&dopt=Abstract

- **Continuous regional anesthesia before surgical peripheral sympathectomy in a patient with severe digital necrosis associated with Raynaud's phenomenon and scleroderma.**
  Author(s): Greengrass RA, Feinglass NG, Murray PM, Trigg SD.
  Source: Regional Anesthesia and Pain Medicine. 2003 July-August; 28(4): 354-8.
  http://www.ncbi.nlm.nih.gov:80/entrez/query.fcgi?cmd=Retrieve&db=PubMed&list_
  uids=12945033&dopt=Abstract

- **Corticosteroid-induced scleroderma renal crisis.**
  Author(s): Lee AT, Burnet S.
  Source: The Medical Journal of Australia. 2002 October 21; 177(8): 459.
  http://www.ncbi.nlm.nih.gov:80/entrez/query.fcgi?cmd=Retrieve&db=PubMed&list_uids=12381259&dopt=Abstract

- **CT and MRI findings in sclerodermatous chronic graft vs. host disease.**
  Author(s): Dumford K, Anderson JC.
  Source: Clinical Imaging. 2001 March-April; 25(2): 138-40.
  http://www.ncbi.nlm.nih.gov:80/entrez/query.fcgi?cmd=Retrieve&db=PubMed&list_uids=11483427&dopt=Abstract

- **CTGF and SMADs, maintenance of scleroderma phenotype is independent of SMAD signaling.**
  Author(s): Holmes A, Abraham DJ, Sa S, Shiwen X, Black CM, Leask A.
  Source: The Journal of Biological Chemistry. 2001 April 6; 276(14): 10594-601. Epub 2001 January 04.
  http://www.ncbi.nlm.nih.gov:80/entrez/query.fcgi?cmd=Retrieve&db=PubMed&list_uids=11152469&dopt=Abstract

- **Current treatment options in systemic Sclerosis (Scleroderma).**
  Author(s): Stummvoll GH.
  Source: Acta Medica Austriaca. 2002; 29(1): 14-9. Review.
  http://www.ncbi.nlm.nih.gov:80/entrez/query.fcgi?cmd=Retrieve&db=PubMed&list_uids=11899748&dopt=Abstract

- **Cutaneous concerns of scleroderma patients.**
  Author(s): Paquette DL, Falanga V.
  Source: The Journal of Dermatology. 2003 June; 30(6): 438-43.
  http://www.ncbi.nlm.nih.gov:80/entrez/query.fcgi?cmd=Retrieve&db=PubMed&list_uids=12810990&dopt=Abstract

- **Cyclooxygenase-2 expression and prostaglandin E2 biosynthesis are enhanced in scleroderma fibroblasts and inhibited by UVA irradiation.**
  Author(s): Kanekura T, Higashi Y, Kanzaki T.
  Source: The Journal of Rheumatology. 2001 July; 28(7): 1568-72.
  http://www.ncbi.nlm.nih.gov:80/entrez/query.fcgi?cmd=Retrieve&db=PubMed&list_uids=11469463&dopt=Abstract

- **Cytochrome P2 polymorphisms and susceptibility to scleroderma following exposure to organic solvents.**
  Author(s): Povey A, Guppy MJ, Wood M, Knight C, Black CM, Silman AJ.
  Source: Arthritis and Rheumatism. 2001 March; 44(3): 662-5.
  http://www.ncbi.nlm.nih.gov:80/entrez/query.fcgi?cmd=Retrieve&db=PubMed&list_uids=11263781&dopt=Abstract

- **Cytochrome P2 polymorphisms and susceptibility to scleroderma: comment on the article by Povey et al.**
  Author(s): Pandey JP, Nietert PJ, Silver RM.
  Source: Arthritis and Rheumatism. 2001 November; 44(11): 2705-6.
  http://www.ncbi.nlm.nih.gov:80/entrez/query.fcgi?cmd=Retrieve&db=PubMed&list_uids=11710729&dopt=Abstract

- **Cytokine directed therapy in scleroderma: rationale, current status, and the future.**
  Author(s): Simms RW, Korn JH.
  Source: Current Opinion in Rheumatology. 2002 November; 14(6): 717-22. Review.
  http://www.ncbi.nlm.nih.gov:80/entrez/query.fcgi?cmd=Retrieve&db=PubMed&list_uids=12410097&dopt=Abstract

- **Deficient Smad7 expression: a putative molecular defect in scleroderma.**
  Author(s): Dong C, Zhu S, Wang T, Yoon W, Li Z, Alvarez RJ, ten Dijke P, White B, Wigley FM, Goldschmidt-Clermont PJ.
  Source: Proceedings of the National Academy of Sciences of the United States of America. 2002 March 19; 99(6): 3908-13.
  http://www.ncbi.nlm.nih.gov:80/entrez/query.fcgi?cmd=Retrieve&db=PubMed&list_uids=11904440&dopt=Abstract

- **Depletion of protein kinase Cepsilon in normal and scleroderma lung fibroblasts has opposite effects on tenascin expression.**
  Author(s): Tourkina E, Hoffman S, Fenton JW 2nd, Lipsitz S, Silver RM, Ludwicka-Bradley A.
  Source: Arthritis and Rheumatism. 2001 June; 44(6): 1370-81.
  http://www.ncbi.nlm.nih.gov:80/entrez/query.fcgi?cmd=Retrieve&db=PubMed&list_uids=11407697&dopt=Abstract

- **Dermal organization in scleroderma: the fast Fourier transform and the laser scatter method objectify fibrosis in nonlesional as well as lesional skin.**
  Author(s): de Vries HJ, Enomoto DN, van Marle J, van Zuijlen PP, Mekkes JR, Bos JD.
  Source: Laboratory Investigation; a Journal of Technical Methods and Pathology. 2000 August; 80(8): 1281-9.
  http://www.ncbi.nlm.nih.gov:80/entrez/query.fcgi?cmd=Retrieve&db=PubMed&list_uids=10950119&dopt=Abstract

- **Dermatomyositis-scleroderma overlap syndrome presenting as autoimmune haemolytic anaemia.**
  Author(s): Andrews J, Hall MA.
  Source: Rheumatology (Oxford, England). 2002 August; 41(8): 956-8.
  http://www.ncbi.nlm.nih.gov:80/entrez/query.fcgi?cmd=Retrieve&db=PubMed&list_uids=12154224&dopt=Abstract

- **Detection of activated complement complex C5b-9 and complement receptor C5a in skin biopsies of patients with systemic sclerosis (scleroderma).**
  Author(s): Sprott H, Muller-Ladner U, Distler O, Gay RE, Barnum SR, Landthaler M, Scholmerich J, Lang B, Gay S.
  Source: The Journal of Rheumatology. 2000 February; 27(2): 402-4.
  http://www.ncbi.nlm.nih.gov:80/entrez/query.fcgi?cmd=Retrieve&db=PubMed&list_uids=10685805&dopt=Abstract

- **Development and evaluation of a patient education program for persons with systemic sclerosis (scleroderma).**
  Author(s): Samuelson UK, Ahlmen EM.
  Source: Arthritis Care and Research : the Official Journal of the Arthritis Health Professions Association. 2000 June; 13(3): 141-8.
  http://www.ncbi.nlm.nih.gov:80/entrez/query.fcgi?cmd=Retrieve&db=PubMed&list_uids=14635287&dopt=Abstract

- **Development of histologic features of scleroderma in congenital lesions.**
  Author(s): Harford R, Smith KJ, Skelton H.
  Source: Journal of Cutaneous Pathology. 2002 April; 29(4): 249-54.
  http://www.ncbi.nlm.nih.gov:80/entrez/query.fcgi?cmd=Retrieve&db=PubMed&list_uids=12028159&dopt=Abstract

- **Different pattern of collagen cross-links in two sclerotic skin diseases: lipodermatosclerosis and circumscribed scleroderma.**
  Author(s): Brinckmann J, Neess CM, Gaber Y, Sobhi H, Notbohm H, Hunzelmann N, Fietzek PP, Muller PK, Risteli J, Gebker R, Scharffetter-Kochanek K.
  Source: The Journal of Investigative Dermatology. 2001 August; 117(2): 269-73.
  http://www.ncbi.nlm.nih.gov:80/entrez/query.fcgi?cmd=Retrieve&db=PubMed&list_uids=11511304&dopt=Abstract

- **Differential expression of nitric oxide by dermal microvascular endothelial cells from patients with scleroderma.**
  Author(s): Romero LI, Zhang DN, Cooke JP, Ho HK, Avalos E, Herrera R, Herron GS.
  Source: Vascular Medicine (London, England). 2000; 5(3): 147-58.
  http://www.ncbi.nlm.nih.gov:80/entrez/query.fcgi?cmd=Retrieve&db=PubMed&list_uids=11104297&dopt=Abstract

- **Diffuse and limited cutaneous systemic scleroderma.**
  Author(s): Foeldvari I.
  Source: Current Opinion in Rheumatology. 2000 September; 12(5): 435-8. Review.
  http://www.ncbi.nlm.nih.gov:80/entrez/query.fcgi?cmd=Retrieve&db=PubMed&list_uids=10990182&dopt=Abstract

- **Diffuse scleroderma occurring after the use of paclitaxel for ovarian cancer.**
  Author(s): De Angelis R, Bugatti L, Cerioni A, Del Medico P, Filosa G.
  Source: Clinical Rheumatology. 2003 February; 22(1): 49-52.
  http://www.ncbi.nlm.nih.gov:80/entrez/query.fcgi?cmd=Retrieve&db=PubMed&list_uids=12605319&dopt=Abstract

- **Digital arterial occlusion in scleroderma: is there a role for digital arterial reconstruction?**
  Author(s): Tomaino MM.
  Source: Journal of Hand Surgery (Edinburgh, Lothian). 2000 December; 25(6): 611-3.
  http://www.ncbi.nlm.nih.gov:80/entrez/query.fcgi?cmd=Retrieve&db=PubMed&list_uids=11106531&dopt=Abstract

- **Disease severity as a predictor of outcome in scleroderma.**
  Author(s): Gelber AC, Wigley FM.
  Source: Lancet. 2002 January 26; 359(9303): 277-9.
  http://www.ncbi.nlm.nih.gov:80/entrez/query.fcgi?cmd=Retrieve&db=PubMed&list_uids=11830191&dopt=Abstract

- **Disseminated scleroderma of a Japanese patient successfully treated with bath PUVA photochemotherapy.**
  Author(s): Aragane Y, Kawada A, Maeda A, Isogai R, Isogai N, Tezuka T.
  Source: Journal of Cutaneous Medicine and Surgery. 2001 March-April; 5(2): 135-9. Epub 2001 March 21.
  http://www.ncbi.nlm.nih.gov:80/entrez/query.fcgi?cmd=Retrieve&db=PubMed&list_uids=11443486&dopt=Abstract

- **Diversity and plasticity of the anti-DNA topoisomerase I autoantibody response in scleroderma.**
  Author(s): Henry PA, Atamas SP, Yurovsky VV, Luzina I, Wigley FM, White B.
  Source: Arthritis and Rheumatism. 2000 December; 43(12): 2733-42.
  http://www.ncbi.nlm.nih.gov:80/entrez/query.fcgi?cmd=Retrieve&db=PubMed&list_uids=11145031&dopt=Abstract

- **Double-blind, placebo-controlled study of oral calcitriol for the treatment of localized and systemic scleroderma.**
  Author(s): Hulshof MM, Bouwes Bavinck JN, Bergman W, Masclee AA, Heickendorff L, Breedveld FC, Dijkmans BA.
  Source: Journal of the American Academy of Dermatology. 2000 December; 43(6): 1017-23.
  http://www.ncbi.nlm.nih.gov:80/entrez/query.fcgi?cmd=Retrieve&db=PubMed&list_uids=11100017&dopt=Abstract

- **D-penicillamine-induced crescentic glomerulonephritis in a patient with scleroderma.**
  Author(s): Garcia-Porrua C, Gonzalez-Gay MA, Bouza P.
  Source: Nephron. 2000 January; 84(1): 101-2. Review.
  http://www.ncbi.nlm.nih.gov:80/entrez/query.fcgi?cmd=Retrieve&db=PubMed&list_uids=10644924&dopt=Abstract

- **Drug treatment of scleroderma.**
  Author(s): Leighton C.
  Source: Drugs. 2001; 61(3): 419-27. Review.
  http://www.ncbi.nlm.nih.gov:80/entrez/query.fcgi?cmd=Retrieve&db=PubMed&list_uids=11293650&dopt=Abstract

- **Dysregulation of transforming growth factor beta signaling in scleroderma: overexpression of endoglin in cutaneous scleroderma fibroblasts.**
  Author(s): Leask A, Abraham DJ, Finlay DR, Holmes A, Pennington D, Shi-Wen X, Chen Y, Venstrom K, Dou X, Ponticos M, Black C, Bernabeu C, Jackman JK, Findell PR, Connolly MK.
  Source: Arthritis and Rheumatism. 2002 July; 46(7): 1857-65. Erratum In: Arthritis Rheum 2002 October; 46(10): 2830.
  http://www.ncbi.nlm.nih.gov:80/entrez/query.fcgi?cmd=Retrieve&db=PubMed&list_uids=12124870&dopt=Abstract

- **Eccrine squamous syringometaplasia and syringomatous hyperplasia in association with linear scleroderma.**
  Author(s): Sakai H, Satoh K, Manabe A, Nakane H, Ishida-Yamamoto A, Iizuka H.
  Source: Dermatology (Basel, Switzerland). 2002; 204(2): 136-8.
  http://www.ncbi.nlm.nih.gov:80/entrez/query.fcgi?cmd=Retrieve&db=PubMed&list_uids=11937740&dopt=Abstract

- **Effect of integrin on procollagen synthesis by fibroblasts from scleroderma.**
  Author(s): Hong W, Chen M, Kong X, Liao W.
  Source: Chinese Medical Journal. 1999 November; 112(11): 1024-7.
  http://www.ncbi.nlm.nih.gov:80/entrez/query.fcgi?cmd=Retrieve&db=PubMed&list_uids=11721465&dopt=Abstract

- **Effects of a nonsurgical exercise program on the decreased mouth opening in patients with systemic scleroderma.**
  Author(s): Pizzo G, Scardina GA, Messina P.
  Source: Clinical Oral Investigations. 2003 September; 7(3): 175-8. Epub 2003 July 09.
  http://www.ncbi.nlm.nih.gov:80/entrez/query.fcgi?cmd=Retrieve&db=PubMed&list_uids=14513305&dopt=Abstract

- **Elevated levels of leukotriene B4 and leukotriene E4 in bronchoalveolar lavage fluid from patients with scleroderma lung disease.**
  Author(s): Kowal-Bielecka O, Distler O, Kowal K, Siergiejko Z, Chwiecko J, Sulik A, Gay RE, Lukaszyk AB, Gay S, Sierakowski S.
  Source: Arthritis and Rheumatism. 2003 June; 48(6): 1639-46.
  http://www.ncbi.nlm.nih.gov:80/entrez/query.fcgi?cmd=Retrieve&db=PubMed&list_uids=12794832&dopt=Abstract

- **Endothelial injury in internal organs of University of California at Davis line 200 (UCD 200) chickens, an animal model for systemic sclerosis (Scleroderma).**
  Author(s): Nguyen VA, Sgonc R, Dietrich H, Wick G.
  Source: Journal of Autoimmunity. 2000 March; 14(2): 143-9.
  http://www.ncbi.nlm.nih.gov:80/entrez/query.fcgi?cmd=Retrieve&db=PubMed&list_uids=10677245&dopt=Abstract

- **Endothelium-dependent regulation of cutaneous microcirculation in patients with systemic scleroderma.**
  Author(s): Schlez A, Kittel M, Braun S, Hafner HM, Junger M.
  Source: The Journal of Investigative Dermatology. 2003 February; 120(2): 332-4.
  http://www.ncbi.nlm.nih.gov:80/entrez/query.fcgi?cmd=Retrieve&db=PubMed&list_uids=12542541&dopt=Abstract

- **Enhanced expression of the receptor for granulocyte macrophage colony stimulating factor on dermal fibroblasts from scleroderma patients.**
  Author(s): Postiglione L, Montagnani S, Riccio A, Montuori N, Sciorio S, Ladogana P, Spigna GD, Castaldo C, Rossi G.
  Source: The Journal of Rheumatology. 2002 January; 29(1): 94-101.
  http://www.ncbi.nlm.nih.gov:80/entrez/query.fcgi?cmd=Retrieve&db=PubMed&list_uids=11824978&dopt=Abstract

- **Enhanced in vivo lipid peroxidation in scleroderma spectrum disorders.**
  Author(s): Cracowski JL, Marpeau C, Carpentier PH, Imbert B, Hunt M, Stanke-Labesque F, Bessard G.
  Source: Arthritis and Rheumatism. 2001 May; 44(5): 1143-8.
  http://www.ncbi.nlm.nih.gov:80/entrez/query.fcgi?cmd=Retrieve&db=PubMed&list_uids=11352247&dopt=Abstract

- **Epidemiology and pathogenesis of scleroderma.**
  Author(s): Chen K, See A, Shumack S.
  Source: The Australasian Journal of Dermatology. 2003 February; 44(1): 1-7; Quiz 8-9. Review.
  http://www.ncbi.nlm.nih.gov:80/entrez/query.fcgi?cmd=Retrieve&db=PubMed&list_uids=12581091&dopt=Abstract

- **Epidermal growth factor up-regulates expression of transforming growth factor beta receptor type II in human dermal fibroblasts by phosphoinositide 3-kinase/Akt signaling pathway: Resistance to epidermal growth factor stimulation in scleroderma fibroblasts.**
  Author(s): Yamane K, Ihn H, Tamaki K.
  Source: Arthritis and Rheumatism. 2003 June; 48(6): 1652-66.
  http://www.ncbi.nlm.nih.gov:80/entrez/query.fcgi?cmd=Retrieve&db=PubMed&list_uids=12794834&dopt=Abstract

- **Epidermolysis bullosa acquisita-like reaction associated with penicillamine therapy for sclerodermatous graft-versus-host disease.**
  Author(s): Cetkovska P, Pizinger K, Skalova A.
  Source: Journal of the American Academy of Dermatology. 2003 December; 49(6): 1157-9.
  http://www.ncbi.nlm.nih.gov:80/entrez/query.fcgi?cmd=Retrieve&db=PubMed&list_uids=14639407&dopt=Abstract

- **European Scleroderma Study Group to define disease activity criteria for systemic sclerosis. III. Assessment of the construct validity of the preliminary activity criteria.**
  Author(s): Valentini G, Bencivelli W, Bombardieri S, D'Angelo S, Della Rossa A, Silman AJ, Black CM, Czirjak L, Nielsen H, Vlachoyiannopoulos PG.
  Source: Annals of the Rheumatic Diseases. 2003 September; 62(9): 901-3.
  http://www.ncbi.nlm.nih.gov:80/entrez/query.fcgi?cmd=Retrieve&db=PubMed&list_uids=12922968&dopt=Abstract

- **European Scleroderma Study Group to define disease activity criteria for systemic sclerosis. IV. Assessment of skin thickening by modified Rodnan skin score.**
  Author(s): Valentini G, D'Angelo S, Della Rossa A, Bencivelli W, Bombardieri S.
  Source: Annals of the Rheumatic Diseases. 2003 September; 62(9): 904-5.
  http://www.ncbi.nlm.nih.gov:80/entrez/query.fcgi?cmd=Retrieve&db=PubMed&list_uids=12922969&dopt=Abstract

- **Evaluation and management of alveolitis and interstitial lung disease in scleroderma.**
  Author(s): Latsi PI, Wells AU.
  Source: Current Opinion in Rheumatology. 2003 November; 15(6): 748-55. Review.
  http://www.ncbi.nlm.nih.gov:80/entrez/query.fcgi?cmd=Retrieve&db=PubMed&list_uids=14569205&dopt=Abstract

- **Evaluation and management of pulmonary fibrosis in scleroderma.**
  Author(s): White B.
  Source: Curr Rheumatol Rep. 2002 April; 4(2): 108-12. Review.
  http://www.ncbi.nlm.nih.gov:80/entrez/query.fcgi?cmd=Retrieve&db=PubMed&list_uids=11890875&dopt=Abstract

- **Evidence of cerebral hypoperfusion in scleroderma patients.**
  Author(s): Cutolo M, Nobili F, Sulli A, Pizzorni C, Briata M, Faelli F, Vitali P, Mariani G, Copello F, Seriolo B, Barone C, Rodriguez G.
  Source: Rheumatology (Oxford, England). 2000 December; 39(12): 1366-73.
  http://www.ncbi.nlm.nih.gov:80/entrez/query.fcgi?cmd=Retrieve&db=PubMed&list_uids=11136880&dopt=Abstract

- **Exposure to solvents in female patients with scleroderma.**
  Author(s): Czirjak L, Kumanovics G.
  Source: Clinical Rheumatology. 2002 May; 21(2): 114-8.
  http://www.ncbi.nlm.nih.gov:80/entrez/query.fcgi?cmd=Retrieve&db=PubMed&list_uids=12086160&dopt=Abstract

- **Expression and regulation of intracellular SMAD signaling in scleroderma skin fibroblasts.**
  Author(s): Mori Y, Chen SJ, Varga J.
  Source: Arthritis and Rheumatism. 2003 July; 48(7): 1964-78.
  http://www.ncbi.nlm.nih.gov:80/entrez/query.fcgi?cmd=Retrieve&db=PubMed&list_uids=12847691&dopt=Abstract

- **Expression of the costimulatory molecule BB-1 and its receptors in patients with scleroderma-polymyositis overlap syndrome.**
  Author(s): Murata KY, Sugie K, Takamure M, Ueno S.
  Source: Journal of the Neurological Sciences. 2002 December 15; 205(1): 65-70.
  http://www.ncbi.nlm.nih.gov:80/entrez/query.fcgi?cmd=Retrieve&db=PubMed&list_uids=12409186&dopt=Abstract

- **Extracorporeal photopheresis for scleroderma.**
  Author(s): Wollina U, Liebold K, Kaatz M.
  Source: Journal of the American Academy of Dermatology. 2001 January; 44(1): 146-8.
  http://www.ncbi.nlm.nih.gov:80/entrez/query.fcgi?cmd=Retrieve&db=PubMed&list_uids=11148498&dopt=Abstract

- **Failure to detect antinucleosome antibodies in scleroderma: comment on the article by Amoura et al.**
  Author(s): Hmida Y, Schmit P, Gilson G, Humbel RL.
  Source: Arthritis and Rheumatism. 2002 January; 46(1): 280-2.
  http://www.ncbi.nlm.nih.gov:80/entrez/query.fcgi?cmd=Retrieve&db=PubMed&list_uids=11817606&dopt=Abstract

- **Familial occurrence frequencies and relative risks for systemic sclerosis (scleroderma) in three United States cohorts.**
  Author(s): Arnett FC, Cho M, Chatterjee S, Aguilar MB, Reveille JD, Mayes MD.
  Source: Arthritis and Rheumatism. 2001 June; 44(6): 1359-62.
  http://www.ncbi.nlm.nih.gov:80/entrez/query.fcgi?cmd=Retrieve&db=PubMed&list_uids=11407695&dopt=Abstract

- **Familial occurrence of scleroderma.**
  Author(s): Jablonska S.
  Source: Journal of the European Academy of Dermatology and Venereology : Jeadv. 2001 January; 15(1): 9-10.
  http://www.ncbi.nlm.nih.gov:80/entrez/query.fcgi?cmd=Retrieve&db=PubMed&list_uids=11451343&dopt=Abstract

- **Familial scleroderma: do environmental factors, genes and microchimerism share the same relevance?**
  Author(s): Del Rosso A, Pignone A, Giacomelli R, Cerinic MM.
  Source: Journal of the European Academy of Dermatology and Venereology : Jeadv. 2001 January; 15(1): 11-4.
  http://www.ncbi.nlm.nih.gov:80/entrez/query.fcgi?cmd=Retrieve&db=PubMed&list_uids=11451311&dopt=Abstract

- **Fatal scleroderma renal crisis caused by gastrointestinal bleeding in a patient with scleroderma, Sjogren's syndrome and primary biliary cirrhosis overlap.**
  Author(s): Szigeti N, Fabian G, Czirjak L.
  Source: Journal of the European Academy of Dermatology and Venereology : Jeadv. 2002 May; 16(3): 276-9.
  http://www.ncbi.nlm.nih.gov:80/entrez/query.fcgi?cmd=Retrieve&db=PubMed&list_uids=12195572&dopt=Abstract

- **Fibrillin-1 protein in tight skin mice and scleroderma.**
  Author(s): Bona C, Saito S.
  Source: Clinical Reviews in Allergy & Immunology. 2000 February; 18(1): 119-26. Review.
  http://www.ncbi.nlm.nih.gov:80/entrez/query.fcgi?cmd=Retrieve&db=PubMed&list_uids=10907111&dopt=Abstract

- **Fibrosis in scleroderma.**
  Author(s): Kissin EY, Korn JH.
  Source: Rheumatic Diseases Clinics of North America. 2003 May; 29(2): 351-69. Review.
  http://www.ncbi.nlm.nih.gov:80/entrez/query.fcgi?cmd=Retrieve&db=PubMed&list_uids=12841299&dopt=Abstract

- **Free tissue transfer in the treatment of linear scleroderma.**
  Author(s): Katarincic JA, Bishop AT, Wood MB.
  Source: Journal of Pediatric Orthopedics. 2000 March-April; 20(2): 255-8.
  http://www.ncbi.nlm.nih.gov:80/entrez/query.fcgi?cmd=Retrieve&db=PubMed&list_uids=10739293&dopt=Abstract

- **Frequency and analysis of factors closely associated with the development of depressive symptoms in patients with scleroderma.**
  Author(s): Matsuura E, Ohta A, Kanegae F, Haruda Y, Ushiyama O, Koarada S, Togashi R, Tada Y, Suzuki N, Nagasawa K.
  Source: The Journal of Rheumatology. 2003 August; 30(8): 1782-7.
  http://www.ncbi.nlm.nih.gov:80/entrez/query.fcgi?cmd=Retrieve&db=PubMed&list_uids=12913935&dopt=Abstract

- **Frontal linear scleroderma (en coup de sabre).**
  Author(s): Katz KA.
  Source: Dermatology Online Journal [electronic Resource]. 2003 October; 9(4): 10.
  http://www.ncbi.nlm.nih.gov:80/entrez/query.fcgi?cmd=Retrieve&db=PubMed&list_uids=14594583&dopt=Abstract

- **Gene expression in bronchoalveolar lavage cells from scleroderma patients.**
  Author(s): Luzina IG, Atamas SP, Wise R, Wigley FM, Xiao HQ, White B.
  Source: American Journal of Respiratory Cell and Molecular Biology. 2002 May; 26(5): 549-57.
  http://www.ncbi.nlm.nih.gov:80/entrez/query.fcgi?cmd=Retrieve&db=PubMed&list_uids=11970906&dopt=Abstract

- **Guess what! Multiple erythemato-hemorrhagic papules on the legs: papular dermatitis induced by Scleroderma domesticum.**
  Author(s): Viglizzo G, Parodi A, Rebora A.
  Source: European Journal of Dermatology : Ejd. 2002 March-April; 12(2): 207-8.
  http://www.ncbi.nlm.nih.gov:80/entrez/query.fcgi?cmd=Retrieve&db=PubMed&list_uids=11872427&dopt=Abstract

- **Hand Mobility in Scleroderma (HAMIS) test: the reliability of a novel hand function test.**
  Author(s): Sandqvist G, Eklund M.
  Source: Arthritis Care and Research : the Official Journal of the Arthritis Health Professions Association. 2000 December; 13(6): 369-74.
  http://www.ncbi.nlm.nih.gov:80/entrez/query.fcgi?cmd=Retrieve&db=PubMed&list_uids=14635312&dopt=Abstract

- **Hemimasticatory spasm associated with localized scleroderma and facial hemiatrophy.**
  Author(s): Kim HJ, Jeon BS, Lee KW.
  Source: Archives of Neurology. 2000 April; 57(4): 576-80.
  http://www.ncbi.nlm.nih.gov:80/entrez/query.fcgi?cmd=Retrieve&db=PubMed&list_uids=10768634&dopt=Abstract

- **High expression and autoinduction of monocyte chemoattractant protein-1 in scleroderma fibroblasts.**
  Author(s): Yamamoto T, Eckes B, Krieg T.
  Source: European Journal of Immunology. 2001 October; 31(10): 2936-41.
  http://www.ncbi.nlm.nih.gov:80/entrez/query.fcgi?cmd=Retrieve&db=PubMed&list_uids=11592069&dopt=Abstract

- **Hodgkin's disease and scleroderma.**
  Author(s): Duggal L, Gupta S, Aggarwal PK, Sachar VP, Bhalla S.
  Source: J Assoc Physicians India. 2002 September; 50: 1186-8.
  http://www.ncbi.nlm.nih.gov:80/entrez/query.fcgi?cmd=Retrieve&db=PubMed&list_uids=12516708&dopt=Abstract

- **Homocysteine plasma concentration is related to severity of lung impairment in scleroderma.**
  Author(s): Caramaschi P, Martinelli N, Biasi D, Carletto A, Faccini G, Volpe A, Ferrari M, Scambi C, Bambara LM.
  Source: The Journal of Rheumatology. 2003 February; 30(2): 298-304.
  http://www.ncbi.nlm.nih.gov:80/entrez/query.fcgi?cmd=Retrieve&db=PubMed&list_uids=12563684&dopt=Abstract

- **Homolateral linear morphea with coarctation of aorta.**
  Author(s): Basu S, Ganguly S.
  Source: Indian Pediatrics. 2003 November; 40(11): 1108-9.
  http://www.ncbi.nlm.nih.gov:80/entrez/query.fcgi?cmd=Retrieve&db=PubMed&list_uids=14660854&dopt=Abstract

- **Human scleroderma sera contain autoantibodies to protein components specific to the U3 small nucleolar RNP complex.**
  Author(s): Yang JM, Hildebrandt B, Luderschmidt C, Pollard KM.
  Source: Arthritis and Rheumatism. 2003 January; 48(1): 210-7.
  http://www.ncbi.nlm.nih.gov:80/entrez/query.fcgi?cmd=Retrieve&db=PubMed&list_uids=12528121&dopt=Abstract

- **Identification of novel targets in scleroderma: update on population studies, cDNA arrays, SNP analysis, and mutations.**
  Author(s): Ahmed SS, Tan FK.
  Source: Current Opinion in Rheumatology. 2003 November; 15(6): 766-71. Review.
  http://www.ncbi.nlm.nih.gov:80/entrez/query.fcgi?cmd=Retrieve&db=PubMed&list_uids=14569208&dopt=Abstract

- **Identification of the mouse beta'-COP Golgi component as a spermatocyte autoantigen in scleroderma and mapping of its gene Copb2 to mouse chromosome 9.**
  Author(s): Tarsounas M, Heng HH, Ye CJ, Pearlman RE, Moens PB.
  Source: Cytogenetics and Cell Genetics. 1999; 87(3-4): 201-4.
  http://www.ncbi.nlm.nih.gov:80/entrez/query.fcgi?cmd=Retrieve&db=PubMed&list_uids=10702668&dopt=Abstract

- **Iloprost suppresses connective tissue growth factor production in fibroblasts and in the skin of scleroderma patients.**
  Author(s): Stratton R, Shiwen X, Martini G, Holmes A, Leask A, Haberberger T, Martin GR, Black CM, Abraham D.
  Source: The Journal of Clinical Investigation. 2001 July; 108(2): 241-50.
  http://www.ncbi.nlm.nih.gov:80/entrez/query.fcgi?cmd=Retrieve&db=PubMed&list_uids=11457877&dopt=Abstract

- **Image of the month: "hide-bound" bowel sign in scleroderma.**
  Author(s): Neef B, Kirsch H, Andus T.
  Source: Gastroenterology. 2003 May; 124(5): 1179, 1567.
  http://www.ncbi.nlm.nih.gov:80/entrez/query.fcgi?cmd=Retrieve&db=PubMed&list_uids=12730856&dopt=Abstract

- **Images in vascular medicine. Limited cutaneous scleroderma.**
  Author(s): Zide RS, Tsapatsaris NP.
  Source: Vascular Medicine (London, England). 2000; 5(1): 61-2.
  http://www.ncbi.nlm.nih.gov:80/entrez/query.fcgi?cmd=Retrieve&db=PubMed&list_uids=10737158&dopt=Abstract

- **Immune stimulation in scleroderma patients treated with thalidomide.**
  Author(s): Oliver SJ, Moreira A, Kaplan G.
  Source: Clinical Immunology (Orlando, Fla.). 2000 November; 97(2): 109-20.
  http://www.ncbi.nlm.nih.gov:80/entrez/query.fcgi?cmd=Retrieve&db=PubMed&list_uids=11027451&dopt=Abstract

- **Immunopathogenesis of scleroderma--evolving concepts.**
  Author(s): Sapadin AN, Esser AC, Fleischmajer R.
  Source: The Mount Sinai Journal of Medicine, New York. 2001 September-October; 68(4-5): 233-42. Review.
  http://www.ncbi.nlm.nih.gov:80/entrez/query.fcgi?cmd=Retrieve&db=PubMed&list_uids=11514910&dopt=Abstract

- **Impaired Smad7-Smurf-mediated negative regulation of TGF-beta signaling in scleroderma fibroblasts.**
  Author(s): Asano Y, Ihn H, Yamane K, Kubo M, Tamaki K.
  Source: The Journal of Clinical Investigation. 2004 January; 113(2): 253-64.
  http://www.ncbi.nlm.nih.gov:80/entrez/query.fcgi?cmd=Retrieve&db=PubMed&list_uids=14722617&dopt=Abstract

- **Implant-supported, long-span fixed partial denture for a scleroderma patient: a clinical report.**
  Author(s): Haas SE.
  Source: The Journal of Prosthetic Dentistry. 2002 February; 87(2): 136-9.
  http://www.ncbi.nlm.nih.gov:80/entrez/query.fcgi?cmd=Retrieve&db=PubMed&list_uids=11854666&dopt=Abstract

- **Increased alpha2-adrenergic constriction of isolated arterioles in diffuse scleroderma.**
  Author(s): Flavahan NA, Flavahan S, Liu Q, Wu S, Tidmore W, Wiener CM, Spence RJ, Wigley FM.
  Source: Arthritis and Rheumatism. 2000 August; 43(8): 1886-90.
  http://www.ncbi.nlm.nih.gov:80/entrez/query.fcgi?cmd=Retrieve&db=PubMed&list_uids=10943881&dopt=Abstract

- **Increased circulating concentrations of the counteradhesive proteins SPARC and thrombospondin-1 in systemic sclerosis (scleroderma). Relationship to platelet and endothelial cell activation.**
  Author(s): Macko RF, Gelber AC, Young BA, Lowitt MH, White B, Wigley FM, Goldblum SE.
  Source: The Journal of Rheumatology. 2002 December; 29(12): 2565-70.
  http://www.ncbi.nlm.nih.gov:80/entrez/query.fcgi?cmd=Retrieve&db=PubMed&list_uids=12465153&dopt=Abstract

- **Increased phosphorylation of transcription factor Sp1 in scleroderma fibroblasts: association with increased expression of the type I collagen gene.**
  Author(s): Ihn H, Tamaki K.
  Source: Arthritis and Rheumatism. 2000 October; 43(10): 2240-7.
  http://www.ncbi.nlm.nih.gov:80/entrez/query.fcgi?cmd=Retrieve&db=PubMed&list_uids=11037883&dopt=Abstract

- **Increased prevalence of scleroderma in southwestern Ontario: a cluster analysis.**
  Author(s): Thompson AE, Pope JE.
  Source: The Journal of Rheumatology. 2002 September; 29(9): 1867-73.
  http://www.ncbi.nlm.nih.gov:80/entrez/query.fcgi?cmd=Retrieve&db=PubMed&list_uids=12233880&dopt=Abstract

- **Increased transcriptional activities of transforming growth factor beta receptors in scleroderma fibroblasts.**
  Author(s): Yamane K, Ihn H, Kubo M, Tamaki K.
  Source: Arthritis and Rheumatism. 2002 September; 46(9): 2421-8.
  http://www.ncbi.nlm.nih.gov:80/entrez/query.fcgi?cmd=Retrieve&db=PubMed&list_uids=12355490&dopt=Abstract

- **Infections in systemic connective tissue diseases: systemic lupus erythematosus, scleroderma, and polymyositis/dermatomyositis.**
  Author(s): Juarez M, Misischia R, Alarcon GS.
  Source: Rheumatic Diseases Clinics of North America. 2003 February; 29(1): 163-84. Review.
  http://www.ncbi.nlm.nih.gov:80/entrez/query.fcgi?cmd=Retrieve&db=PubMed&list_uids=12635506&dopt=Abstract

- **Inflammatory myopathy associated with mixed connective tissue disease and scleroderma renal crisis.**
  Author(s): Greenberg SA, Amato AA.
  Source: Muscle & Nerve. 2001 November; 24(11): 1562-6.
  http://www.ncbi.nlm.nih.gov:80/entrez/query.fcgi?cmd=Retrieve&db=PubMed&list_uids=11745962&dopt=Abstract

- **Integrin signaling in fibrosis and scleroderma.**
  Author(s): Gardner HA.
  Source: Curr Rheumatol Rep. 1999 October; 1(1): 28-33. Review.
  http://www.ncbi.nlm.nih.gov:80/entrez/query.fcgi?cmd=Retrieve&db=PubMed&list_uids=11123011&dopt=Abstract

- **Interstitial lung disease in scleroderma.**
  Author(s): White B.
  Source: Rheumatic Diseases Clinics of North America. 2003 May; 29(2): 371-90. Review.
  http://www.ncbi.nlm.nih.gov:80/entrez/query.fcgi?cmd=Retrieve&db=PubMed&list_uids=12841300&dopt=Abstract

- **Intestinal obstruction associated with scleroderma: not always pseudo-obstruction.**
  Author(s): Hung SC, Lin HY.
  Source: Clin Exp Rheumatol. 2000 January-February; 18(1): 112. No Abstract Available.
  http://www.ncbi.nlm.nih.gov:80/entrez/query.fcgi?cmd=Retrieve&db=PubMed&list_uids=10728459&dopt=Abstract

- **Intestinal perforation associated with octreotide therapy in scleroderma.**
  Author(s): Malcolm A, Ellard K.
  Source: The American Journal of Gastroenterology. 2001 November; 96(11): 3206-8.
  http://www.ncbi.nlm.nih.gov:80/entrez/query.fcgi?cmd=Retrieve&db=PubMed&list_uids=11721779&dopt=Abstract

- **Juvenile scleroderma.**
  Author(s): Athreya BH.
  Source: Current Opinion in Rheumatology. 2002 September; 14(5): 553-61. Review.
  http://www.ncbi.nlm.nih.gov:80/entrez/query.fcgi?cmd=Retrieve&db=PubMed&list_uids=12192254&dopt=Abstract

- **Juvenile systemic scleroderma.**
  Author(s): Martini A.
  Source: Curr Rheumatol Rep. 2001 October; 3(5): 387-90. Review.
  http://www.ncbi.nlm.nih.gov:80/entrez/query.fcgi?cmd=Retrieve&db=PubMed&list_uids=11564369&dopt=Abstract

- **Juvenile-onset localized scleroderma activity detection by infrared thermography.**
  Author(s): Martini G, Murray KJ, Howell KJ, Harper J, Atherton D, Woo P, Zulian F, Black CM.
  Source: Rheumatology (Oxford, England). 2002 October; 41(10): 1178-82.
  http://www.ncbi.nlm.nih.gov:80/entrez/query.fcgi?cmd=Retrieve&db=PubMed&list_uids=12364640&dopt=Abstract

- **Keloid morphea and nodular scleroderma: two distinct clinical variants of scleroderma?**
  Author(s): Rencic A, Brinster N, Nousari CH.
  Source: Journal of Cutaneous Medicine and Surgery. 2003 January-February; 7(1): 20-4. Epub 2002 October 09. Review.
  http://www.ncbi.nlm.nih.gov:80/entrez/query.fcgi?cmd=Retrieve&db=PubMed&list_uids=12362259&dopt=Abstract

- **Keloidal scleroderma.**
  Author(s): Ling TC, Herrick AL, Andrew SM, Brammah T, Griffiths CE.
  Source: Clinical and Experimental Dermatology. 2003 March; 28(2): 171-3.
  http://www.ncbi.nlm.nih.gov:80/entrez/query.fcgi?cmd=Retrieve&db=PubMed&list_uids=12653707&dopt=Abstract

- **Keloid-like scleroderma.**
  Author(s): Barzilai A, Lyakhovitsky A, Horowitz A, Trau H.
  Source: The American Journal of Dermatopathology. 2003 August; 25(4): 327-30.
  http://www.ncbi.nlm.nih.gov:80/entrez/query.fcgi?cmd=Retrieve&db=PubMed&list_uids=12876490&dopt=Abstract

- **Lack of association of a functionally relevant single nucleotide polymorphism of matrix metalloproteinase-1 promoter with systemic sclerosis (scleroderma).**
  Author(s): Johnson RW, Reveille JD, McNearney T, Fischbach M, Friedman AW, Ahn C, Arnett FC, Tan FK.
  Source: Genes and Immunity. 2001 August; 2(5): 273-5.
  http://www.ncbi.nlm.nih.gov:80/entrez/query.fcgi?cmd=Retrieve&db=PubMed&list_uids=11528521&dopt=Abstract

- **Lichen planopilaris and scleroderma en coup de sabre.**
  Author(s): Munoz-Perez MA, Camacho F.
  Source: Journal of the European Academy of Dermatology and Venereology : Jeadv. 2002 September; 16(5): 542-4.
  http://www.ncbi.nlm.nih.gov:80/entrez/query.fcgi?cmd=Retrieve&db=PubMed&list_uids=12428864&dopt=Abstract

- **Life with a rare chronic disease: the scleroderma experience.**
  Author(s): Joachim G, Acorn S.
  Source: Journal of Advanced Nursing. 2003 June; 42(6): 598-606. Review.
  http://www.ncbi.nlm.nih.gov:80/entrez/query.fcgi?cmd=Retrieve&db=PubMed&list_uids=12787233&dopt=Abstract

- **Linear scleroderma "en coup de sabre" coexisting with plaque-morphea: neuroradiological manifestation and response to corticosteroids.**
  Author(s): Unterberger I, Trinka E, Engelhardt K, Muigg A, Eller P, Wagner M, Sepp N, Bauer G.
  Source: Journal of Neurology, Neurosurgery, and Psychiatry. 2003 May; 74(5): 661-4.
  http://www.ncbi.nlm.nih.gov:80/entrez/query.fcgi?cmd=Retrieve&db=PubMed&list_uids=12700315&dopt=Abstract

- **Linear scleroderma "en coup de sabre" of the cheek.**
  Author(s): Demir Y, Karaaslan T, Aktepe F, Yucel A, Demir S.
  Source: Journal of Oral and Maxillofacial Surgery : Official Journal of the American Association of Oral and Maxillofacial Surgeons. 2003 September; 61(9): 1091-4.
  http://www.ncbi.nlm.nih.gov:80/entrez/query.fcgi?cmd=Retrieve&db=PubMed&list_uids=12966486&dopt=Abstract

- **Linear scleroderma and autoimmune hemolytic anaemia.**
  Author(s): Wanchu A, Sud A, Bambery P.
  Source: J Assoc Physicians India. 2002 March; 50: 441-2.
  http://www.ncbi.nlm.nih.gov:80/entrez/query.fcgi?cmd=Retrieve&db=PubMed&list_uids=11922240&dopt=Abstract

- **Linear scleroderma associated with hypertrichosis in the absence of melorheostosis.**
  Author(s): Juhn BJ, Cho YH, Lee MH.
  Source: Acta Dermato-Venereologica. 2000 January-February; 80(1): 62-3.
  http://www.ncbi.nlm.nih.gov:80/entrez/query.fcgi?cmd=Retrieve&db=PubMed&list_uids=10721844&dopt=Abstract

- **Linear scleroderma associated with progressive brain atrophy.**
  Author(s): Grosso S, Fioravanti A, Biasi G, Conversano E, Marcolongo R, Morgese G, Balestri P.
  Source: Brain & Development. 2003 January; 25(1): 57-61.
  http://www.ncbi.nlm.nih.gov:80/entrez/query.fcgi?cmd=Retrieve&db=PubMed&list_uids=12536035&dopt=Abstract

- **Linear scleroderma en coup de sabre and brain calcification: is there a pathogenic relationship?**
  Author(s): Flores-Alvarado DE, Esquivel-Valerio JA, Garza-Elizondo M, Espinoza LR.
  Source: The Journal of Rheumatology. 2003 January; 30(1): 193-5.
  http://www.ncbi.nlm.nih.gov:80/entrez/query.fcgi?cmd=Retrieve&db=PubMed&list_uids=12508412&dopt=Abstract

- **Linear scleroderma 'en coup de sabre' treated with topical calcipotriol and cream psoralen plus ultraviolet A.**
  Author(s): Gambichler T, Kreuter A, Rotterdam S, Altmeyer P, Hoffmann K.
  Source: Journal of the European Academy of Dermatology and Venereology : Jeadv. 2003 September; 17(5): 601-2.
  http://www.ncbi.nlm.nih.gov:80/entrez/query.fcgi?cmd=Retrieve&db=PubMed&list_uids=12941109&dopt=Abstract

- **Localized and systemic scleroderma show different histological responses to methotrexate therapy.**
  Author(s): Seyger MM, van den Hoogen FH, van Vlijmen-Willems IM, van de Kerkhof PC, de Jong EM.
  Source: The Journal of Pathology. 2001 April; 193(4): 511-6.
  http://www.ncbi.nlm.nih.gov:80/entrez/query.fcgi?cmd=Retrieve&db=PubMed&list_uids=11276011&dopt=Abstract

- **Localized and systemic scleroderma.**
  Author(s): Hawk A, English JC 3rd.
  Source: Semin Cutan Med Surg. 2001 March; 20(1): 27-37. Review.
  http://www.ncbi.nlm.nih.gov:80/entrez/query.fcgi?cmd=Retrieve&db=PubMed&list_uids=11308134&dopt=Abstract

- **Localized linear scleroderma with cutaneous calcinosis.**
  Author(s): Yamamoto A, Morita A, Shintani Y, Sakakibara S, Tsuji T.
  Source: The Journal of Dermatology. 2002 February; 29(2): 112-4.
  http://www.ncbi.nlm.nih.gov:80/entrez/query.fcgi?cmd=Retrieve&db=PubMed&list_uids=11890294&dopt=Abstract

- **Localized scleroderma in a 12-year-old girl presenting as gingival recession. A case report and literature review.**
  Author(s): Baxter AM, Roberts A, Shaw L, Chapple IL.
  Source: Dent Update. 2001 November; 28(9): 458-62. Review.
  http://www.ncbi.nlm.nih.gov:80/entrez/query.fcgi?cmd=Retrieve&db=PubMed&list_uids=11806189&dopt=Abstract

- **Localized scleroderma in a woman irradiated at two sites for endometrial and breast carcinoma: a case history and a review of the literature.**
  Author(s): Ullen H, Bjorkholm E.
  Source: International Journal of Gynecological Cancer : Official Journal of the International Gynecological Cancer Society. 2003 January-February; 13(1): 77-82. Review.
  http://www.ncbi.nlm.nih.gov:80/entrez/query.fcgi?cmd=Retrieve&db=PubMed&list_uids=12631225&dopt=Abstract

- **Localized scleroderma in adults and children. Clinical and laboratory investigations on 239 cases.**
  Author(s): Marzano AV, Menni S, Parodi A, Borghi A, Fuligni A, Fabbri P, Caputo R.
  Source: European Journal of Dermatology : Ejd. 2003 March-April; 13(2): 171-6.
  http://www.ncbi.nlm.nih.gov:80/entrez/query.fcgi?cmd=Retrieve&db=PubMed&list_uids=12695134&dopt=Abstract

- **Localized scleroderma of the breast.**
  Author(s): Opere E, Oleaga L, Ibanez T, Grande D.
  Source: European Radiology. 2002 June; 12(6): 1483-5. Epub 2001 November 20.
  http://www.ncbi.nlm.nih.gov:80/entrez/query.fcgi?cmd=Retrieve&db=PubMed&list_uids=12042958&dopt=Abstract

- **Localized scleroderma or morphea?**
  Author(s): Greenberg JE, Schachner LA.
  Source: Dermatology Nursing / Dermatology Nurses' Association. 2001 October; 13(5): 335-8, 342; Quiz 343-4.
  http://www.ncbi.nlm.nih.gov:80/entrez/query.fcgi?cmd=Retrieve&db=PubMed&list_uids=11917622&dopt=Abstract

- **Localized scleroderma/morphea.**
  Author(s): Sehgal VN, Srivastava G, Aggarwal AK, Behl PN, Choudhary M, Bajaj P.
  Source: International Journal of Dermatology. 2002 August; 41(8): 467-75. Review.
  http://www.ncbi.nlm.nih.gov:80/entrez/query.fcgi?cmd=Retrieve&db=PubMed&list_uids=12207760&dopt=Abstract

- **Long-term outcomes of scleroderma renal crisis.**
  Author(s): Steen VD, Medsger TA Jr.
  Source: Annals of Internal Medicine. 2000 October 17; 133(8): 600-3.
  http://www.ncbi.nlm.nih.gov:80/entrez/query.fcgi?cmd=Retrieve&db=PubMed&list_uids=11033587&dopt=Abstract

- **Male microchimerism in healthy women and women with scleroderma: cells or circulating DNA? A quantitative answer.**
  Author(s): Lambert NC, Lo YM, Erickson TD, Tylee TS, Guthrie KA, Furst DE, Nelson JL.
  Source: Blood. 2002 October 15; 100(8): 2845-51.
  http://www.ncbi.nlm.nih.gov:80/entrez/query.fcgi?cmd=Retrieve&db=PubMed&list_uids=12351394&dopt=Abstract

- **Management of Raynaud's phenomenon and digital ischemic lesions in scleroderma.**
  Author(s): Hummers LK, Wigley FM.
  Source: Rheumatic Diseases Clinics of North America. 2003 May; 29(2): 293-313. Review.
  http://www.ncbi.nlm.nih.gov:80/entrez/query.fcgi?cmd=Retrieve&db=PubMed&list_uids=12841296&dopt=Abstract

- **Measuring disease activity and functional status in patients with scleroderma and Raynaud's phenomenon.**
  Author(s): Merkel PA, Herlyn K, Martin RW, Anderson JJ, Mayes MD, Bell P, Korn JH, Simms RW, Csuka ME, Medsger TA Jr, Rothfield NF, Ellman MH, Collier DH, Weinstein A, Furst DE, Jimenez SA, White B, Seibold JR, Wigley FM; Scleroderma Clinical Trials Consortium.
  Source: Arthritis and Rheumatism. 2002 September; 46(9): 2410-20.
  http://www.ncbi.nlm.nih.gov:80/entrez/query.fcgi?cmd=Retrieve&db=PubMed&list_uids=12355489&dopt=Abstract

- **Mechanical properties of the gastro-esophageal junction in health, achalasia, and scleroderma.**
  Author(s): Mearin F, Fonollosa V, Vilardell M, Malagelada JR.
  Source: Scandinavian Journal of Gastroenterology. 2000 July; 35(7): 705-10.
  http://www.ncbi.nlm.nih.gov:80/entrez/query.fcgi?cmd=Retrieve&db=PubMed&list_uids=10972173&dopt=Abstract

- **Medical pearl: Scleroderma-like skin changes in patients with diabetes mellitus.**
  Author(s): Yosipovitch G, Loh KC, Hock OB.
  Source: Journal of the American Academy of Dermatology. 2003 July; 49(1): 109-11.
  http://www.ncbi.nlm.nih.gov:80/entrez/query.fcgi?cmd=Retrieve&db=PubMed&list_
  uids=12833019&dopt=Abstract

- **Medium-dose UVA1 phototherapy in localized scleroderma and its effect in CD34-positive dendritic cells.**
  Author(s): Camacho NR, Sanchez JE, Martin RF, Gonzalez JR, Sanchez JL.
  Source: Journal of the American Academy of Dermatology. 2001 November; 45(5): 697-9.
  http://www.ncbi.nlm.nih.gov:80/entrez/query.fcgi?cmd=Retrieve&db=PubMed&list_
  uids=11606918&dopt=Abstract

- **Methotrexate and corticosteroid therapy for pediatric localized scleroderma.**
  Author(s): Uziel Y, Feldman BM, Krafchik BR, Yeung RS, Laxer RM.
  Source: The Journal of Pediatrics. 2000 January; 136(1): 91-5.
  http://www.ncbi.nlm.nih.gov:80/entrez/query.fcgi?cmd=Retrieve&db=PubMed&list_
  uids=10636981&dopt=Abstract

- **Methotrexate for the treatment of early diffuse scleroderma: comment on the article by Pope et al.**
  Author(s): Lehman TJ.
  Source: Arthritis and Rheumatism. 2002 March; 46(3): 845.
  http://www.ncbi.nlm.nih.gov:80/entrez/query.fcgi?cmd=Retrieve&db=PubMed&list_
  uids=11920427&dopt=Abstract

- **Methotrexate shows marginal clinical efficiency in early scleroderma.**
  Author(s): Varga J.
  Source: Curr Rheumatol Rep. 2002 April; 4(2): 97-8. No Abstract Available.
  http://www.ncbi.nlm.nih.gov:80/entrez/query.fcgi?cmd=Retrieve&db=PubMed&list_
  uids=11890873&dopt=Abstract

- **MHC class II associations with autoantibody and T cell immune responses to the scleroderma autoantigen topoisomerase I.**
  Author(s): Rands AL, Whyte J, Cox B, Hall ND, McHugh NJ.
  Source: Journal of Autoimmunity. 2000 December; 15(4): 451-8.
  http://www.ncbi.nlm.nih.gov:80/entrez/query.fcgi?cmd=Retrieve&db=PubMed&list_
  uids=11090244&dopt=Abstract

- **Microchimerism and scleroderma.**
  Author(s): Nelson JL.
  Source: Curr Rheumatol Rep. 1999 October; 1(1): 15-21. Review.
  http://www.ncbi.nlm.nih.gov:80/entrez/query.fcgi?cmd=Retrieve&db=PubMed&list_
  uids=11123009&dopt=Abstract

- **Microchimerism and scleroderma: an update.**
  Author(s): Artlett CM.
  Source: Curr Rheumatol Rep. 2003 April; 5(2): 154-9. Review.
  http://www.ncbi.nlm.nih.gov:80/entrez/query.fcgi?cmd=Retrieve&db=PubMed&list_
  uids=12628047&dopt=Abstract

- **Microsatellites and intragenic polymorphisms of transforming growth factor beta and platelet-derived growth factor and their receptor genes in Native Americans with systemic sclerosis (scleroderma): a preliminary analysis showing no genetic association.**
  Author(s): Zhou X, Tan FK, Stivers DN, Arnett FC.
  Source: Arthritis and Rheumatism. 2000 May; 43(5): 1068-73.
  http://www.ncbi.nlm.nih.gov:80/entrez/query.fcgi?cmd=Retrieve&db=PubMed&list_uids=10817561&dopt=Abstract

- **Molecular aspects of scleroderma.**
  Author(s): Trojanowska M.
  Source: Frontiers in Bioscience : a Journal and Virtual Library. 2002 March 1; 7: D608-18. Review.
  http://www.ncbi.nlm.nih.gov:80/entrez/query.fcgi?cmd=Retrieve&db=PubMed&list_uids=11861221&dopt=Abstract

- **Murine sclerodermatous graft-versus-host disease, a model for human scleroderma: cutaneous cytokines, chemokines, and immune cell activation.**
  Author(s): Zhang Y, McCormick LL, Desai SR, Wu C, Gilliam AC.
  Source: Journal of Immunology (Baltimore, Md. : 1950). 2002 March 15; 168(6): 3088-98.
  http://www.ncbi.nlm.nih.gov:80/entrez/query.fcgi?cmd=Retrieve&db=PubMed&list_uids=11884483&dopt=Abstract

- **Musculoskeletal involvement in scleroderma.**
  Author(s): Pope JE.
  Source: Rheumatic Diseases Clinics of North America. 2003 May; 29(2): 391-408. Review.
  http://www.ncbi.nlm.nih.gov:80/entrez/query.fcgi?cmd=Retrieve&db=PubMed&list_uids=12841301&dopt=Abstract

- **Myasthenia gravis associated with limited scleroderma (CREST syndrome)**
  Author(s): Kambara C, Kinoshita I, Amenomori T, Eguchi K, Yoshimura T.
  Source: Journal of Neurology. 2000 January; 247(1): 61-2.
  http://www.ncbi.nlm.nih.gov:80/entrez/query.fcgi?cmd=Retrieve&db=PubMed&list_uids=10701901&dopt=Abstract

- **Necrobiotic xanthogranuloma with scleroderma.**
  Author(s): Russo GG.
  Source: Cutis; Cutaneous Medicine for the Practitioner. 2002 December; 70(6): 311-6. Review.
  http://www.ncbi.nlm.nih.gov:80/entrez/query.fcgi?cmd=Retrieve&db=PubMed&list_uids=12502118&dopt=Abstract

- **Nerve growth factor and neuropeptides circulating levels in systemic sclerosis (scleroderma).**
  Author(s): Matucci-Cerinic M, Giacomelli R, Pignone A, Cagnoni ML, Generini S, Casale R, Cipriani P, Del Rosso A, Tirassa P, Konttinen YT, Kahaleh BM, Fan PS, Paoletti M, Marchesi C, Cagnoni M, Aloe L.
  Source: Annals of the Rheumatic Diseases. 2001 May; 60(5): 487-94.
  http://www.ncbi.nlm.nih.gov:80/entrez/query.fcgi?cmd=Retrieve&db=PubMed&list_uids=11302871&dopt=Abstract

- **Nevus lipomatosus cutaneous superficialis (Hoffmann-Zurhelle) with localized scleroderma like appearance.**
  Author(s): Ioannidou DJ, Stefanidou MP, Panayiotides JG, Tosca AD.
  Source: International Journal of Dermatology. 2001 January; 40(1): 54-7.
  http://www.ncbi.nlm.nih.gov:80/entrez/query.fcgi?cmd=Retrieve&db=PubMed&list_uids=11277956&dopt=Abstract

- **New treatments in scleroderma: dermatologic perspective.**
  Author(s): Jablonska S, Blaszczyk M.
  Source: Journal of the European Academy of Dermatology and Venereology : Jeadv. 2002 September; 16(5): 433-5.
  http://www.ncbi.nlm.nih.gov:80/entrez/query.fcgi?cmd=Retrieve&db=PubMed&list_uids=12428831&dopt=Abstract

- **New treatments in scleroderma: the rheumatologic perspective.**
  Author(s): Righi A, Cerinic MM.
  Source: Journal of the European Academy of Dermatology and Venereology : Jeadv. 2002 September; 16(5): 431-2.
  http://www.ncbi.nlm.nih.gov:80/entrez/query.fcgi?cmd=Retrieve&db=PubMed&list_uids=12428830&dopt=Abstract

- **New trends in the treatment of scleroderma renal crisis.**
  Author(s): Shor R, Halabe A.
  Source: Nephron. 2002; 92(3): 716-8. Review.
  http://www.ncbi.nlm.nih.gov:80/entrez/query.fcgi?cmd=Retrieve&db=PubMed&list_uids=12372964&dopt=Abstract

- **Nodular scleroderma: case report and literature review.**
  Author(s): Cannick L 3rd, Douglas G, Crater S, Silver R.
  Source: The Journal of Rheumatology. 2003 November; 30(11): 2500-2. Review.
  http://www.ncbi.nlm.nih.gov:80/entrez/query.fcgi?cmd=Retrieve&db=PubMed&list_uids=14677198&dopt=Abstract

- **Novel therapeutic strategies in scleroderma.**
  Author(s): Denton CP, Black CM.
  Source: Curr Rheumatol Rep. 1999 October; 1(1): 22-7. Review.
  http://www.ncbi.nlm.nih.gov:80/entrez/query.fcgi?cmd=Retrieve&db=PubMed&list_uids=11123010&dopt=Abstract

- **Novel therapy in the treatment of scleroderma.**
  Author(s): Wigley FM, Sule SD.
  Source: Expert Opinion on Investigational Drugs. 2001 January; 10(1): 31-48. Review.
  Erratum In: Expert Opin Investig Drugs 2001 February; 10(2): 407.
  http://www.ncbi.nlm.nih.gov:80/entrez/query.fcgi?cmd=Retrieve&db=PubMed&list_uids=11116279&dopt=Abstract

- **Occurrence of an activated, profibrotic pattern of gene expression in lung CD8+ T cells from scleroderma patients.**
  Author(s): Luzina IG, Atamas SP, Wise R, Wigley FM, Choi J, Xiao HQ, White B.
  Source: Arthritis and Rheumatism. 2003 August; 48(8): 2262-74.
  http://www.ncbi.nlm.nih.gov:80/entrez/query.fcgi?cmd=Retrieve&db=PubMed&list_uids=12905481&dopt=Abstract

- **Occurrence of scleroderma in monozygotic twins.**
  Author(s): De Keyser F, Peene I, Joos R, Naeyaert JM, Messiaen L, Veys EM.
  Source: The Journal of Rheumatology. 2000 September; 27(9): 2267-9.
  http://www.ncbi.nlm.nih.gov:80/entrez/query.fcgi?cmd=Retrieve&db=PubMed&list_uids=10990246&dopt=Abstract

- **Open label trial of tamoxifen in scleroderma.**
  Author(s): Thomas-Golbanov CK, Wilke WS, Fessler BJ, Hoffman GS.
  Source: Clin Exp Rheumatol. 2003 January-February; 21(1): 99-102.
  http://www.ncbi.nlm.nih.gov:80/entrez/query.fcgi?cmd=Retrieve&db=PubMed&list_uids=12673898&dopt=Abstract

- **Osteoporosis--less than expected in patients with scleroderma?**
  Author(s): Neumann K, Wallace DJ, Metzger AL.
  Source: The Journal of Rheumatology. 2000 July; 27(7): 1822-3.
  http://www.ncbi.nlm.nih.gov:80/entrez/query.fcgi?cmd=Retrieve&db=PubMed&list_uids=10914882&dopt=Abstract

- **Other rheumatic diseases in adolescence. Dermatomyositis, scleroderma, overlap syndromes, systemic vasculitis, and panniculitis.**
  Author(s): Hom C, Ilowite NT.
  Source: Adolescent Medicine (Philadelphia, Pa.). 1998 February; 9(1): 69-83, Vi. Review.
  http://www.ncbi.nlm.nih.gov:80/entrez/query.fcgi?cmd=Retrieve&db=PubMed&list_uids=10961253&dopt=Abstract

- **Overlap of idiopathic portal hypertension and scleroderma: report of two autopsy cases and a review of literature.**
  Author(s): Tsuneyama K, Harada K, Katayanagi K, Watanabe K, Kurumaya H, Minato H, Nakanuma Y.
  Source: Journal of Gastroenterology and Hepatology. 2002 February; 17(2): 217-23. Review.
  http://www.ncbi.nlm.nih.gov:80/entrez/query.fcgi?cmd=Retrieve&db=PubMed&list_uids=11966956&dopt=Abstract

- **Oxidative stress in scleroderma: maintenance of scleroderma fibroblast phenotype by the constitutive up-regulation of reactive oxygen species generation through the NADPH oxidase complex pathway.**
  Author(s): Sambo P, Baroni SS, Luchetti M, Paroncini P, Dusi S, Orlandini G, Gabrielli A.
  Source: Arthritis and Rheumatism. 2001 November; 44(11): 2653-64.
  http://www.ncbi.nlm.nih.gov:80/entrez/query.fcgi?cmd=Retrieve&db=PubMed&list_uids=11710721&dopt=Abstract

- **Pancytopenia in a patient with scleroderma treated with infliximab.**
  Author(s): Menon Y, Cucurull E, Espinoza LR.
  Source: Rheumatology (Oxford, England). 2003 October; 42(10): 1273-4; Author Reply 1274.
  http://www.ncbi.nlm.nih.gov:80/entrez/query.fcgi?cmd=Retrieve&db=PubMed&list_uids=14508054&dopt=Abstract

- **Paraspinal cervical calcifications associated with scleroderma.**
  Author(s): Van de Perre S, Vanhoenacker FM, Op de Beeck B, Gielen JL, De Schepper AM.
  Source: Jbr-Btr. 2003 March-April; 86(2): 80-2.
  http://www.ncbi.nlm.nih.gov:80/entrez/query.fcgi?cmd=Retrieve&db=PubMed&list_uids=12839421&dopt=Abstract

- **Parry Romberg syndrome: a close differential diagnosis of linear scleroderma en coup de sabre.**
  Author(s): Wakhlu A, Agarwal V, Aggarwal A, Misra R.
  Source: J Assoc Physicians India. 2003 October; 51: 980. No Abstract Available.
  http://www.ncbi.nlm.nih.gov:80/entrez/query.fcgi?cmd=Retrieve&db=PubMed&list_uids=14719588&dopt=Abstract

- **Partitioning of alveolar and conducting airway nitric oxide in scleroderma lung disease.**
  Author(s): Girgis RE, Gugnani MK, Abrams J, Mayes MD.
  Source: American Journal of Respiratory and Critical Care Medicine. 2002 June 15; 165(12): 1587-91.
  http://www.ncbi.nlm.nih.gov:80/entrez/query.fcgi?cmd=Retrieve&db=PubMed&list_uids=12070057&dopt=Abstract

- **Patterns of hospital admissions and emergency room visits among patients with scleroderma in South Carolina, USA.**
  Author(s): Nietert PJ, Silver RM.
  Source: The Journal of Rheumatology. 2003 June; 30(6): 1238-43.
  http://www.ncbi.nlm.nih.gov:80/entrez/query.fcgi?cmd=Retrieve&db=PubMed&list_uids=12784396&dopt=Abstract

- **Peripheral neuropathy in scleroderma.**
  Author(s): Poncelet AN, Connolly MK.
  Source: Muscle & Nerve. 2003 September; 28(3): 330-5.
  http://www.ncbi.nlm.nih.gov:80/entrez/query.fcgi?cmd=Retrieve&db=PubMed&list_uids=12929193&dopt=Abstract

- **Persistent down-regulation of Fli1, a suppressor of collagen transcription, in fibrotic scleroderma skin.**
  Author(s): Kubo M, Czuwara-Ladykowska J, Moussa O, Markiewicz M, Smith E, Silver RM, Jablonska S, Blaszczyk M, Watson DK, Trojanowska M.
  Source: American Journal of Pathology. 2003 August; 163(2): 571-81.
  http://www.ncbi.nlm.nih.gov:80/entrez/query.fcgi?cmd=Retrieve&db=PubMed&list_uids=12875977&dopt=Abstract

- **Photo quiz. Linear Scleroderma.**
  Author(s): Osswald SS, Pak HS, Elston DM.
  Source: Cutis; Cutaneous Medicine for the Practitioner. 2002 June; 69(6): 426, 433-4.
  http://www.ncbi.nlm.nih.gov:80/entrez/query.fcgi?cmd=Retrieve&db=PubMed&list_uids=12078841&dopt=Abstract

- **Phototherapy for scleroderma: biologic rationale, results, and promise.**
  Author(s): Fisher GJ, Kang S.
  Source: Current Opinion in Rheumatology. 2002 November; 14(6): 723-6. Review.
  http://www.ncbi.nlm.nih.gov:80/entrez/query.fcgi?cmd=Retrieve&db=PubMed&list_uids=12410098&dopt=Abstract

- **Pitting oedema in early diffuse systemic scleroderma.**
  Author(s): Englert H, Low S.
  Source: Annals of the Rheumatic Diseases. 2001 November; 60(11): 1079-80.
  http://www.ncbi.nlm.nih.gov:80/entrez/query.fcgi?cmd=Retrieve&db=PubMed&list_uids=11688491&dopt=Abstract

- **Polymorphic fibrosing reaction mimicking keloidal scleroderma but without associated classic scleroderma.**
  Author(s): Labandeira J, Leon-Mateos A, Suarez-Penaranda JM, Garea MT, Toribio J.
  Source: Dermatology (Basel, Switzerland). 2003; 207(2): 204-5.
  http://www.ncbi.nlm.nih.gov:80/entrez/query.fcgi?cmd=Retrieve&db=PubMed&list_uids=12920378&dopt=Abstract

- **Predictors and outcomes of scleroderma renal crisis: data from the high-dose versus low-dose D-penicillamine in early diffuse systemic sclerosis trial.**
  Author(s): Strand V.
  Source: Arthritis and Rheumatism. 2002 November; 46(11): 2836-7.
  http://www.ncbi.nlm.nih.gov:80/entrez/query.fcgi?cmd=Retrieve&db=PubMed&list_uids=12428222&dopt=Abstract

- **Predictors and outcomes of scleroderma renal crisis: the high-dose versus low-dose D-penicillamine in early diffuse systemic sclerosis trial.**
  Author(s): DeMarco PJ, Weisman MH, Seibold JR, Furst DE, Wong WK, Hurwitz EL, Mayes M, White B, Wigley F, Barr W, Moreland L, Medsger TA Jr, Steen V, Martin RW, Collier D, Weinstein A, Lally E, Varga J, Weiner SR, Andrews B, Abeles M, Clements PJ.
  Source: Arthritis and Rheumatism. 2002 November; 46(11): 2983-9.
  http://www.ncbi.nlm.nih.gov:80/entrez/query.fcgi?cmd=Retrieve&db=PubMed&list_uids=12428241&dopt=Abstract

- **Predictors of end stage lung disease in a cohort of patients with scleroderma.**
  Author(s): Morgan C, Knight C, Lunt M, Black CM, Silman AJ.
  Source: Annals of the Rheumatic Diseases. 2003 February; 62(2): 146-50.
  http://www.ncbi.nlm.nih.gov:80/entrez/query.fcgi?cmd=Retrieve&db=PubMed&list_uids=12525384&dopt=Abstract

- **Prescleroderma: a distinct stage of systemic sclerosis.**
  Author(s): Amato L, Gallerani I, Berti S, Fabbri P.
  Source: Skinmed. 2003 January-February; 2(1): 59-61. No Abstract Available.
  http://www.ncbi.nlm.nih.gov:80/entrez/query.fcgi?cmd=Retrieve&db=PubMed&list_
  uids=14673329&dopt=Abstract

- **Prevention of vascular damage in scleroderma with angiotensin-converting enzyme (ACE) inhibition.**
  Author(s): Maddison P.
  Source: Rheumatology (Oxford, England). 2002 September; 41(9): 965-71. Review.
  http://www.ncbi.nlm.nih.gov:80/entrez/query.fcgi?cmd=Retrieve&db=PubMed&list_
  uids=12209028&dopt=Abstract

- **Primary pulmonary hypertension is not associated with scleroderma-like changes in nailfold capillaries.**
  Author(s): Greidinger EL, Gaine SP, Wise RA, Boling C, Housten-Harris T, Wigley FM.
  Source: Chest. 2001 September; 120(3): 796-800.
  http://www.ncbi.nlm.nih.gov:80/entrez/query.fcgi?cmd=Retrieve&db=PubMed&list_
  uids=11555512&dopt=Abstract

- **Progressive facial hemiatrophy: central nervous system involvement and relationship with scleroderma en coup de sabre.**
  Author(s): Blaszczyk M, Krolicki L, Krasu M, Glinska O, Jablonska S.
  Source: The Journal of Rheumatology. 2003 September; 30(9): 1997-2004.
  http://www.ncbi.nlm.nih.gov:80/entrez/query.fcgi?cmd=Retrieve&db=PubMed&list_
  uids=12966605&dopt=Abstract

- **Pseudoscleroderma associated with transforming growth factor beta1-producing advanced gastric carcinoma: comment on the article by Varga.**
  Author(s): Fujii T, Mimori T, Kimura N, Satoh S, Hirakata M.
  Source: Arthritis and Rheumatism. 2003 June; 48(6): 1766-7; Author Repy 1767-8.
  http://www.ncbi.nlm.nih.gov:80/entrez/query.fcgi?cmd=Retrieve&db=PubMed&list_
  uids=12794850&dopt=Abstract

- **Pulmonary hypertension in scleroderma spectrum of disease: lack of bone morphogenetic protein receptor 2 mutations.**
  Author(s): Morse J, Barst R, Horn E, Cuervo N, Deng Z, Knowles J.
  Source: The Journal of Rheumatology. 2002 November; 29(11): 2379-81.
  http://www.ncbi.nlm.nih.gov:80/entrez/query.fcgi?cmd=Retrieve&db=PubMed&list_
  uids=12415595&dopt=Abstract

- **Rationale for and efficacy of digital arterial reconstruction in scleroderma: report of two cases.**
  Author(s): Tomaino MM, King J, Medsger T.
  Source: Journal of Reconstructive Microsurgery. 2002 May; 18(4): 263-8.
  http://www.ncbi.nlm.nih.gov:80/entrez/query.fcgi?cmd=Retrieve&db=PubMed&list_
  uids=12022030&dopt=Abstract

- **Raynaud's phenomenon affecting the tongue of a patient with scleroderma.**
  Author(s): Bridges MJ, Kelly CA.
  Source: Annals of the Rheumatic Diseases. 2002 May; 61(5): 472.
  http://www.ncbi.nlm.nih.gov:80/entrez/query.fcgi?cmd=Retrieve&db=PubMed&list_
  uids=11959778&dopt=Abstract

- **Raynaud's phenomenon, anticentromere antibodies, and digital necrosis without sclerodactyly: an entity independent of scleroderma?**
  Author(s): Sachsenberg-Studer EM, Prins C, Saurat JH, Salomon D.
  Source: Journal of the American Academy of Dermatology. 2000 October; 43(4): 631-4.
  http://www.ncbi.nlm.nih.gov:80/entrez/query.fcgi?cmd=Retrieve&db=PubMed&list_
  uids=11004618&dopt=Abstract

- **Raynaud's phenomenon, scleroderma, overlap syndromes, and other fibrosing syndromes.**
  Author(s): Korn JH.
  Source: Current Opinion in Rheumatology. 2000 November; 12(6): 509-10.
  http://www.ncbi.nlm.nih.gov:80/entrez/query.fcgi?cmd=Retrieve&db=PubMed&list_
  uids=11092200&dopt=Abstract

- **Re: Tager and Tikly. Clinical and laboratory manifestations of systemic sclerosis (scleroderma) in black South Africans.**
  Author(s): Rozman B, Kveder T.
  Source: Rheumatology (Oxford, England). 2000 February; 39(2): 220-2.
  http://www.ncbi.nlm.nih.gov:80/entrez/query.fcgi?cmd=Retrieve&db=PubMed&list_
  uids=10725083&dopt=Abstract

- **Recognition and management of scleroderma in children.**
  Author(s): Foeldvari I, Wulffraat N.
  Source: Paediatric Drugs. 2001; 3(8): 575-83. Review.
  http://www.ncbi.nlm.nih.gov:80/entrez/query.fcgi?cmd=Retrieve&db=PubMed&list_
  uids=11577922&dopt=Abstract

- **Recognition of Granzyme B-generated autoantigen fragments in scleroderma patients with ischemic digital loss.**
  Author(s): Schachna L, Wigley FM, Morris S, Gelber AC, Rosen A, Casciola-Rosen L.
  Source: Arthritis and Rheumatism. 2002 July; 46(7): 1873-84.
  http://www.ncbi.nlm.nih.gov:80/entrez/query.fcgi?cmd=Retrieve&db=PubMed&list_
  uids=12124872&dopt=Abstract

- **Recombinant human relaxin in the treatment of scleroderma. A randomized, double-blind, placebo-controlled trial.**
  Author(s): Seibold JR, Korn JH, Simms R, Clements PJ, Moreland LW, Mayes MD, Furst DE, Rothfield N, Steen V, Weisman M, Collier D, Wigley FM, Merkel PA, Csuka ME, Hsu V, Rocco S, Erikson M, Hannigan J, Harkonen WS, Sanders ME.
  Source: Annals of Internal Medicine. 2000 June 6; 132(11): 871-9.
  http://www.ncbi.nlm.nih.gov:80/entrez/query.fcgi?cmd=Retrieve&db=PubMed&list_
  uids=10836913&dopt=Abstract

- **Reflux esophagitis and scleroderma.**
  Author(s): Martin J, Ferraro P, Duranceau A.
  Source: Chest Surg Clin N Am. 2001 August; 11(3): 619-38, Viii. Review.
  http://www.ncbi.nlm.nih.gov:80/entrez/query.fcgi?cmd=Retrieve&db=PubMed&list_
  uids=11787971&dopt=Abstract

- **Reliability and validity of the Arthritis Hand Function Test in adults with systemic sclerosis (scleroderma).**
  Author(s): Poole JL, Gallegos M, O'Linc S.
  Source: Arthritis Care and Research : the Official Journal of the Arthritis Health Professions Association. 2000 April; 13(2): 69-73.
  http://www.ncbi.nlm.nih.gov:80/entrez/query.fcgi?cmd=Retrieve&db=PubMed&list_
  uids=14635280&dopt=Abstract

- **Remodeling of elastic fiber components in scleroderma skin.**
  Author(s): Davis EC, Blattel SA, Mecham RP.
  Source: Connective Tissue Research. 1999; 40(2): 113-21.
  http://www.ncbi.nlm.nih.gov:80/entrez/query.fcgi?cmd=Retrieve&db=PubMed&list_
  uids=10761636&dopt=Abstract

- **Renal crisis in asclerodermic scleroderma--lupus overlap syndrome.**
  Author(s): Horn HC, Ottosen P, Junker P.
  Source: Lupus. 2001; 10(12): 886-8. Review.
  http://www.ncbi.nlm.nih.gov:80/entrez/query.fcgi?cmd=Retrieve&db=PubMed&list_
  uids=11787881&dopt=Abstract

- **Renal failure due to scleroderma with thrombotic microangiopathy developing in a woman treated with carboplatin for ovarian cancer.**
  Author(s): Karim M, Vaux E, Davies DR, Mason PD.
  Source: Clinical Nephrology. 2002 November; 58(5): 384-8.
  http://www.ncbi.nlm.nih.gov:80/entrez/query.fcgi?cmd=Retrieve&db=PubMed&list_
  uids=12425490&dopt=Abstract

- **Reproductive factors and the risk of scleroderma: an Italian case-control study.**
  Author(s): Pisa FE, Bovenzi M, Romeo L, Tonello A, Biasi D, Bambara LM, Betta A, Barbone F.
  Source: Arthritis and Rheumatism. 2002 February; 46(2): 451-6.
  http://www.ncbi.nlm.nih.gov:80/entrez/query.fcgi?cmd=Retrieve&db=PubMed&list_
  uids=11840448&dopt=Abstract

- **Risk of cancer in patients with scleroderma.**
  Author(s): Pearson JE, Silman AJ.
  Source: Annals of the Rheumatic Diseases. 2003 August; 62(8): 697-9.
  http://www.ncbi.nlm.nih.gov:80/entrez/query.fcgi?cmd=Retrieve&db=PubMed&list_
  uids=12860720&dopt=Abstract

- **Risk of cancer in patients with scleroderma: a population based cohort study.**
  Author(s): Hill CL, Nguyen AM, Roder D, Roberts-Thomson P.
  Source: Annals of the Rheumatic Diseases. 2003 August; 62(8): 728-31.
  http://www.ncbi.nlm.nih.gov:80/entrez/query.fcgi?cmd=Retrieve&db=PubMed&list_
  uids=12860727&dopt=Abstract

- **Role of p38 MAPK in transforming growth factor beta stimulation of collagen production by scleroderma and healthy dermal fibroblasts.**
  Author(s): Sato M, Shegogue D, Gore EA, Smith EA, McDermott PJ, Trojanowska M.
  Source: The Journal of Investigative Dermatology. 2002 April; 118(4): 704-11.
  http://www.ncbi.nlm.nih.gov:80/entrez/query.fcgi?cmd=Retrieve&db=PubMed&list_
  uids=11918720&dopt=Abstract

- **Role of profibrogenic cytokines secreted by T cells in fibrotic processes in scleroderma.**
  Author(s): McGaha TL, Bona CA.
  Source: Autoimmunity Reviews. 2002 May; 1(3): 174-81. Review.
  http://www.ncbi.nlm.nih.gov:80/entrez/query.fcgi?cmd=Retrieve&db=PubMed&list_
  uids=12849012&dopt=Abstract

- **Role of protein kinase C-delta in the regulation of collagen gene expression in scleroderma fibroblasts.**
  Author(s): Jimenez SA, Gaidarova S, Saitta B, Sandorfi N, Herrich DJ, Rosenbloom JC, Kucich U, Abrams WR, Rosenbloom J.
  Source: The Journal of Clinical Investigation. 2001 November; 108(9): 1395-403.
  http://www.ncbi.nlm.nih.gov:80/entrez/query.fcgi?cmd=Retrieve&db=PubMed&list_
  uids=11696585&dopt=Abstract

- **Scleroderma and solvent exposure among women.**
  Author(s): Garabrant DH, Lacey JV Jr, Laing TJ, Gillespie BW, Mayes MD, Cooper BC, Schottenfeld D.
  Source: American Journal of Epidemiology. 2003 March 15; 157(6): 493-500.
  http://www.ncbi.nlm.nih.gov:80/entrez/query.fcgi?cmd=Retrieve&db=PubMed&list_
  uids=12631538&dopt=Abstract

- **Scleroderma en coup de sabre with central nervous system and ophthalmologic involvement: treatment of ocular symptoms with interferon gamma.**
  Author(s): Obermoser G, Pfausler BE, Linder DM, Sepp NT.
  Source: Journal of the American Academy of Dermatology. 2003 September; 49(3): 543-6.
  http://www.ncbi.nlm.nih.gov:80/entrez/query.fcgi?cmd=Retrieve&db=PubMed&list_
  uids=12963929&dopt=Abstract

- **Scleroderma epidemiology.**
  Author(s): Mayes MD.
  Source: Rheumatic Diseases Clinics of North America. 2003 May; 29(2): 239-54. Review.
  http://www.ncbi.nlm.nih.gov:80/entrez/query.fcgi?cmd=Retrieve&db=PubMed&list_
  uids=12841293&dopt=Abstract

- **Scleroderma patients with combined pulmonary hypertension and interstitial lung disease.**
  Author(s): Chang B, Wigley FM, White B, Wise RA.
  Source: The Journal of Rheumatology. 2003 November; 30(11): 2398-405.
  http://www.ncbi.nlm.nih.gov:80/entrez/query.fcgi?cmd=Retrieve&db=PubMed&list_uids=14677184&dopt=Abstract

- **Scleroderma renal crisis in pregnancy associated with massive proteinuria.**
  Author(s): Brown AN, Bolster MB.
  Source: Clin Exp Rheumatol. 2003 January-February; 21(1): 114-6.
  http://www.ncbi.nlm.nih.gov:80/entrez/query.fcgi?cmd=Retrieve&db=PubMed&list_uids=12673902&dopt=Abstract

- **Scleroderma renal crisis sine scleroderma during pregnancy.**
  Author(s): Mok CC, Kwan TH, Chow L.
  Source: Scandinavian Journal of Rheumatology. 2003; 32(1): 55-7.
  http://www.ncbi.nlm.nih.gov:80/entrez/query.fcgi?cmd=Retrieve&db=PubMed&list_uids=12635948&dopt=Abstract

- **Scleroderma renal crisis.**
  Author(s): Adams BD.
  Source: Annals of Emergency Medicine. 2003 November; 42(5): 713-4.
  http://www.ncbi.nlm.nih.gov:80/entrez/query.fcgi?cmd=Retrieve&db=PubMed&list_uids=14596246&dopt=Abstract

- **Scleroderma renal crisis.**
  Author(s): Steen VD.
  Source: Rheumatic Diseases Clinics of North America. 2003 May; 29(2): 315-33. Review.
  http://www.ncbi.nlm.nih.gov:80/entrez/query.fcgi?cmd=Retrieve&db=PubMed&list_uids=12841297&dopt=Abstract

- **Scleroderma renal crisis.**
  Author(s): Prisant LM, Loebl DH, Mulloy LL.
  Source: Journal of Clinical Hypertension (Greenwich, Conn.). 2003 March-April; 5(2): 168-70, 176.
  http://www.ncbi.nlm.nih.gov:80/entrez/query.fcgi?cmd=Retrieve&db=PubMed&list_uids=12671333&dopt=Abstract

- **Scleroderma renal crisis: poor outcome despite aggressive antihypertensive treatment.**
  Author(s): Walker JG, Ahern MJ, Smith MD, Coleman M, Pile K, Rischmueller M, Cleland L, Roberts-Thomson PJ.
  Source: Internal Medicine Journal. 2003 May-June; 33(5-6): 216-20.
  http://www.ncbi.nlm.nih.gov:80/entrez/query.fcgi?cmd=Retrieve&db=PubMed&list_uids=12752889&dopt=Abstract

- **Scleroderma.**
  Author(s): Schmults CA.
  Source: Dermatology Online Journal [electronic Resource]. 2003 October; 9(4): 11.
  http://www.ncbi.nlm.nih.gov:80/entrez/query.fcgi?cmd=Retrieve&db=PubMed&list_uids=14594584&dopt=Abstract

- **Scleroderma.**
  Author(s): Leininger SM.
  Source: Rn. 2003 July; 66(7): 35-40; Quiz 42. Review.
  http://www.ncbi.nlm.nih.gov:80/entrez/query.fcgi?cmd=Retrieve&db=PubMed&list_
  uids=12900996&dopt=Abstract

- **Scleroderma: a case report of possible cause of restricted movement of the temporomandibular joint with effects on facial development.**
  Author(s): Defabianis P.
  Source: J Clin Pediatr Dent. 2003 Fall; 28(1): 33-8.
  http://www.ncbi.nlm.nih.gov:80/entrez/query.fcgi?cmd=Retrieve&db=PubMed&list_
  uids=14604139&dopt=Abstract

- **Scleroderma: a treatable disease.**
  Author(s): Korn JH.
  Source: Cleve Clin J Med. 2003 November; 70(11): 954, 956, 958 Passim.
  http://www.ncbi.nlm.nih.gov:80/entrez/query.fcgi?cmd=Retrieve&db=PubMed&list_
  uids=14650470&dopt=Abstract

- **Scleroderma: living with unpredictability.**
  Author(s): Acorn S, Joachim G, Wachs JE.
  Source: Aaohn Journal : Official Journal of the American Association of Occupational Health Nurses. 2003 August; 51(8): 353-7; Quiz 358-9. Review.
  http://www.ncbi.nlm.nih.gov:80/entrez/query.fcgi?cmd=Retrieve&db=PubMed&list_
  uids=12934863&dopt=Abstract

- **Selective stimulation of collagen synthesis in the presence of costimulatory insulin signaling by connective tissue growth factor in scleroderma fibroblasts.**
  Author(s): Gore-Hyer E, Pannu J, Smith EA, Grotendorst G, Trojanowska M.
  Source: Arthritis and Rheumatism. 2003 March; 48(3): 798-806.
  http://www.ncbi.nlm.nih.gov:80/entrez/query.fcgi?cmd=Retrieve&db=PubMed&list_
  uids=12632435&dopt=Abstract

- **Serum levels of tumor necrosis factor and interleukin-13 are elevated in patients with localized scleroderma.**
  Author(s): Hasegawa M, Sato S, Nagaoka T, Fujimoto M, Takehara K.
  Source: Dermatology (Basel, Switzerland). 2003; 207(2): 141-7.
  http://www.ncbi.nlm.nih.gov:80/entrez/query.fcgi?cmd=Retrieve&db=PubMed&list_
  uids=12920362&dopt=Abstract

- **Sildenafil improved pulmonary hypertension and peripheral blood flow in a patient with scleroderma-associated lung fibrosis and the raynaud phenomenon.**
  Author(s): Rosenkranz S, Diet F, Karasch T, Weihrauch J, Wassermann K, Erdmann E.
  Source: Annals of Internal Medicine. 2003 November 18; 139(10): 871-3.
  http://www.ncbi.nlm.nih.gov:80/entrez/query.fcgi?cmd=Retrieve&db=PubMed&list_
  uids=14623635&dopt=Abstract

- **Systemic and cell type-specific gene expression patterns in scleroderma skin.**
  Author(s): Whitfield ML, Finlay DR, Murray JI, Troyanskaya OG, Chi JT, Pergamenschikov A, McCalmont TH, Brown PO, Botstein D, Connolly MK.
  Source: Proceedings of the National Academy of Sciences of the United States of America. 2003 October 14; 100(21): 12319-24. Epub 2003 Oct 06.
  http://www.ncbi.nlm.nih.gov:80/entrez/query.fcgi?cmd=Retrieve&db=PubMed&list_uids=14530402&dopt=Abstract

- **Systemic scleroderma patients have improved skin perfusion after the transdermal application of PGE1 ethyl ester.**
  Author(s): Schlez A, Hafner HM, Kittel M, Braun S, Diehm C, Junger M.
  Source: Vasa. Zeitschrift Fur Gefasskrankheiten. Journal for Vascular Diseases. 2003 May; 32(2): 83-6.
  http://www.ncbi.nlm.nih.gov:80/entrez/query.fcgi?cmd=Retrieve&db=PubMed&list_uids=12945100&dopt=Abstract

- **Targeting mediators of vascular injury in scleroderma.**
  Author(s): Schachna L, Wigley FM.
  Source: Current Opinion in Rheumatology. 2002 November; 14(6): 686-93. Review.
  http://www.ncbi.nlm.nih.gov:80/entrez/query.fcgi?cmd=Retrieve&db=PubMed&list_uids=12410092&dopt=Abstract

- **The assessment of anti-endothelial cell antibodies in scleroderma-associated pulmonary fibrosis. A study of indirect immunofluorescent and western blot analysis in 49 patients with scleroderma.**
  Author(s): Wusirika R, Ferri C, Marin M, Knight DA, Waldman WJ, Ross P Jr, Magro CM.
  Source: American Journal of Clinical Pathology. 2003 October; 120(4): 596-606.
  http://www.ncbi.nlm.nih.gov:80/entrez/query.fcgi?cmd=Retrieve&db=PubMed&list_uids=14560571&dopt=Abstract

- **The association of serum matrix metalloproteinases and their tissue inhibitor levels with scleroderma disease severity.**
  Author(s): Toubi E, Kessel A, Grushko G, Sabo E, Rozenbaum M, Rosner I.
  Source: Clin Exp Rheumatol. 2002 March-April; 20(2): 221-4.
  http://www.ncbi.nlm.nih.gov:80/entrez/query.fcgi?cmd=Retrieve&db=PubMed&list_uids=12051403&dopt=Abstract

- **The clinical relevance of autoantibodies in scleroderma.**
  Author(s): Ho KT, Reveille JD.
  Source: Arthritis Research & Therapy. 2003; 5(2): 80-93. Epub 2003 February 12. Review.
  http://www.ncbi.nlm.nih.gov:80/entrez/query.fcgi?cmd=Retrieve&db=PubMed&list_uids=12718748&dopt=Abstract

- **The complex genetics of scleroderma.**
  Author(s): Ahmed SS, Tan FK, Arnett FC.
  Source: The American Journal of Medicine. 2002 May; 112(7): 584-6.
  http://www.ncbi.nlm.nih.gov:80/entrez/query.fcgi?cmd=Retrieve&db=PubMed&list_uids=12015255&dopt=Abstract

- **The impact of pain and symptoms of depression in scleroderma.**
  Author(s): Benrud-Larson LM, Haythornthwaite JA, Heinberg LJ, Boling C, Reed J, White B, Wigley FM.
  Source: Pain. 2002 February; 95(3): 267-75.
  http://www.ncbi.nlm.nih.gov:80/entrez/query.fcgi?cmd=Retrieve&db=PubMed&list_uids=11839426&dopt=Abstract

- **The major histopathologic pattern of pulmonary fibrosis in scleroderma is nonspecific interstitial pneumonia.**
  Author(s): Kim DS, Yoo B, Lee JS, Kim EK, Lim CM, Lee SD, Koh Y, Kim WS, Kim WD, Colby TV, Kitiaichi M.
  Source: Sarcoidosis Vasc Diffuse Lung Dis. 2002 June; 19(2): 121-7.
  http://www.ncbi.nlm.nih.gov:80/entrez/query.fcgi?cmd=Retrieve&db=PubMed&list_uids=12108451&dopt=Abstract

- **The role of chemokines in the pathogenesis of scleroderma.**
  Author(s): Atamas SP, White B.
  Source: Current Opinion in Rheumatology. 2003 November; 15(6): 772-7. Review.
  http://www.ncbi.nlm.nih.gov:80/entrez/query.fcgi?cmd=Retrieve&db=PubMed&list_uids=14569209&dopt=Abstract

- **The role of leukotrienes in alveolitis associated with scleroderma.**
  Author(s): Simms RW, Korn JH.
  Source: Arthritis and Rheumatism. 2003 June; 48(6): 1478-80. Review.
  http://www.ncbi.nlm.nih.gov:80/entrez/query.fcgi?cmd=Retrieve&db=PubMed&list_uids=12794812&dopt=Abstract

- **The role of TGF-beta signaling in the pathogenesis of fibrosis in scleroderma.**
  Author(s): Ihn H.
  Source: Arch Immunol Ther Exp (Warsz). 2002; 50(5): 325-31. Review.
  http://www.ncbi.nlm.nih.gov:80/entrez/query.fcgi?cmd=Retrieve&db=PubMed&list_uids=12455866&dopt=Abstract

- **The roles of transforming growth factor type beta3 (TGF-beta3) and mast cells in the pathogenesis of scleroderma.**
  Author(s): Ozbilgin MK, Inan S.
  Source: Clinical Rheumatology. 2003 September; 22(3): 189-95.
  http://www.ncbi.nlm.nih.gov:80/entrez/query.fcgi?cmd=Retrieve&db=PubMed&list_uids=14505209&dopt=Abstract

- **The vasculopathy of Raynaud's phenomenon and scleroderma.**
  Author(s): Flavahan NA, Flavahan S, Mitra S, Chotani MA.
  Source: Rheumatic Diseases Clinics of North America. 2003 May; 29(2): 275-91, Vi. Review.
  http://www.ncbi.nlm.nih.gov:80/entrez/query.fcgi?cmd=Retrieve&db=PubMed&list_uids=12841295&dopt=Abstract

- **Thirteen-megahertz ultrasound probe: its role in diagnosing localized scleroderma.**
  Author(s): Cosnes A, Anglade MC, Revuz J, Radier C.
  Source: The British Journal of Dermatology. 2003 April; 148(4): 724-9.
  http://www.ncbi.nlm.nih.gov:80/entrez/query.fcgi?cmd=Retrieve&db=PubMed&list_uids=12752130&dopt=Abstract

- **Thrombotic thrombocytopenic purpura in a case of scleroderma renal crisis treated with twice-daily therapeutic plasma exchange.**
  Author(s): Kfoury Baz EM, Mahfouz RA, Masri AF, Jamaleddine GW.
  Source: Renal Failure. 2001 September; 23(5): 737-42.
  http://www.ncbi.nlm.nih.gov:80/entrez/query.fcgi?cmd=Retrieve&db=PubMed&list_uids=11725922&dopt=Abstract

- **Transcriptional inhibition of type I collagen gene expression in scleroderma fibroblasts by the antineoplastic drug ecteinascidin 743.**
  Author(s): Louneva N, Saitta B, Herrick DJ, Jimenez SA.
  Source: The Journal of Biological Chemistry. 2003 October 10; 278(41): 40400-7. Epub 2003 July 24.
  http://www.ncbi.nlm.nih.gov:80/entrez/query.fcgi?cmd=Retrieve&db=PubMed&list_uids=12881530&dopt=Abstract

- **Transdermal application of prostaglandin E1 ethyl ester for the treatment of trophic acral skin lesions in a patient with systemic scleroderma.**
  Author(s): Schlez A, Kittel M, Scheurle B, Diehm C, Junger M.
  Source: Journal of the European Academy of Dermatology and Venereology : Jeadv. 2002 September; 16(5): 526-8.
  http://www.ncbi.nlm.nih.gov:80/entrez/query.fcgi?cmd=Retrieve&db=PubMed&list_uids=12428854&dopt=Abstract

- **Treatment of atrophies secondary to trilinear scleroderma en coup de sabre by autologous tissue cocktail injection.**
  Author(s): Oh CK, Lee J, Jang BS, Kang YS, Bae YC, Kwon KS, Jang HS.
  Source: Dermatologic Surgery : Official Publication for American Society for Dermatologic Surgery [et Al.]. 2003 October; 29(10): 1073-5.
  http://www.ncbi.nlm.nih.gov:80/entrez/query.fcgi?cmd=Retrieve&db=PubMed&list_uids=12974710&dopt=Abstract

- **Treatment of GI dysmotility in scleroderma with the new enterokinetic agent prucalopride.**
  Author(s): Boeckxstaens GE, Bartelsman JF, Lauwers L, Tytgat GN.
  Source: The American Journal of Gastroenterology. 2002 January; 97(1): 194-7.
  http://www.ncbi.nlm.nih.gov:80/entrez/query.fcgi?cmd=Retrieve&db=PubMed&list_uids=11811166&dopt=Abstract

- **Treatment of scleroderma skin ulcers using becaplermin gel and hydrocolloid membrane.**
  Author(s): Yoon J, Giacopelli J, Granoff D, Kobayashi W.
  Source: Journal of the American Podiatric Medical Association. 2002 June; 92(6): 350-4.
  http://www.ncbi.nlm.nih.gov:80/entrez/query.fcgi?cmd=Retrieve&db=PubMed&list_uids=12070235&dopt=Abstract

- **Treatment of scleroderma.**
  Author(s): Sapadin AN, Fleischmajer R.
  Source: Archives of Dermatology. 2002 January; 138(1): 99-105. Review.
  http://www.ncbi.nlm.nih.gov:80/entrez/query.fcgi?cmd=Retrieve&db=PubMed&list_uids=11790173&dopt=Abstract

- **U3 snoRNP associates with fibrillarin a component of the scleroderma clumpy nucleolar domain.**
  Author(s): Herrera-Esparza R, Kruse L, von Essen M, Campos L, Barbosa O, Bollain JJ, Badillo I, Avalos-Diaz E.
  Source: Archives of Dermatological Research. 2002 October; 294(7): 310-7. Epub 2002 September 05.
  http://www.ncbi.nlm.nih.gov:80/entrez/query.fcgi?cmd=Retrieve&db=PubMed&list_uids=12373336&dopt=Abstract

- **Ulcerated dystrophic calcinosis cutis secondary to localised linear scleroderma.**
  Author(s): Vereecken P, Stallenberg B, Tas S, de Dobbeleer G, Heenen M.
  Source: Int J Clin Pract. 1998 November-December; 52(8): 593-4.
  http://www.ncbi.nlm.nih.gov:80/entrez/query.fcgi?cmd=Retrieve&db=PubMed&list_uids=10622063&dopt=Abstract

- **Ulnar artery involvement in systemic sclerosis (scleroderma).**
  Author(s): Taylor MH, McFadden JA, Bolster MB, Silver RM.
  Source: The Journal of Rheumatology. 2002 January; 29(1): 102-6.
  http://www.ncbi.nlm.nih.gov:80/entrez/query.fcgi?cmd=Retrieve&db=PubMed&list_uids=11824945&dopt=Abstract

- **Ultraviolet A sunbed used for the treatment of scleroderma.**
  Author(s): Oikarinen A, Knuutinen A.
  Source: Acta Dermato-Venereologica. 2001 November-December; 81(6): 432-3.
  http://www.ncbi.nlm.nih.gov:80/entrez/query.fcgi?cmd=Retrieve&db=PubMed&list_uids=11859951&dopt=Abstract

- **Ultraviolet A1 (340-400 nm) phototherapy for scleroderma in systemic sclerosis.**
  Author(s): Morita A, Kobayashi K, Isomura I, Tsuji T, Krutmann J.
  Source: Journal of the American Academy of Dermatology. 2000 October; 43(4): 670-4.
  http://www.ncbi.nlm.nih.gov:80/entrez/query.fcgi?cmd=Retrieve&db=PubMed&list_uids=11004624&dopt=Abstract

- **Understanding the special needs of the patient with scleroderma.**
  Author(s): Rossiter RC.
  Source: Australian Nursing Journal (July 1993). 2000 September; 8(3): Suppl 1-4. Review.
  http://www.ncbi.nlm.nih.gov:80/entrez/query.fcgi?cmd=Retrieve&db=PubMed&list_uids=11894369&dopt=Abstract

- **Unusual overlap of systemic lupus erythematosus and diffuse scleroderma.**
  Author(s): Mok CC, Cheung JC, Yee YK, Szeto ML.
  Source: Clin Exp Rheumatol. 2001 January-February; 19(1): 113-4. No Abstract Available.
  http://www.ncbi.nlm.nih.gov:80/entrez/query.fcgi?cmd=Retrieve&db=PubMed&list_uids=11247318&dopt=Abstract

- **Update on management of scleroderma.**
  Author(s): Sule SD, Wigley FM.
  Source: Bulletin on the Rheumatic Diseases. 2000; 49(10): 1-4. Review. Erratum In: Bull Rheum Dis 2001; 50(5): 4.
  http://www.ncbi.nlm.nih.gov:80/entrez/query.fcgi?cmd=Retrieve&db=PubMed&list_uids=11286150&dopt=Abstract

- **Updating the American College of Rheumatology preliminary classification criteria for systemic sclerosis: addition of severe nailfold capillaroscopy abnormalities markedly increases the sensitivity for limited scleroderma.**
  Author(s): Lonzetti LS, Joyal F, Raynauld JP, Roussin A, Goulet JR, Rich E, Choquette D, Raymond Y, Senecal JL.
  Source: Arthritis and Rheumatism. 2001 March; 44(3): 735-6.
  http://www.ncbi.nlm.nih.gov:80/entrez/query.fcgi?cmd=Retrieve&db=PubMed&list_uids=11263791&dopt=Abstract

- **Up-regulated expression of transforming growth factor beta receptors in dermal fibroblasts in skin sections from patients with localized scleroderma.**
  Author(s): Kubo M, Ihn H, Yamane K, Tamaki K.
  Source: Arthritis and Rheumatism. 2001 March; 44(3): 731-4.
  http://www.ncbi.nlm.nih.gov:80/entrez/query.fcgi?cmd=Retrieve&db=PubMed&list_uids=11263790&dopt=Abstract

- **Upregulation of histidine decarboxylase mRNA expression in scleroderma skin.**
  Author(s): Ohtsuka T, Ohtake H, Matsuzaki S, Ichimura K, Ichikawa A, Yamakage A, Yamazaki S.
  Source: Archives of Dermatological Research. 2001 April; 293(4): 171-7.
  http://www.ncbi.nlm.nih.gov:80/entrez/query.fcgi?cmd=Retrieve&db=PubMed&list_uids=11380149&dopt=Abstract

- **Validity of HAMIS: a test of hand mobility in scleroderma.**
  Author(s): Sandqvist G, Eklund M.
  Source: Arthritis Care and Research : the Official Journal of the Arthritis Health Professions Association. 2000 December; 13(6): 382-7.
  http://www.ncbi.nlm.nih.gov:80/entrez/query.fcgi?cmd=Retrieve&db=PubMed&list_uids=14635314&dopt=Abstract

- **Vascular and connective tissue histopathologic alterations of the female lower genital tract in scleroderma.**
  Author(s): Doss BJ, Qureshi F, Mayes MD, Jacques SM.
  Source: The Journal of Rheumatology. 2002 July; 29(7): 1384-7.
  http://www.ncbi.nlm.nih.gov:80/entrez/query.fcgi?cmd=Retrieve&db=PubMed&list_uids=12136892&dopt=Abstract

- **Von Willebrand factor propeptide as a marker of disease activity in systemic sclerosis (scleroderma).**
  Author(s): Scheja A, Akesson A, Geborek P, Wildt M, Wollheim CB, Wollheim FA, Vischer UM.
  Source: Arthritis Research. 2001; 3(3): 178-82. Epub 2001 February 19.
  http://www.ncbi.nlm.nih.gov:80/entrez/query.fcgi?cmd=Retrieve&db=PubMed&list_uids=11299058&dopt=Abstract

- **What is nodular-keloidal scleroderma?**
  Author(s): Labandeira J, Leon-Mateos A, Suarez-Penaranda JM, Garea MT, Toribio J.
  Source: Dermatology (Basel, Switzerland). 2003; 207(2): 130-2.
  http://www.ncbi.nlm.nih.gov:80/entrez/query.fcgi?cmd=Retrieve&db=PubMed&list_uids=12920359&dopt=Abstract

- **When is scleroderma really scleroderma?**
  Author(s): Wigley FM.
  Source: The Journal of Rheumatology. 2001 July; 28(7): 1471-3. Review.
  http://www.ncbi.nlm.nih.gov:80/entrez/query.fcgi?cmd=Retrieve&db=PubMed&list_uids=11469447&dopt=Abstract

CHAPTER 2. NUTRITION AND SCLERODERMA

Overview

In this chapter, we will show you how to find studies dedicated specifically to nutrition and scleroderma.

Finding Nutrition Studies on Scleroderma

The National Institutes of Health's Office of Dietary Supplements (ODS) offers a searchable bibliographic database called the IBIDS (International Bibliographic Information on Dietary Supplements; National Institutes of Health, Building 31, Room 1B29, 31 Center Drive, MSC 2086, Bethesda, Maryland 20892-2086, Tel: 301-435-2920, Fax: 301-480-1845, E-mail: ods@nih.gov). The IBIDS contains over 460,000 scientific citations and summaries about dietary supplements and nutrition as well as references to published international, scientific literature on dietary supplements such as vitamins, minerals, and botanicals.[7] The IBIDS includes references and citations to both human and animal research studies.

As a service of the ODS, access to the IBIDS database is available free of charge at the following Web address: **http://ods.od.nih.gov/databases/ibids.html**. After entering the search area, you have three choices: (1) IBIDS Consumer Database, (2) Full IBIDS Database, or (3) Peer Reviewed Citations Only.

Now that you have selected a database, click on the "Advanced" tab. An advanced search allows you to retrieve up to 100 fully explained references in a comprehensive format. Type "scleroderma" (or synonyms) into the search box, and click "Go." To narrow the search, you can also select the "Title" field.

---

[7] Adapted from **http://ods.od.nih.gov**. IBIDS is produced by the Office of Dietary Supplements (ODS) at the National Institutes of Health to assist the public, healthcare providers, educators, and researchers in locating credible, scientific information on dietary supplements. IBIDS was developed and will be maintained through an interagency partnership with the Food and Nutrition Information Center of the National Agricultural Library, U.S. Department of Agriculture.

The following information is typical of that found when using the "Full IBIDS Database" to search for "scleroderma" (or a synonym):

- **A case of multicentric reticulohistiocytosis, systemic sclerosis and Sjogren syndrome.**
  Author(s): Department of Dermatology, Mie University, Faculty of Medicine, Tsu, Japan.
  Source: Takahashi, M Mizutani, H Nakamura, Y Shimizu, M J-Dermatol. 1997 August; 24(8): 530-4 0385-2407

- **A double-blind placebo-controlled trial of antioxidant therapy in limited cutaneous systemic sclerosis.**
  Author(s): University of Manchester Rheumatic Diseases Centre, Hope Hospital, Salford, UK. aherrick@fs1.ho.man.ac.uk
  Source: Herrick, A L Hollis, S Schofield, D Rieley, F Blann, A Griffin, K Moore, T Braganza, J M Jayson, M I Clin-Exp-Rheumatol. 2000 May-June; 18(3): 349-56 0392-856X

- **A randomised, double-blind study of cicaprost, an oral prostacyclin analogue, in the treatment of Raynaud's phenomenon secondary to systemic sclerosis.**
  Author(s): University Department of Medicine, Ninewells Hospital and Medical School, Dundee, Scotland.
  Source: Lau, C S Belch, J J Madhok, R Cappell, H Herrick, A Jayson, M Thompson, J M Clin-Exp-Rheumatol. 1993 Jan-February; 11(1): 35-40 0392-856X

- **Abnormal lymphocyte function in scleroderma: a study on identical twins.**
  Source: Dustoor, M M McInerney, M M Mazanec, D J Cathcart, M K Clin-Immunol-Immunopathol. 1987 July; 44(1): 20-30 0090-1229

- **Acute effects of nebulised epoprostenol in pulmonary hypertension due to systemic sclerosis.**
  Author(s): Department of Respiratory Medicine, Royal Sunderland Hospital, U.K. parames@fhs.mcmaster.ca
  Source: Parameswaran, K Purcell, I Farrer, M Holland, C Taylor, I K Keaney, N P Respir-Med. 1999 February; 93(2): 75-8 0954-6111

- **Acute estrogen administration can reverse cold-induced coronary Raynaud's phenomenon in systemic sclerosis.**
  Author(s): Department of Clinical Therapeutics, Alexandra University Hospital, Athens, Greece.
  Source: Lekakis, J Mavrikakis, M Emmanuel, M Prassopoulos, V Papamichael, C Moulopoulou, D Ziaga, A Kostamis, P Moulopoulos, S Clin-Exp-Rheumatol. 1996 Jul-August; 14(4): 421-4 0392-856X

- **Antiphospholipid syndrome associated with progressive systemic sclerosis.**
  Author(s): Department of Dermatology, Yonsei University College of Medicine, Seoul, Korea.
  Source: Chun, W H Bang, D Lee, S K J-Dermatol. 1996 May; 23(5): 347-51 0385-2407

- **Autologous bone marrow transplantation in the treatment of refractory systemic sclerosis: early results from a French multicentre phase I-II study.**
  Author(s): Service de Medecine Interne, site transfusionnel de Saint-Louis, France. dominique.farge-bancel@sls.ap-hop-paris.fr
  Source: Farge, D Marolleau, J P Zohar, S Marjanovic, Z Cabane, J Mounier, N Hachulla, E Philippe, P Sibilia, J Rabian, C Chevret, S Gluckman, E Br-J-Haematol. 2002 December; 119(3): 726-39 0007-1048

- **Benign breast disease in systemic sclerosis (SSc). A case-control study.**
  Author(s): Rheumatic Diseases Unit, Ottawa General Hospital, University of Ottawa, Ontario, Canada.
  Source: McKendry, R J Cyr, M Dale, P Clin-Exp-Rheumatol. 1992 May-June; 10(3): 235-9 0392-856X

- **Calcium influx into red blood cells: the effect of sera from patients with systemic sclerosis.**
  Author(s): Department of Dermatology, St. Bartholomew's Hospital, London, U.K.
  Source: Rademaker, M Thomas, R H Kirby, J D Kovacs, I B Clin-Exp-Rheumatol. 1991 May-June; 9(3): 247-51 0392-856X

- **Calculated glomerular filtration rate is a useful screening tool to identify scleroderma patients with renal impairment.**
  Author(s): Centre for Nephrology, Royal Free and University College Medical School, University College London, Rowland Hill Street, London NW3 2PF, UK. kingdon@rfc.ucl.ac.uk
  Source: Kingdon, E J Knight, C J Dustan, K Irwin, A G Thomas, M Powis, S H Burns, A Hilson, A J Black, C M Rheumatology-(Oxford). 2003 January; 42(1): 26-33 1462-0324

- **Carnitine deficiency in scleroderma.**
  Source: Famularo, G De Simone, C Danese, C Immunol-Today. 1999 May; 20(5): 246 0167-5699

- **Chromosome abnormalities in peripheral lymphocytes from patients with progressive systemic sclerosis.**
  Author(s): Department of Medicine and Physical Therapy, Faculty of Medicine, University of Tokyo, Japan.
  Source: Takeuchi, F Nakano, K Yamada, H Kosuge, E Hirai, M Maeda, H Moroi, Y Rheumatol-Int. 1993; 12(6): 243-6 0172-8172

- **Clinical trials for the treatment of systemic sclerosis/scleroderma.**
  Author(s): Department of Medicine, University of Illinois at Chicago College of Medicine, Chicago, IL, USA.
  Source: Varga, J Ponor, I Curr-Rheumatol-Repage 1999 October; 1(1): 13-4 1523-3774

- **Coagulative modifications in patients with systemic sclerosis treated with iloprost or nifedipine.**
  Author(s): Istituto di Clinica Medica Generale, Ematologia ed Immunologia Clinica, Universita degli Studi, Azienda Ospedaliera Umberto I di Ancona.
  Source: Candela, M Pansoni, A Jannino, L Menditto, V G Natalini, M Ravaglia, F Da Lio, L Scorza, R Gabrielli, A Danieli, G Ann-Ital-Med-Int. 2001 Jul-September; 16(3): 170-4 0393-9340

- **Coexistence of morphea and psoriasis responding to acitretin treatment.**
  Author(s): Department of Dermatology, Kocaeli University, Faculty of Medicine, Izmit, Turkey.
  Source: Bilen, N Apaydin, R Ercin, C Harova, G Basdas, F Bayramgurler, D J-Eur-Acad-Dermatol-Venereol. 1999 September; 13(2): 113-7 0926-9959

- **Collagen in the extracellular matrix of cultured scleroderma skin fibroblasts: changes related to ascorbic acid-treatment.**
  Author(s): Department of Medical Biochemistry, University of Turku, Finland.
  Source: Heino, J Kahari, V M Jaakkola, S Peltonen, J Matrix. 1989 January; 9(1): 34-9 0934-8832

- **Combination therapies for systemic sclerosis.**
  Author(s): Center for Rheumatology, Royal Free Campus, University College London, Rowland Hill Street, Hampstead, NW3 2PF, UK.
  Source: Denton, C P Black, C M Springer-Semin-Immunopathol. 2001; 23(1-2): 109-29 0172-6641

- **CT and MRI findings in sclerodermatous chronic graft vs. host disease.**
  Author(s): NHS-Department of Radiology, 981045 Nebraska Medical Center, Omaha, NE 68198-1045, USA. kdumford@hotmail.com
  Source: Dumford, K Anderson, J C Clin-Imaging. 2001 Mar-April; 25(2): 138-40 0899-7071

- **Current treatment options in systemic Sclerosis (Scleroderma).**
  Author(s): Division of Rheumatology, Department of Internal Medicine III, University of Vienna, Wahringer Gurtel 18-20, A-1090 Vienna. Georg.Stummvoll@akh-wien.ac.at
  Source: Stummvoll, G H Acta-Med-Austriaca. 2002; 29(1): 14-9 0303-8173

- **Cyclosporin A and iloprost treatment of systemic sclerosis: clinical results and interleukin-6 serum changes after 12 months of therapy.**
  Author(s): Division of Internal Medicine, Department of Internal Medicine, University of Genoa, Genoa, Italy.
  Source: Filaci, G Cutolo, M Scudeletti, M Castagneto, C Derchi, L Gianrossi, R Ropolo, F Zentilin, P Sulli, A Murdaca, G Ghio, M Indiveri, F Puppo, F Rheumatology-(Oxford). 1999 October; 38(10): 992-6 1462-0324

- **Cystic lung disease in systemic sclerosis: a case report with high resolution computed tomography findings.**
  Author(s): Department of Medicine, Baragwanath Hospital, Johannesburg, South Africa.
  Source: Bergemann, A Tikly, M Rev-Rhum-Engl-Ed. 1996 March; 63(3): 213-5 1169-8446

- **Cytokine production in scleroderma patients: effects of therapy with either iloprost or nifedipine.**
  Author(s): Institute of Internal Medicine, Infectious Diseases and Immunopathology, IRCCS Ospedale Maggiore di Milano, Italy.
  Source: Della Bella, S Molteni, M Mascagni, B Zulian, C Compasso, S Scorza, R Clin-Exp-Rheumatol. 1997 Mar-April; 15(2): 135-41 0392-856X

- **Deconjugation ability of bacteria isolated from the jejunal fluid of patients with progressive systemic sclerosis and its gastric pH.**
  Author(s): The First Department of Internal Medicine, Yokohama City University School of Medicine, Yokohama, Japan.
  Source: Shindo, K Machida, M Koide, K Fukumura, M Yamazaki, R Hepatogastroenterology. 1998 Sep-October; 45(23): 1643-50 0172-6390

- **Decorin and glycosaminoglycan synthesis in skin fibroblasts from patients with systemic sclerosis.**
  Author(s): Department of Dermatology, School of Medicine, Chiba University, Japan.
  Source: Kuroda, K Shinkai, H Arch-Dermatol-Res. 1997 July; 289(8): 481-5 0340-3696

- **Dermal elastin and collagen in systemic sclerosis. Effect of D-penicillamine treatment.**
  Author(s): Institute of General Pathology, University of Modena.
  Source: Pasquali Ronchetti, I Guerra, D Quaglino, D Vincenzi, D Manzini, E Canossi, B Manzini, C U Clin-Exp-Rheumatol. 1989 Jul-August; 7(4): 373-83 0392-856X

- **Effect of D-penicillamine on the T cell phenotype in scleroderma. Comparison between treated and untreated patients.**
Author(s): Division of Rheumatology, University of Padova, Italy.
Source: Rosada, M Fiocco, U De Silvestro, G Doria, A Cozzi, L Favaretto, M Todesco, S Clin-Exp-Rheumatol. 1993 Mar-April; 11(2): 143-8 0392-856X

- **Effects of cytokine application on glucocorticoid secretion in an animal model for systemic scleroderma.**
Author(s): Institute for General and Experimental Pathology, University of Innsbruck, Medical School, Austria.
Source: Brezinschek, H P Gruschwitz, M Sgonc, R Moormann, S Herold, M Gershwin, M E Wick, G J-Autoimmun. 1993 December; 6(6): 719-33 0896-8411

- **Effects of famotidine on upper gastrointestinal motility in patients with progressive systemic sclerosis.**
Author(s): First Department of Internal Medicine, Gunma University School of Medicine, Maebashi, Japan.
Source: Horikoshi, T Sekiguchi, T Kusano, M Matsuzaki, T Gastroenterol-Jpn. 1991 April; 26(2): 145-50 0435-1339

- **Effects of five-day versus one-day infusion of iloprost on the peripheral microcirculation in patients with systemic sclerosis.**
Author(s): Institute of Internal Medicine, Policlinico Borgo Roma, University of Verona, Italy.
Source: Ceru, S Pancera, P Sansone, S Sfondrini, G Codella, O De Sandre, G Lechi, A Lunardi, C Clin-Exp-Rheumatol. 1997 Jul-August; 15(4): 381-5 0392-856X

- **Effects of long-term cyclic iloprost therapy in systemic sclerosis with Raynaud's phenomenon. A randomized, controlled study.**
Author(s): Clinical Immunology and Allergy, University of Milan, IRCCS Ospedale Maggiore, Milan, Italy. raffaella.scorza@unimi.it
Source: Scorza, R Caronni, M Mascagni, B Berruti, V Bazzi, S Micallef, E Arpaia, G Sardina, M Origgi, L Vanoli, M Clin-Exp-Rheumatol. 2001 Sep-October; 19(5): 503-8 0392-856X

- **Essential fatty acid and prostaglandin metabolism in Sjogren's syndrome, systemic sclerosis and rheumatoid arthritis.**
Source: Horrobin, D F Scand-J-Rheumatol-Suppl. 1986; 61: 242-5 0301-3847

- **Iloprost and cisaprost for Raynaud's phenomenon in progressive systemic sclerosis.**
Author(s): Medicine (Division of Rheumatology), University of Western Ontario, LHSC-South Campus, 375 South Street Room 309;Colborne Bldg., London, Ontario, Canada, N6A 4G5. jpope@julian.uwo.ca
Source: Pope, J Fenlon, D Thompson, A Shea, B Furst, D Wells, G Silman, A Cochrane-Database-Syst-Revolume 2000; (2): CD000953 1469-493X

- **Iloprost as cyclic five-day infusions in the treatment of scleroderma. An open pilot study in 20 patients treated for one year.**
Author(s): Special Medical Pathology Institute, Verona, Italy.
Source: Biasi, D Carletto, A Caramaschi, P Zeminian, S Pacor, M L Corrocher, R Bambara, L M Rev-Rhum-Engl-Ed. 1998 December; 65(12): 745-50 1169-8446

- **Juvenile systemic scleroderma.**
Author(s): Dipartimento di Scienze Pediatriche, Universita di Pavia, IRCCS Policlinico S. Matteo, 27100, Pavia, Italy. amartini@smatteo.pv.it
Source: Martini, A Curr-Rheumatol-Repage 2001 October; 3(5): 387-90 1523-3774

- **Localized and systemic scleroderma.**
  Author(s): Department of Dermatology, University of Virginia School of Medicine, Charlottesville 22908-0718, USA.
  Source: Hawk, A English, J C 3rd Semin-Cutan-Med-Surg. 2001 March; 20(1): 27-37 1085-5629

- **Long-term therapy with plasma exchange in systemic sclerosis: effects on laboratory markers reflecting disease activity.**
  Author(s): Division of Rheumatology, Universita di Padova, Italy. fcozzi@ux1.unipd.it
  Source: Cozzi, F Marson, P Rosada, M De Silvestro, G Bullo, A Punzi, L Todesco, S Transfus-Apheresis-Sci. 2001 August; 25(1): 25-31 1473-0502

- **L-tryptophan syndrome: histologic features of scleroderma-like skin changes.**
  Author(s): Denver General Hospital, Colorado 80204.
  Source: Guerin, S B Schmidt, J J Kulik, J E Golitz, L E J-Cutan-Pathol. 1992 June; 19(3): 207-11 0303-6987

- **Marked and sustained improvement of systemic sclerosis following polychemotherapy for coexistent multiple myeloma.**
  Author(s): Department of Internal Medicine I, University of Vienna, Austria.
  Source: Bachleitner Hofmann, T Machold, K Knobler, R Drach, J Grumbeck, E Gisslinger, H Clin-Exp-Rheumatol. 2002 Jan-February; 20(1): 85-8 0392-856X

- **Monocytes of patients wiht systemic sclerosis (scleroderma spontaneously release in vitro increased amounts of superoxide anion.**
  Author(s): Institute of Internal Medicine, Hematology and Clinical Immunology, University of Ancona, Italy.
  Source: Sambo, P Jannino, L Candela, M Salvi, A Donini, M Dusi, S Luchetti, M M Gabrielli, A J-Invest-Dermatol. 1999 Jan; 112(1): 78-84 0022-202X

- **Morphea and localized scleroderma in children.**
  Author(s): Department of Medicine (Dermatology), University of California at San Diego, Children's Hospital and Health Center, USA.
  Source: Vierra, E Cunningham, B B Semin-Cutan-Med-Surg. 1999 September; 18(3): 210-25 1085-5629

- **Neural blockade, urokinase and prostaglandin E1 combination therapy for acute digital ischemia of progressive systemic sclerosis.**
  Author(s): Department of Dermatology, Mie University, Faculty of Medicine, Tsu, Japan.
  Source: Shimizu, Y Mizutani, H Inachi, S Tsuchibashi, T Shimizu, M J-Dermatol. 1994 October; 21(10): 755-9 0385-2407

- **Nodular scleroderma in systemic sclerosis under D-penicillamine therapy.**
  Author(s): Department of Dermatology, Yokohama City University School of Medicine, Japan.
  Source: Sasaki, T Denpo, K Ono, H Nakajima, H J-Dermatol. 1992 December; 19(12): 968-71 0385-2407

- **Nodular scleroderma: focally increased tenascin expression differing from that in the surrounding scleroderma skin.**
  Author(s): Department of Dermatology, Mie University Faculty of Medicine, Tsu, Japan.
  Source: Mizutani, H Taniguchi, H Sakakura, T Shimizu, M J-Dermatol. 1995 April; 22(4): 267-71 0385-2407

- **Novel therapeutic strategies in scleroderma.**
  Author(s): Centre for Rheumatology, Royal Free and University College Medical School, Royal Free Campus, London NW3, UK.
  Source: Denton, C P Black, C M Curr-Rheumatol-Repage 1999 October; 1(1): 22-7 1523-3774

- **Overlap syndrome of progressive systemic sclerosis and polymyositis: report of 40 cases.**
  Author(s): PUMC Hospital, CAMS, Beijing.
  Source: Yuan, X Chen, M Chin-Med-Sci-J. 1991 June; 6(2): 107-9 1001-9294

- **Palindromic morphea: multiple recurrence of morphea lesions in a case of systemic sclerosis.**
  Author(s): Department of Dermatology, Mie University School of Medicine, Japan.
  Source: Mizutani, H Tanaka, H Okada, H Mizutani, T Shimizu, M J-Dermatol. 1992 May; 19(5): 298-301 0385-2407

- **Penicillamine in systemic sclerosis: a reappraisal.**
  Author(s): Department of Medicine, Faculty of Medicine, Kuwait University.
  Source: Sattar, M A Guindi, R T Sugathan, T N Clin-Rheumatol. 1990 December; 9(4): 517-22 0770-3198

- **Penicillamine in the treatment of systemic sclerosis.**
  Author(s): University of California at Los Angeles, School of Medicine, Department of Medicine, Division of Rheumatology, Los Angeles, California, USA.
  Source: Clements, P J Curr-Rheumatol-Repage 1999 October; 1(1): 38-42 1523-3774

- **Pentoxyfilline treatment does not influence the plasma levels of IL-2 and sIL-2R in limited scleroderma patients.**
  Author(s): Department of Dermatology, Medical University, ul. Radziwillowska 13, 20-250 Lublin, Poland.
  Source: Chibowska, M Krasowska, D Weglarz, J Med-Sci-Monit. 2001 Mar-April; 7(2): 282-8 1234-1010

- **Peripheral blood T lymphocytes from systemic sclerosis patients show both Th1 and Th2 activation.**
  Author(s): Rheumatology Unit, Second University of Naples, Italy. gabriele.valentini@unina2.it
  Source: Valentini, G Baroni, A Esposito, K Naclerio, C Buommino, E Farzati, A Cuomo, G Farzati, B J-Clin-Immunol. 2001 May; 21(3): 210-7 0271-9142

- **Pharmacokinetics of oral iloprost in patients with Raynaud's phenomenon secondary to systemic sclerosis.**
  Author(s): Department of Medicine, Division of General Internal Medicine, University Hospital Nijmegen, P.O. Box 9101, 6500 HB, Nijmegen, The Netherlands.
  Source: Janssena, M C Wollersheim, H Kraus, C Hildebrand, M Watson, H R Thien, T Prostaglandins-Other-Lipid-Mediat. 2000 March; 60(4-6): 153-60 1098-8823

- **Pilot study of anti-thymocyte globulin plus mycophenolate mofetil in recent-onset diffuse scleroderma.**
  Author(s): Royal Free Hospital, London NW3 2QG, UK.
  Source: Stratton, R J Wilson, H Black, C M Rheumatology-(Oxford). 2001 January; 40(1): 84-8 1462-0324

- **Polyclonal B lymphocyte activation in progressive systemic sclerosis.**
  Author(s): Clinica Medica, University of L'Aquila, Italy.

Source: Famularo, G Giacomelli, R Alesse, E Cifone, M G Morrone, S Boirivant, M Danese, C Perego, M A Santoni, A Tonietti, G J-Clin-Lab-Immunol. 1989 June; 29(2): 59-63 0141-2760

- **Pregnancy in mixed connective tissue disease, poly/dermatomyositis and scleroderma.**
  Author(s): LAC/USC Medical Center 90033.
  Source: Kitridou, R C Clin-Exp-Rheumatol. 1988 Apr-June; 6(2): 173-8 0392-856X

- **Progressive systemic sclerosis: intrathecal pain management.**
  Author(s): Department of Anesthesia and Intensive Care, Sahlgrenska University Hospital, Gothenburg, Sweden.
  Source: Lundborg, C N Nitescu, P V Appelgren, L K Curelaru, I D Reg-Anesth-Pain-Med. 1999 Jan-February; 24(1): 89-93 1098-7339

- **Pseudoscleroderma secondary to phytomenadione (vitamin K1) injections: Texier's disease.**
  Author(s): Department of Dermatology, St Vincent's Hospital, Darlinghurst, New South Wales, Australia.
  Source: Pang, B K Munro, V Kossard, S Australas-J-Dermatol. 1996 February; 37(1): 44-7 0004-8380

- **Pulmonary hypertension in systemic sclerosis: bete noire no more?**
  Source: Varga, J Curr-Opin-Rheumatol. 2002 November; 14(6): 666-70 1040-8711

- **Recognition and management of scleroderma in children.**
  Author(s): Paediatric Rheumatology Clinic, AK-Eilbek, Hamburg, Germany.
  Source: Foeldvari, I Wulffraat, N Paediatr-Drugs. 2001; 3(8): 575-83 1174-5878

- **Retrospective studies in scleroderma: skin response to potassium para-aminobenzoate therapy.**
  Author(s): Department of Internal Medicine, University of Michigan Medical School, Ann Arbor.
  Source: Zarafonetis, C J Dabich, L Skovronski, J J DeVol, E B Negri, D Yuan, W Wolfe, R Clin-Exp-Rheumatol. 1988 Jul-September; 6(3): 261-8 0392-856X

- **Scleroderma in a child after chemotherapy for cancer.**
  Author(s): Department of Pediatric Oncology, Hacettepe University Faculty of Medicine, Ankara, Turkey.
  Source: Emir, S Kutluk, T Topaloglu, R Bakkaloglu, A Buyukpamukcu, M Clin-Exp-Rheumatol. 2001 Mar-April; 19(2): 221-3 0392-856X

- **Scleroderma in association with the use of docetaxel (taxotere) for breast cancer.**
  Author(s): Department of Rheumatology, Westmead Hospital, Australia.
  Source: Hassett, G Harnett, P Manolios, N Clin-Exp-Rheumatol. 2001 Mar-April; 19(2): 197-200 0392-856X

- **Scleroderma.**
  Author(s): Department of Dermatology, New York University, USA.
  Source: Frank, P J Dermatol-Online-J. 2001 February; 7(1): 16 1087-2108

- **Selective stimulation of collagen synthesis in the presence of costimulatory insulin signaling by connective tissue growth factor in scleroderma fibroblasts.**
  Author(s): Medical University of South Carolina, Charleston, 29425, USA.
  Source: Gore Hyer, E Pannu, J Smith, E A Grotendorst, G Trojanowska, M Arthritis-Rheum. 2003 March; 48(3): 798-806 0004-3591

- **Serum xylosyltransferase: a new biochemical marker of the sclerotic process in systemic sclerosis.**
Author(s): Institut fur Laboratoriums-und Transfusionsmedizin, Herz-und Diabeteszentrum, Nodrhein-Westfalen, Universitatsklinik der Ruhr-Universitat Bochum, Bad Oeynhausen, Germany.
Source: Gotting, C Sollberg, S Kuhn, J Weilke, C Huerkamp, C Brinkmann, T Krieg, T Kleesiek, K J-Invest-Dermatol. 1999 June; 112(6): 919-24 0022-202X

- **Systemic sclerosis therapy with iloprost: a prospective observational study of 30 patients treated for a median of 3 years.**
Author(s): Servizio di Reumatologia ed Immunologia Clinica, Spedali Civili and University, I-25124 Brescia, Italy.
Source: Bettoni, L Geri, A Airo, P Danieli, E Cavazzana, I Antonioli, C Chiesa, L Franceschini, F Grottolo, A Zambruni, A Radaeli, E Cattaneo, R Clin-Rheumatol. 2002 June; 21(3): 244-50 0770-3198

- **The emerging problem of oxidative stress and the role of antioxidants in systemic sclerosis.**
Source: Herrick, A L Matucci Cerinic, M Clin-Exp-Rheumatol. 2001 Jan-February; 19(1): 4-8 0392-856X

- **The inhibitory effects of camptothecin, a topoisomerase I inhibitor, on collagen synthesis in fibroblasts from patients with systemic sclerosis.**
Author(s): Department of Medicine, Division of Rheumatology and Immunology, Medical University of South Carolina, 96 Jonathan Lucas Street, Charleston, SC 29425, USA. czuwaraj@musc.edu
Source: Czuwara Ladykowska, J Makiela, B Smith, E A Trojanowska, M Rudnicka, L Arthritis-Res. 2001; 3(5): 311-8 1465-9905

- **The pharmacological effects of cicaprost, an oral prostacyclin analogue, in patients with Raynaud's syndrome secondary to systemic sclerosis--a preliminary study.**
Author(s): University Department of Medicine, Ninewells Hospital and Medical School, Dundee, Scotland, UK.
Source: Lau, C S McLaren, M Saniabadi, A Scott, N Belch, J J Clin-Exp-Rheumatol. 1991 May-June; 9(3): 271-3 0392-856X

- **Theophylline-resistant and theophylline-sensitive "active" and "total" E rosette-forming lymphocytes in patients with systemic scleroderma.**
Author(s): Department of Laboratory Diagnostics and Clinical Immunology, Warsaw Medical Academy, Poland.
Source: Skopinska Rozewska, E Majewski, S Blaszczyk, M Wlodarska, B Jablonska, S J-Invest-Dermatol. 1988 June; 90(6): 851-6 0022-202X

- **Thrombocytopenia responsive to warfarin in a patient with systemic sclerosis--systemic lupus erythematosus overlap.**
Author(s): Department of Medicine and Transfusion Center, Keio University School of Medicine, Tokyo, Japan.
Source: Kuwana, M Kaburaki, J Hirakata, M Tojo, T Handa, M Ikeda, Y Clin-Exp-Rheumatol. 1995 Jan-February; 13(1): 103-6 0392-856X

- **Topical tocoretinate improved hypertrophic scar, skin sclerosis in systemic sclerosis and morphea.**
Author(s): Department of Dermatology, Mie University, Faculty of Medicine, Japan.
Source: Mizutani, H Yoshida, T Nouchi, N Hamanaka, H Shimizu, M J-Dermatol. 1999 January; 26(1): 11-7 0385-2407

- **Transdermal application of prostaglandin E1 ethyl ester for the treatment of trophic acral skin lesions in a patient with systemic scleroderma.**
  Author(s): Department of Dermatology, University Tubingen, Germany. anja.schlez@med.uni-tuebingen.de
  Source: Schlez, A Kittel, M Scheurle, B Diehm, C Junger, M J-Eur-Acad-Dermatol-Venereol. 2002 September; 16(5): 526-8 0926-9959

- **Treating systemic sclerosis in 2001.**
  Author(s): Internal Medicine Department, Hjpital Avicenne, Universite Paris-Nord, Bobigny France. luc.mouthon@avc.ap-hop-paris.fr
  Source: Moutho, L Agard, C Joint-Bone-Spine. 2001 October; 68(5): 393-402 1297-319X

- **Treatment of scleroderma.**
  Author(s): Johns Hopkins University School of Medicine, Division of Molecular and Clinical Rheumatology, Baltimore, MD 21205, USA.
  Source: Gelber, A C Wigley, F M Curr-Opin-Rheumatol. 1995 November; 7(6): 551-9 1040-8711

- **Trigeminal and peripheral neuropathy in a patient with systemic sclerosis and silicosis.**
  Author(s): Department of Medicine, All India Institute of Medical Sciences, New Delhi.
  Source: Agarwal, R Vasan, R S Singh, R R Saxena, S P Bhadoria, D P Srivastava, A K Verma, A Tiwari, S C Malaviya, A N Clin-Exp-Rheumatol. 1987 Oct-December; 5(4): 375-6 0392-856X

- **Unilateral generalized morphea in childhood.**
  Author(s): Division of Dermatology, Tone Central Hospital, Numata, Gunma, Japan.
  Source: Nagai, Y Hattori, T Ishikawa, O J-Dermatol. 2002 July; 29(7): 435-8 0385-2407

Federal Resources on Nutrition

In addition to the IBIDS, the United States Department of Health and Human Services (HHS) and the United States Department of Agriculture (USDA) provide many sources of information on general nutrition and health. Recommended resources include:

- healthfinder®, HHS's gateway to health information, including diet and nutrition: **http://www.healthfinder.gov/scripts/SearchContext.asp?topic=238&page=0**

- The United States Department of Agriculture's Web site dedicated to nutrition information: **www.nutrition.gov**

- The Food and Drug Administration's Web site for federal food safety information: **www.foodsafety.gov**

- The National Action Plan on Overweight and Obesity sponsored by the United States Surgeon General: **http://www.surgeongeneral.gov/topics/obesity/**

- The Center for Food Safety and Applied Nutrition has an Internet site sponsored by the Food and Drug Administration and the Department of Health and Human Services: **http://vm.cfsan.fda.gov/**

- Center for Nutrition Policy and Promotion sponsored by the United States Department of Agriculture: **http://www.usda.gov/cnpp/**

- Food and Nutrition Information Center, National Agricultural Library sponsored by the United States Department of Agriculture: **http://www.nal.usda.gov/fnic/**

- Food and Nutrition Service sponsored by the United States Department of Agriculture: **http://www.fns.usda.gov/fns/**

Additional Web Resources

A number of additional Web sites offer encyclopedic information covering food and nutrition. The following is a representative sample:

- AOL: **http://search.aol.com/cat.adp?id=174&layer=&from=subcats**

- Family Village: **http://www.familyvillage.wisc.edu/med_nutrition.html**

- Google: **http://directory.google.com/Top/Health/Nutrition/**

- Healthnotes: **http://www.healthnotes.com/**

- Open Directory Project: **http://dmoz.org/Health/Nutrition/**

- Yahoo.com: **http://dir.yahoo.com/Health/Nutrition/**

- WebMD®Health: **http://my.webmd.com/nutrition**

- WholeHealthMD.com: **http://www.wholehealthmd.com/reflib/0,1529,00.html**

The following is a specific Web list relating to scleroderma; please note that any particular subject below may indicate either a therapeutic use, or a contraindication (potential danger), and does not reflect an official recommendation:

- **Vitamins**

    Provitamin A
    Source: Integrative Medicine Communications; www.drkoop.com

    Vitamin E
    Alternative names: Alpha-Tocopherol, Beta-Tocopherol, D-Alpha-Tocopherol, Delta-Tocopherol, Gamma-Tocopherol
    Source: Integrative Medicine Communications; www.drkoop.com

- **Minerals**

    Alpha-tocopherol
    Source: Integrative Medicine Communications; www.drkoop.com

    Beta-tocopherol
    Source: Integrative Medicine Communications; www.drkoop.com

    D-alpha-tocopherol
    Source: Integrative Medicine Communications; www.drkoop.com

    Delta-tocopherol
    Source: Integrative Medicine Communications; www.drkoop.com

Gamma-tocopherol
Source: Integrative Medicine Communications; www.drkoop.com

CHAPTER 3. ALTERNATIVE MEDICINE AND SCLERODERMA

Overview

In this chapter, we will begin by introducing you to official information sources on complementary and alternative medicine (CAM) relating to scleroderma. At the conclusion of this chapter, we will provide additional sources.

National Center for Complementary and Alternative Medicine

The National Center for Complementary and Alternative Medicine (NCCAM) of the National Institutes of Health (**http://nccam.nih.gov/**) has created a link to the National Library of Medicine's databases to facilitate research for articles that specifically relate to scleroderma and complementary medicine. To search the database, go to the following Web site: **http://www.nlm.nih.gov/nccam/camonpubmed.html**. Select "CAM on PubMed." Enter "scleroderma" (or synonyms) into the search box. Click "Go." The following references provide information on particular aspects of complementary and alternative medicine that are related to scleroderma:

- **"Paul Klee and the hypothesis of morphic resonance". Adjustment to illness and life history of patients with progressive systemic scleroderma]**
  Author(s): Morscher C.
  Source: Psychotherapie, Psychosomatik, Medizinische Psychologie. 1994 June; 44(6): 200-6. German.
  http://www.ncbi.nlm.nih.gov:80/entrez/query.fcgi?cmd=Retrieve&db=PubMed&list_uids=8066164&dopt=Abstract

- **A bioactive triterpenoid and vulpinic acid derivatives from the mushroom Scleroderma citrinum.**
  Author(s): Kanokmedhakul S, Kanokmedhakul K, Prajuabsuk T, Soytong K, Kongsaeree P, Suksamrarn A.
  Source: Planta Medica. 2003 June; 69(6): 568-71.
  http://www.ncbi.nlm.nih.gov:80/entrez/query.fcgi?cmd=Retrieve&db=PubMed&list_uids=12865983&dopt=Abstract

- Activin, a grape seed-derived proanthocyanidin extract, reduces plasma levels of oxidative stress and adhesion molecules (ICAM-1, VCAM-1 and E-selectin) in systemic sclerosis.
  Author(s): Kalin R, Righi A, Del Rosso A, Bagchi D, Generini S, Cerinic MM, Das DK.
  Source: Free Radical Research. 2002 August; 36(8): 819-25.
  http://www.ncbi.nlm.nih.gov:80/entrez/query.fcgi?cmd=Retrieve&db=PubMed&list_uids=12420739&dopt=Abstract

- An objective evaluation of the treatment of systemic scleroderma with disodium EDTA, pyridoxine and reserpine.
  Author(s): Fuleihan FJ, Kurban AK, Abboud RT, Beidas-Jubran N, Farah FS.
  Source: The British Journal of Dermatology. 1968 March; 80(3): 184-9.
  http://www.ncbi.nlm.nih.gov:80/entrez/query.fcgi?cmd=Retrieve&db=PubMed&list_uids=4967134&dopt=Abstract

- Avocado/soybean unsaponifiables in the treatment of scleroderma: comment on the article by Maheu et al.
  Author(s): Jablonska S.
  Source: Arthritis and Rheumatism. 1998 September; 41(9): 1705.
  http://www.ncbi.nlm.nih.gov:80/entrez/query.fcgi?cmd=Retrieve&db=PubMed&list_uids=9751109&dopt=Abstract

- Behavioral treatment of Raynaud's phenomenon in scleroderma.
  Author(s): Freedman RR, Ianni P, Wenig P.
  Source: Journal of Behavioral Medicine. 1984 December; 7(4): 343-53.
  http://www.ncbi.nlm.nih.gov:80/entrez/query.fcgi?cmd=Retrieve&db=PubMed&list_uids=6520866&dopt=Abstract

- Calculated glomerular filtration rate is a useful screening tool to identify scleroderma patients with renal impairment.
  Author(s): Kingdon EJ, Knight CJ, Dustan K, Irwin AG, Thomas M, Powis SH, Burns A, Hilson AJ, Black CM.
  Source: Rheumatology (Oxford, England). 2003 January; 42(1): 26-33.
  http://www.ncbi.nlm.nih.gov:80/entrez/query.fcgi?cmd=Retrieve&db=PubMed&list_uids=12509609&dopt=Abstract

- Diffuse scleroderma occurring after the use of paclitaxel for ovarian cancer.
  Author(s): De Angelis R, Bugatti L, Cerioni A, Del Medico P, Filosa G.
  Source: Clinical Rheumatology. 2003 February; 22(1): 49-52.
  http://www.ncbi.nlm.nih.gov:80/entrez/query.fcgi?cmd=Retrieve&db=PubMed&list_uids=12605319&dopt=Abstract

- Disease severity of 100 patients with systemic sclerosis over a period of 14 years: using a modified Medsger scale.
  Author(s): Geirsson AJ, Wollheim FA, Akesson A.
  Source: Annals of the Rheumatic Diseases. 2001 December; 60(12): 1117-22.
  http://www.ncbi.nlm.nih.gov:80/entrez/query.fcgi?cmd=Retrieve&db=PubMed&list_uids=11709453&dopt=Abstract

- **Disseminated scleroderma of a Japanese patient successfully treated with bath PUVA photochemotherapy.**
  Author(s): Aragane Y, Kawada A, Maeda A, Isogai R, Isogai N, Tezuka T.
  Source: Journal of Cutaneous Medicine and Surgery. 2001 March-April; 5(2): 135-9. Epub 2001 March 21.
  http://www.ncbi.nlm.nih.gov:80/entrez/query.fcgi?cmd=Retrieve&db=PubMed&list_uids=11443486&dopt=Abstract

- **Docetaxel (Taxotere) associated scleroderma-like changes of the lower extremities. A report of three cases.**
  Author(s): Battafarano DF, Zimmerman GC, Older SA, Keeling JH, Burris HA.
  Source: Cancer. 1995 July 1; 76(1): 110-5.
  http://www.ncbi.nlm.nih.gov:80/entrez/query.fcgi?cmd=Retrieve&db=PubMed&list_uids=8630861&dopt=Abstract

- **Effect of ethylenediaminetetraacetic acid (EDTA) and tetrahydroxyquinone on sclerodermatous skin. Histologic and chemical studies.**
  Author(s): Keech MK, McCann DS, Boyle AJ, Pinkus H.
  Source: The Journal of Investigative Dermatology. 1966 September; 47(3): 235-46.
  http://www.ncbi.nlm.nih.gov:80/entrez/query.fcgi?cmd=Retrieve&db=PubMed&list_uids=4958819&dopt=Abstract

- **Effect of transcutaneous nerve stimulation on esophageal motility in patients with achalasia and scleroderma.**
  Author(s): Mearin F, Zacchi P, Armengol JR, Vilardell M, Malagelada JR.
  Source: Scandinavian Journal of Gastroenterology. 1990 October; 25(10): 1018-23.
  http://www.ncbi.nlm.nih.gov:80/entrez/query.fcgi?cmd=Retrieve&db=PubMed&list_uids=2263874&dopt=Abstract

- **Efficacy of physiatric management of linear scleroderma.**
  Author(s): Rudolph RI, Leyden JJ, Berger BJ.
  Source: Archives of Physical Medicine and Rehabilitation. 1974 September; 55(9): 428-31.
  http://www.ncbi.nlm.nih.gov:80/entrez/query.fcgi?cmd=Retrieve&db=PubMed&list_uids=4413188&dopt=Abstract

- **Increased transcriptional activities of transforming growth factor beta receptors in scleroderma fibroblasts.**
  Author(s): Yamane K, Ihn H, Kubo M, Tamaki K.
  Source: Arthritis and Rheumatism. 2002 September; 46(9): 2421-8.
  http://www.ncbi.nlm.nih.gov:80/entrez/query.fcgi?cmd=Retrieve&db=PubMed&list_uids=12355490&dopt=Abstract

- **Inhibition of collagen production by traditional Chinese herbal medicine in scleroderma fibroblast cultures.**
  Author(s): Sheng FY, Ohta A, Yamaguchi M.
  Source: Intern Med. 1994 August; 33(8): 466-71.
  http://www.ncbi.nlm.nih.gov:80/entrez/query.fcgi?cmd=Retrieve&db=PubMed&list_uids=7803912&dopt=Abstract

- **Kinetochore structure, duplication, and distribution in mammalian cells: analysis by human autoantibodies from scleroderma patients.**
  Author(s): Brenner S, Pepper D, Berns MW, Tan E, Brinkley BR.
  Source: The Journal of Cell Biology. 1981 October; 91(1): 95-102.
  http://www.ncbi.nlm.nih.gov:80/entrez/query.fcgi?cmd=Retrieve&db=PubMed&list_uids=7298727&dopt=Abstract

- **Lichen sclerosus et atrophicus and morphea.**
  Author(s): Grekin J, Schwartz O, Mehregan A, Mendelson C, Burnham T.
  Source: Archives of Dermatology. 1967 July; 96(1): 106.
  http://www.ncbi.nlm.nih.gov:80/entrez/query.fcgi?cmd=Retrieve&db=PubMed&list_uids=4165766&dopt=Abstract

- **Management of finger ulcers in scleroderma.**
  Author(s): Ward WA, Van Moore A.
  Source: The Journal of Hand Surgery. 1995 September; 20(5): 868-72.
  http://www.ncbi.nlm.nih.gov:80/entrez/query.fcgi?cmd=Retrieve&db=PubMed&list_uids=8522759&dopt=Abstract

- **Marked and sustained improvement of systemic sclerosis following polychemotherapy for coexistent multiple myeloma.**
  Author(s): Bachleitner-Hofmann T, Machold K, Knobler R, Drach J, Grumbeck E, Gisslinger H.
  Source: Clin Exp Rheumatol. 2002 January-February; 20(1): 85-8.
  http://www.ncbi.nlm.nih.gov:80/entrez/query.fcgi?cmd=Retrieve&db=PubMed&list_uids=11892717&dopt=Abstract

- **Marked digital skin temperature increase mediated by thermal biofeedback in advanced scleroderma.**
  Author(s): Wilson E, Belar CD, Panush RS, Ettinger MP.
  Source: The Journal of Rheumatology. 1983 February; 10(1): 167-8.
  http://www.ncbi.nlm.nih.gov:80/entrez/query.fcgi?cmd=Retrieve&db=PubMed&list_uids=6842480&dopt=Abstract

- **Of faddism, toxic oil, and scleroderma.**
  Author(s): Berry CL.
  Source: The Journal of Pathology. 1993 August; 170(4): 419-20.
  http://www.ncbi.nlm.nih.gov:80/entrez/query.fcgi?cmd=Retrieve&db=PubMed&list_uids=8410491&dopt=Abstract

- **Oxidative stress in scleroderma: maintenance of scleroderma fibroblast phenotype by the constitutive up-regulation of reactive oxygen species generation through the NADPH oxidase complex pathway.**
  Author(s): Sambo P, Baroni SS, Luchetti M, Paroncini P, Dusi S, Orlandini G, Gabrielli A.
  Source: Arthritis and Rheumatism. 2001 November; 44(11): 2653-64.
  http://www.ncbi.nlm.nih.gov:80/entrez/query.fcgi?cmd=Retrieve&db=PubMed&list_uids=11710721&dopt=Abstract

- **Pharmacodynamic effect of dipyridamole on thallium-201 myocardial perfusion in progressive systemic sclerosis with diffuse scleroderma.**

Author(s): Kahan A, Devaux JY, Amor B, Menkes CJ, Weber S, Foult JM, Venot A, Guerin F, Degeorges M, Roucayrol JC.
Source: Annals of the Rheumatic Diseases. 1986 September; 45(9): 718-25.
http://www.ncbi.nlm.nih.gov:80/entrez/query.fcgi?cmd=Retrieve&db=PubMed&list_uids=3490227&dopt=Abstract

- **Raynaud's phenomenon in scleroderma treated with hyperbaric oxygen.**
  Author(s): Dowling GB, Copeman PW, Ashfield R.
  Source: Proc R Soc Med. 1967 December; 60(12): 1268-9. No Abstract Available.
  http://www.ncbi.nlm.nih.gov:80/entrez/query.fcgi?cmd=Retrieve&db=PubMed&list_uids=6066573&dopt=Abstract

- **Remission of scleroderma during chemotherapy for lymphoma.**
  Author(s): Comer M, Harvey AR.
  Source: Annals of the Rheumatic Diseases. 1992 August; 51(8): 998-1000.
  http://www.ncbi.nlm.nih.gov:80/entrez/query.fcgi?cmd=Retrieve&db=PubMed&list_uids=1417129&dopt=Abstract

- **Scleroderma (acrosclerosis). I. Treatment of three cases of the non-calcific variety by Chelation (EDTA).**
  Author(s): RUKAVINA JG, MENDELSON C, PRICE JM, BROWN RR, JOHNSON SA.
  Source: The Journal of Investigative Dermatology. 1957 October; 29(4): 273-88.
  http://www.ncbi.nlm.nih.gov:80/entrez/query.fcgi?cmd=Retrieve&db=PubMed&list_uids=13491891&dopt=Abstract

- **Scleroderma (acrosclerosis). II. Tryptophan metabolism before and during treatment by Chelaton (EDTA).**
  Author(s): PRICE JM, BROWN RR, RUKAVINA JG, MENDELSON C, JOHNSON SA.
  Source: The Journal of Investigative Dermatology. 1957 October; 29(4): 289-98.
  http://www.ncbi.nlm.nih.gov:80/entrez/query.fcgi?cmd=Retrieve&db=PubMed&list_uids=13491892&dopt=Abstract

- **Scleroderma and sclerotic skin conditions: unapproved treatments.**
  Author(s): Jablonska S, Blaszczyk M.
  Source: Clinics in Dermatology. 2002 November-December; 20(6): 634-7. Review.
  http://www.ncbi.nlm.nih.gov:80/entrez/query.fcgi?cmd=Retrieve&db=PubMed&list_uids=12490356&dopt=Abstract

- **Scleroderma in a child after chemotherapy for cancer.**
  Author(s): Emir S, Kutluk T, Topaloglu R, Bakkaloglu A, Buyukpamukcu M.
  Source: Clin Exp Rheumatol. 2001 March-April; 19(2): 221-3.
  http://www.ncbi.nlm.nih.gov:80/entrez/query.fcgi?cmd=Retrieve&db=PubMed&list_uids=11326490&dopt=Abstract

- **Scleroderma in association with the use of docetaxel (taxotere) for breast cancer.**
  Author(s): Hassett G, Harnett P, Manolios N.
  Source: Clin Exp Rheumatol. 2001 March-April; 19(2): 197-200.
  http://www.ncbi.nlm.nih.gov:80/entrez/query.fcgi?cmd=Retrieve&db=PubMed&list_uids=11326485&dopt=Abstract

- **Scleroderma overlap syndromes.**
  Author(s): Jablonska S, Blaszczyk M.
  Source: Advances in Experimental Medicine and Biology. 1999; 455: 85-92.
  http://www.ncbi.nlm.nih.gov:80/entrez/query.fcgi?cmd=Retrieve&db=PubMed&list_
  uids=10599327&dopt=Abstract

- **Scleroderma. 1. Clinical features, course of illness and response to treatment in 61 cases.**
  Author(s): Barnett AJ, Coventry DA.
  Source: The Medical Journal of Australia. 1969 May 10; 1(19): 992-1001.
  http://www.ncbi.nlm.nih.gov:80/entrez/query.fcgi?cmd=Retrieve&db=PubMed&list_
  uids=4978080&dopt=Abstract

- **Scleroderma: the more you know, the more you can help.**
  Author(s): Zalac CJ.
  Source: J Pract Nurs. 1979 August; 29(8): 23-5. No Abstract Available.
  http://www.ncbi.nlm.nih.gov:80/entrez/query.fcgi?cmd=Retrieve&db=PubMed&list_
  uids=257011&dopt=Abstract

- **Scleroderma-like cutaneous lesions induced by paclitaxel: a case study.**
  Author(s): Kupfer I, Balguerie X, Courville P, Chinet P, Joly P.
  Source: Journal of the American Academy of Dermatology. 2003 February; 48(2): 279-81.
  http://www.ncbi.nlm.nih.gov:80/entrez/query.fcgi?cmd=Retrieve&db=PubMed&list_
  uids=12582404&dopt=Abstract

- **Scleroderma-like drug reaction to paclitaxel (Taxol).**
  Author(s): Lauchli S, Trueb RM, Fehr M, Hafner J.
  Source: The British Journal of Dermatology. 2002 September; 147(3): 619-21.
  http://www.ncbi.nlm.nih.gov:80/entrez/query.fcgi?cmd=Retrieve&db=PubMed&list_
  uids=12207621&dopt=Abstract

- **Stem cell therapy in scleroderma.**
  Author(s): Braun-Moscovici Y, Furst DE.
  Source: Current Opinion in Rheumatology. 2002 November; 14(6): 711-6. Review.
  http://www.ncbi.nlm.nih.gov:80/entrez/query.fcgi?cmd=Retrieve&db=PubMed&list_
  uids=12410096&dopt=Abstract

- **Stimulating circulation to end stasis in scleroderma.**
  Author(s): Yuan X, Li JD, Chen WJ, Li ZS, Zhu HT, Liu JW, Zhu MJ.
  Source: Chinese Medical Journal. 1981 February; 94(2): 85-93.
  http://www.ncbi.nlm.nih.gov:80/entrez/query.fcgi?cmd=Retrieve&db=PubMed&list_
  uids=6786844&dopt=Abstract

- **The inhibitory effects of camptothecin, a topoisomerase I inhibitor, on collagen synthesis in fibroblasts from patients with systemic sclerosis.**
  Author(s): Czuwara-Ladykowska J, Makiela B, Smith EA, Trojanowska M, Rudnicka L.
  Source: Arthritis Research. 2001; 3(5): 311-8. Epub 2001 August 02.
  http://www.ncbi.nlm.nih.gov:80/entrez/query.fcgi?cmd=Retrieve&db=PubMed&list_
  uids=11549373&dopt=Abstract

- **Transcutaneous electrical nerve stimulation and extensor splint in linear scleroderma knee contracture.**
  Author(s): Rizk TE, Park SJ.
  Source: Archives of Physical Medicine and Rehabilitation. 1981 February; 62(2): 86-8.
  http://www.ncbi.nlm.nih.gov:80/entrez/query.fcgi?cmd=Retrieve&db=PubMed&list_uids=6972203&dopt=Abstract

- **Treatment of generalized scleroderma with combined traditional Chinese and western medicine: report of 30 cases.**
  Author(s): Dexin W.
  Source: Chinese Medical Journal. 1979 June; 92(6): 427-30.
  http://www.ncbi.nlm.nih.gov:80/entrez/query.fcgi?cmd=Retrieve&db=PubMed&list_uids=110556&dopt=Abstract

- **Treatment of generalized scleroderma with inhibitors of collagen synthesis.**
  Author(s): Asboe-Hansen G.
  Source: International Journal of Dermatology. 1982 April; 21(3): 159-61.
  http://www.ncbi.nlm.nih.gov:80/entrez/query.fcgi?cmd=Retrieve&db=PubMed&list_uids=7085173&dopt=Abstract

- **Treatment of localised scleroderma with PUVA bath photochemotherapy.**
  Author(s): Kerscher M, Volkenandt M, Meurer M, Lehmann P, Plewig G, Rocken M.
  Source: Lancet. 1994 May 14; 343(8907): 1233. Erratum In: Lancet 1994 June 18; 343(8912): 1580.
  http://www.ncbi.nlm.nih.gov:80/entrez/query.fcgi?cmd=Retrieve&db=PubMed&list_uids=7909904&dopt=Abstract

- **Treatment of scleroderma, sclerodactylia and calcinosis by chelation (EDTA).**
  Author(s): KLEIN R, HARRIS SB.
  Source: The American Journal of Medicine. 1955 November; 19(5): 798-807.
  http://www.ncbi.nlm.nih.gov:80/entrez/query.fcgi?cmd=Retrieve&db=PubMed&list_uids=13268481&dopt=Abstract

- **Tryptophan metabolism in man (with special reference to rheumatoid arthritis and scleroderma).**
  Author(s): Houpt JB, Ogryzlo MA, Hunt M.
  Source: Seminars in Arthritis and Rheumatism. 1973; 2(4): 333-53.
  http://www.ncbi.nlm.nih.gov:80/entrez/query.fcgi?cmd=Retrieve&db=PubMed&list_uids=4267284&dopt=Abstract

- **Understanding the special needs of the patient with scleroderma.**
  Author(s): Rossiter RC.
  Source: Australian Nursing Journal (July 1993). 2000 September; 8(3): Suppl 1-4. Review.
  http://www.ncbi.nlm.nih.gov:80/entrez/query.fcgi?cmd=Retrieve&db=PubMed&list_uids=11894369&dopt=Abstract

Additional Web Resources

A number of additional Web sites offer encyclopedic information covering CAM and related topics. The following is a representative sample:

- Alternative Medicine Foundation, Inc.: **http://www.herbmed.org/**

- AOL: **http://search.aol.com/cat.adp?id=169&layer=&from=subcats**

- Chinese Medicine: **http://www.newcenturynutrition.com/**

- drkoop.com®: **http://www.drkoop.com/InteractiveMedicine/IndexC.html**

- Family Village: **http://www.familyvillage.wisc.edu/med_altn.htm**

- Google: **http://directory.google.com/Top/Health/Alternative/**

- Healthnotes: **http://www.healthnotes.com/**

- MedWebPlus: **http://medwebplus.com/subject/Alternative_and_Complementary_Medicine**

- Open Directory Project: **http://dmoz.org/Health/Alternative/**

- HealthGate: **http://www.tnp.com/**

- WebMD®Health: **http://my.webmd.com/drugs_and_herbs**

- WholeHealthMD.com: **http://www.wholehealthmd.com/reflib/0,1529,00.html**

- Yahoo.com: **http://dir.yahoo.com/Health/Alternative_Medicine/**

The following is a specific Web list relating to scleroderma; please note that any particular subject below may indicate either a therapeutic use, or a contraindication (potential danger), and does not reflect an official recommendation:

- **General Overview**

    Dupuytren's Contracture
    Source: Healthnotes, Inc.; www.healthnotes.com

    Scleroderma
    Source: Integrative Medicine Communications; www.drkoop.com

    Vitiligo
    Source: Healthnotes, Inc.; www.healthnotes.com

- **Herbs and Supplements**

    5-HTP
    Alternative names: 5-Hydroxytryptophan (5-HTP)
    Source: Integrative Medicine Communications; www.drkoop.com

    5-HTP (5-Hydroxytryptophan)
    Source: Prima Communications, Inc.www.personalhealthzone.com

5-Hydroxytryptophan
Source: Healthnotes, Inc.; www.healthnotes.com

5-Hydroxytryptophan (5-HTP)
Source: Integrative Medicine Communications; www.drkoop.com

Ananas Comosus
Source: Integrative Medicine Communications; www.drkoop.com

B-carotene
Source: Integrative Medicine Communications; www.drkoop.com

Beta-carotene
Alternative names: b-carotene, Trans-beta Carotene; Provitamin A, Betacarotenum
Source: Integrative Medicine Communications; www.drkoop.com

Betacarotenum
Source: Integrative Medicine Communications; www.drkoop.com

Brahmi
Alternative names: Centella asiatica, Centella, March Pennywort, Indian Pennywort, Hydrocotyle, Brahmi (Sanskrit), Luei Gong Gen (Chinese)(Note: Gotu kola should not be confused with kola nut.)
Source: Integrative Medicine Communications; www.drkoop.com

Bromelain
Alternative names: Ananas comosus, Bromelainum
Source: Integrative Medicine Communications; www.drkoop.com

Bromelainum
Source: Integrative Medicine Communications; www.drkoop.com

Carbidopa
Source: Healthnotes, Inc.; www.healthnotes.com

Carbidopa/Levodopa
Source: Healthnotes, Inc.; www.healthnotes.com

Centella
Alternative names: Gotu Kola; Centella asiatica (Linn.)
Source: Alternative Medicine Foundation, Inc.; www.amfoundation.org

Centella
Source: Integrative Medicine Communications; www.drkoop.com

Centella Asiatica
Alternative names: Centella asiatica, Centella, March Pennywort, Indian Pennywort, Hydrocotyle, Brahmi (Sanskrit), Luei Gong Gen (Chinese)(Note: Gotu kola should not be confused with kola nut.)
Source: Integrative Medicine Communications; www.drkoop.com

Dmso
Source: Healthnotes, Inc.; www.healthnotes.com

Fiber
Source: Healthnotes, Inc.; www.healthnotes.com

Gotu Kola
Alternative names: Centella asiatica
Source: Healthnotes, Inc.; www.healthnotes.com

Gotu Kola
Alternative names: Centella asiatica , Centella, March Pennywort, Indian
Pennywort, Hydrocotyle, Brahmi (Sanskrit), Luei Gong Gen (Chinese)(Note: Gotu
kola should not be confused with kola nut.)
Source: Integrative Medicine Communications; www.drkoop.com

Gotu Kola
Source: Prima Communications, Inc.www.personalhealthzone.com

Gotu Kola
Source: WholeHealthMD.com, LLC.; www.wholehealthmd.com
Hyperlink:
http://www.wholehealthmd.com/refshelf/substances_view/0,1525,10031,00.html

Hydrocotyle
Source: Integrative Medicine Communications; www.drkoop.com

Indian Pennywort
Source: Integrative Medicine Communications; www.drkoop.com

Levodopa/carbidopa
Alternative names: Sinemet
Source: Prima Communications, Inc.www.personalhealthzone.com

Marsh Pennywort
Alternative names: Centella asiatica , Centella, March Pennywort, Indian
Pennywort, Hydrocotyle, Brahmi (Sanskrit), Luei Gong Gen (Chinese)(Note: Gotu
kola should not be confused with kola nut.)
Source: Integrative Medicine Communications; www.drkoop.com

PABA
Source: Healthnotes, Inc.; www.healthnotes.com

PABA
Source: WholeHealthMD.com, LLC.; www.wholehealthmd.com
Hyperlink:
http://www.wholehealthmd.com/refshelf/substances_view/0,1525,10049,00.html

PABA (Para-Aminobenzoic Acid)
Source: Prima Communications, Inc.www.personalhealthzone.com

Pregnenolone
Source: Healthnotes, Inc.; www.healthnotes.com

Trans-beta-carotene
Source: Integrative Medicine Communications; www.drkoop.com

General References

A good place to find general background information on CAM is the National Library of Medicine. It has prepared within the MEDLINEplus system an information topic page dedicated to complementary and alternative medicine. To access this page, go to the MEDLINEplus site at **http://www.nlm.nih.gov/medlineplus/alternativemedicine.html.** This Web site provides a general overview of various topics and can lead to a number of general sources.

CHAPTER 4. DISSERTATIONS ON SCLERODERMA

Overview

In this chapter, we will give you a bibliography on recent dissertations relating to scleroderma. We will also provide you with information on how to use the Internet to stay current on dissertations. **IMPORTANT NOTE:** When following the search strategy described below, you may discover <u>non-medical dissertations</u> that use the generic term "scleroderma" (or a synonym) in their titles. To accurately reflect the results that you might find while conducting research on scleroderma, <u>we have not necessarily excluded non-medical dissertations</u> in this bibliography.

Dissertations on Scleroderma

ProQuest Digital Dissertations, the largest archive of academic dissertations available, is located at the following Web address: **http://wwwlib.umi.com/dissertations**. From this archive, we have compiled the following list covering dissertations devoted to scleroderma. You will see that the information provided includes the dissertation's title, its author, and the institution with which the author is associated. The following covers recent dissertations found when using this search procedure:

- **Pulmonary Disease in Scleroderma: Combined Interstitial Lung Disease and Pulmonary Hypertension and Predictors of Pulmonary Hypertension** by Chang, Betty, PhD from The Johns Hopkins University, 2003, 72 pages
  http://wwwlib.umi.com/dissertations/fullcit/3068129

Keeping Current

Ask the medical librarian at your library if it has full and unlimited access to the *ProQuest Digital Dissertations* database. From the library, you should be able to do more complete searches via **http://wwwlib.umi.com/dissertations**.

CHAPTER 5. CLINICAL TRIALS AND SCLERODERMA

Overview

In this chapter, we will show you how to keep informed of the latest clinical trials concerning scleroderma.

Recent Trials on Scleroderma

The following is a list of recent trials dedicated to scleroderma.[8] Further information on a trial is available at the Web site indicated.

- **Autologous Stem Cell Transplant For Systemic Sclerosis**

   Condition(s): Scleroderma, Systemic

   Study Status: This study is currently recruiting patients.

   Sponsor(s): National Institute of Arthritis and Musculoskeletal and Skin Diseases (NIAMS); University of Pittsburgh Cancer Institute; Amgen; Sangstat Medical Corporation

   Purpose - Excerpt: Patients with **systemic sclerosis** undergo tests,sign informed consent. Patients are admitted to hospital for a day of chemotherapy. Patients go home and receive a shot of G-CSF for about 10 days, then a procedure called Leukapheresis begins and is done as outpatient for up to 4 days. Chemotherapy is given for 5 days. The doses of chemotherapy will be increased after every three patients if there are no serious side effects. Thymoglobulin, an immunosuppressing drug, will be given for 3 days. On day 0 patient receive infusion of stem cells. It will take 2-4 weeks to recover from side effects of this treatment. Patient Involvement:Patients must be stay in the Pittsburgh area for their treatment, are required to use appropriate birth control to prevent pregnancy.Patients will have blood sample 16 times during first 2 years of treatment and return to Pittsburgh 12, 18, and 24 months after the transplant to be evaluated and to give blood samples.

   Phase(s): Phase I

   Study Type: Interventional

---

[8] These are listed at **www.ClinicalTrials.gov**.

Contact(s): see Web site below

Web Site: http://clinicaltrials.gov/ct/show/NCT00040651

- **Efficacy and safety of oral bosentan in pulmonary fibrosis associated with scleroderma**

  Condition(s): Pulmonary Fibrosis; Scleroderma, Systemic

  Study Status: This study is currently recruiting patients.

  Sponsor(s): Actelion

  Purpose - Excerpt: Clinical and experimental studies suggest that bosentan could delay the progression of interstitial lung disease (ILD) associated with systemic sclerosis (SSc), a condition for which no established efficacious treatment is available. The present trial investigates a possible use of oral bosentan, which is currently approved for the treatment of symptoms of pulmonary arterial hypertension (PAH) WHO Class III and IV, to a new category of patients suffering from ILD associated with SSc.

  Phase(s): Phase II; Phase III

  Study Type: Interventional

  Contact(s): see Web site below

  Web Site: http://clinicaltrials.gov/ct/show/NCT00070590

- **Efficacy and Safety of Oral Bosentan on Healing/Prevention of Digital (Finger) Ulcers in Scleroderma Patients**

  Condition(s): Systemic Sclerosis; Scleroderma

  Study Status: This study is currently recruiting patients.

  Sponsor(s): Actelion

  Purpose - Excerpt: To date, one clinical trial, RAPIDS-1, was performed in Scleroderma patients with or without digital ulcers at baseline. The RAPIDS-1 study results showed that Bosentan significantly reduced the number of new digital ulcers versus placebo. The purpose of this trial is to evaluate the prevention and healing effects of bosentan versus placebo on digital ulcers over a 24 week treatment period.

  Phase(s): Phase III

  Study Type: Interventional

  Contact(s): see Web site below

  Web Site: http://clinicaltrials.gov/ct/show/NCT00077584

- **Genetic Study of the FBN1 Gene and Fibrillin-1 Abnormalities in Choctaw Native Americans and Other Patients with Systemic Sclerosis**

  Condition(s): Systemic Sclerosis

  Study Status: This study is currently recruiting patients.

  Sponsor(s): National Center for Research Resources (NCRR); University of Texas

  Purpose - Excerpt: Objectives: I. Determine whether defects in fibrillin-1 cellular processing are present in the tsk1 mouse model that carries a known FBN1 gene rearrangement and in a population of Choctaw Native American patients with **systemic sclerosis** who have a strong genetic predisposition to the disease. II. Determine the ultrastructural features of fibrillin-1 in these patients. III. Screen the FBN1 gene for mutations beginning at the regions homologous to the tsk1 duplication and latent transforming growth factor binding proteins in these patients and in an unaffected Choctaw control group. IV. Determine the correlation between fibrillin-1 abnormalities and clinical presentation, autoantibodies, and ethnicity.

Study Type: Observational

Contact(s): see Web site below

Web Site: http://clinicaltrials.gov/ct/show/NCT00006393

- **Oral Type I Collagen in Scleroderma**

  Condition(s): Scleroderma

  Study Status: This study is currently recruiting patients.

  Sponsor(s): National Institute of Arthritis and Musculoskeletal and Skin Diseases (NIAMS)

  Purpose - Excerpt: This is a 15-month study to find out if taking type I collagen by mouth will improve diffuse systemic sclerosis (scleroderma). We will randomly assign 168 patients to receive type I collagen from cows or a placebo (inactive treatment) for 12 months. We will examine patients and do laboratory tests once every 4 months during the 12-month treatment period and once more at 15 months.

  Phase(s): Phase II

  Study Type: Interventional

  Contact(s): see Web site below

  Web Site: http://clinicaltrials.gov/ct/show/NCT00005675

- **Pilot Study of Total Body Irradiation in Combination With Cyclophosphamide, Anti-thymocyte Globulin, and Autologous CD34-Selected Peripheral Blood Stem Cell Transplantation in Children With Refractory Autoimmune Disorders**

  Condition(s): Systemic Sclerosis; Systemic Lupus Erythematosus; Dermatomyositis; Juvenile Rheumatoid Arthritis; Autoimmune Diseases

  Study Status: This study is currently recruiting patients.

  Sponsor(s): Fred Hutchinson Cancer Research Center

  Purpose - Excerpt: Objectives: I. Determine the safety and long term complications of total body irradiation in combination with cyclophosphamide, anti-thymocyte globulin, and autologous CD34-selected peripheral blood stem cell (PBSC) transplantation in children with refractory autoimmune disorders. II. Determine the efficacy of this treatment regimen in these patients. III. Determine the reconstitution of immunity after autologous CD34-selected PBSC transplantation in these patients. IV. Determine engraftment of autologous CD34-selected PBSC in these patients.

  Study Type: Interventional

  Contact(s): see Web site below

  Web Site: http://clinicaltrials.gov/ct/show/NCT00010335

- **Psychological Treatments for Scleroderma**

  Condition(s): Pain; Depression; Scleroderma; Systemic Sclerosis

Study Status: This study is currently recruiting patients.

Sponsor(s): National Institute of Arthritis and Musculoskeletal and Skin Diseases (NIAMS)

Purpose - Excerpt: This study will examine the effectiveness of two psychological treatment approaches designed to help people who have scleroderma with three important areas of daily living: pain, depression, and distress about changes in appearance. We will also study the impact of depression on the psychological treatments. Because psychological approaches requiring a trained professional can be expensive and are often not available to most patients, we will also look at the effectiveness of a self-help treatment approach.

Phase(s): Phase II

Study Type: Interventional

Contact(s): see Web site below

Web Site: http://clinicaltrials.gov/ct/show/NCT00007267

- **Scleroderma Lung Study**

  Condition(s): Lung Diseases; Pulmonary Fibrosis; Systemic Scleroderma; Scleroderma, Systemic

  Study Status: This study is currently recruiting patients.

  Sponsor(s): National Heart, Lung, and Blood Institute (NHLBI)

  Purpose - Excerpt: To evaluate the efficacy and safety of cyclophosphamide versus placebo for the prevention and progression of symptomatic pulmonary disease in patients with systemic sclerosis.

  Phase(s): Phase III

  Study Type: Interventional

  Contact(s): see Web site below

  Web Site: http://clinicaltrials.gov/ct/show/NCT00004563

- **Scleroderma Registry**

  Condition(s): Systemic Sclerosis; Scleroderma

  Study Status: This study is currently recruiting patients.

  Sponsor(s): National Institute of Arthritis and Musculoskeletal and Skin Diseases (NIAMS)

  Purpose - Excerpt: Scleroderma is likely caused by a combination of factors, including an external trigger (infection or other exposure) and a genetic predisposition. The Scleroderma Registry will conduct genetic analyses for disease-related genes in patients with scleroderma and their family members (parents, brothers, and sisters).

  Study Type: Observational

  Contact(s): see Web site below

  Web Site: http://clinicaltrials.gov/ct/show/NCT00074568

- **Six month clinical research study for patients with moderate or severe dry eye syndrome**

  Condition(s): Keratoconjunctivitis Sicca; Sjogren's Syndrome; Lupus Erythematosus, Systemic; Arthritis, Rheumatoid; Scleroderma, Systemic

  Study Status: This study is currently recruiting patients.

  Sponsor(s): Allergan

  Purpose - Excerpt: A six-month clinical research trial to evaluate the effectiveness of an investigational medication for the treatment of dry eye syndrome in patients that have been diagnosed with moderate to severe dry eye syndrome, an autoimmune disorder AND/OR females 65 years of age or older.

  Phase(s): Phase III

  Study Type: Interventional

  Contact(s): Rheumatology Research International 1-888-297-4247 info@dryeyestudy.com

  Web Site: http://clinicaltrials.gov/ct/show/NCT00025818

- **Stem Cell Transplant to Treat Patients with Systemic Sclerosis.**

  Condition(s): Systemic Sclerosis

  Study Status: This study is currently recruiting patients.

  Sponsor(s): Baylor College of Medicine; The Methodist Hospital

  Purpose - Excerpt: Systemic Sclerosis is a disease that may be caused by the immune system reacting against skin and certain organs. It is possible, that by changing the immune system we can modify the progression of this disease. Stem cells are created in the bone marrow. They mature into different types of blood cells that are needed including red blood cells, white blood cells, and platelets. In this study, we will stimulate the bone marrow to make extra stem cells. Next we will collect the stem cells, select specific cells, and store them. We will then give high dose chemotherapy that will destroy the patients immune system. We will then give back the selected stem cells we collected. We believe that these selected stem cells may be able to "re-create" the immune system without the portion that causes **Systemic Sclerosis**. The purpose of this study is to try to discover if stem cell transplantation can help patients with **Systemic Sclerosis**. We will also try to learn what the side effects are of this treatment in patients with **Systemic Sclerosis**. We hope that this treatment will help to relieve the symptoms patients are experiencing, although we do not know if it will.

  Phase(s): Phase I

  Study Type: Interventional

  Contact(s): see Web site below

  Web Site: http://clinicaltrials.gov/ct/show/NCT00058578

- **Study of Families with Twins or Siblings Discordant for Rheumatic Disorders**

  Condition(s): Rheumatic Diseases; Rheumatoid Arthritis; Systemic Lupus Erythematosus; Scleroderma; Dermatomyositis; Myositis

  Study Status: This study is currently recruiting patients.

  Sponsor(s): National Institute of Environmental Health Sciences (NIEHS)

Purpose - Excerpt: This study will examine families in which one sibling of a sibling pair, or twin pair, has developed a systemic rheumatic disease and one has not, to see if and how the two differ in the following: - Blood cell metabolism; - Types of cells in the blood; - Environmental exposures or genetic factors that might explain why one developed disease and the other did not. Families in which one sibling has developed a systemic rheumatic disease, rheumatoid arthritis, systemic lupus erythematosus, **scleroderma**, dermatomyositis, or myositis, and the other has not, are eligible for this study. The siblings may or may not be twins, but must be of the same gender and be within a 3-year age difference. Biological parents, or, in some cases, children, will also be included in the study. Normal, healthy volunteers will serve as control subjects. Participants will undergo some or all of the following tests and procedures: - Medical history and physical examination. Participants will also be asked permission to obtain medical records for review. - Questionnaires about environmental exposures at work, at home, and elsewhere. Probands (participants with rheumatic disease) and their healthy siblings will also answer questions about infections, vaccinations, medications or dietary supplements, sun exposure, and stressful events during the year before disease diagnosis in the affected sibling. - Blood and urine collection for the following tests: - Routine blood chemistries and other studies to rule out certain diseases or medical problems; - Evidence of past toxic exposures and certain infections; - Presence of cells from the mother in the child's blood and vice versa. (Recent studies suggest that during pregnancy or delivery, cells from the mother and baby may be exchanged and circulate in the body for many years, possibly causing problems); - In twin or sibling pairs, presence of certain genes that may be more common in patients with systematic rheumatic diseases as compared with their unaffected siblings and normal volunteers; - In identical twins, comparison of their blood cell metabolism to see if and how the metabolism differs in people with rheumatic disease. Participants may be asked for permission to have some of their blood and urine samples stored and to obtain previously collected blood or tissue biopsy specimens that are no longer needed for clinical care, for research purposes. They may also be asked to give additional blood or urine samples. Participants will be followed every year for 5 years (either in person or by questionnaire) to evaluate any changes in their condition. The final 5-year evaluation will repeat some of the questionnaires and procedures described above.

Study Type: Observational

Contact(s): see Web site below

Web Site: http://clinicaltrials.gov/ct/show/NCT00055055

- **Phase II Pilot Study of Cyclophosphamide and Rabbit Anti-Thymocyte Globulin as Salvage Therapy in Patients With Diffuse Systemic Sclerosis**

  Condition(s): Systemic Sclerosis

  Study Status: This study is no longer recruiting patients.

  Sponsor(s): Fred Hutchinson Cancer Research Center

  Purpose - Excerpt: Objectives: I. Determine the toxicity of cyclophosphamide and rabbit anti-thymocyte globulin in patients with diffuse **systemic sclerosis**. II. Determine the efficacy of this regimen in terms of controlling disease in these patients.

  Phase(s): Phase II

  Study Type: Interventional

  Contact(s): see Web site below

  Web Site: http://clinicaltrials.gov/ct/show/NCT00016458

- **Safety, Tolerability, and Pharmacokinetics of CAT-192 (Human Anti-TGF-Beta1 Monoclonal Antibody) in Patients with Early Stage Diffuse Systemic Sclerosis**

  Condition(s): Systemic Sclerosis; Scleroderma

  Study Status: This study is no longer recruiting patients.

  Sponsor(s): Genzyme; Cambridge Antibody Technology

  Purpose - Excerpt: Systemic Sclerosis (also known as Scleroderma) is a chronic, autoimmune disease of the connective tissue generally classified as one of the rheumatic diseases. **Systemic Sclerosis** causes fibrosis (scar tissue) to be formed in the skin and internal organs. The fibrosis eventually causes the involved skin to harden, limiting mobility, and can also damage other organs. Excess Transforming Growth Factor Beta-1 (TGF-beta1) activity may result in the abnormal fibrosis characteristic of **Systemic Sclerosis**. An antibody against TGF-beta1 may modify pathologic processes characterized by inappropriate fibrosis. Genzyme Corporation is currently investigating a human monoclonal antibody (CAT-192) that neutralizes active TGF-beta1. This study is being conducted in the U.S. and Europe to evaluate the safety, tolerability, and pharmacokinetics of repeated treatments with CAT-192 in patients with early stage diffuse **Systemic Sclerosis.**

  Phase(s): Phase I; Phase II

  Study Type: Interventional

  Contact(s): see Web site below

  Web Site: http://clinicaltrials.gov/ct/show/NCT00043706

- **Idiopathic Pulmonary Fibrosis--Pathogenesis and Staging - SCOR in Occupational and Immunological Lung Diseases**

  Condition(s): Lung Diseases; Pulmonary Fibrosis; Lung Diseases, Interstitial; Scleroderma, Systemic

  Study Status: This study is completed.

  Sponsor(s): National Heart, Lung, and Blood Institute (NHLBI)

  Purpose - Excerpt: To conduct cross-sectional and longitudinal studies of patients with idiopathic pulmonary fibrosis (IPF) and patients with progressive **systemic sclerosis** (PSS), with and without associated lung disease.

  Study Type: Observational

  Contact(s): see Web site below

  Web Site: http://clinicaltrials.gov/ct/show/NCT00005317

- **Phase II Study of Recombinant Relaxin for Progressive Systemic Sclerosis**

  Condition(s): Systemic Sclerosis

  Study Status: This study is completed.

  Sponsor(s): National Center for Research Resources (NCRR); National Institute of Arthritis and Musculoskeletal and Skin Diseases (NIAMS); Stanford University

  Purpose - Excerpt: Objectives: I. Determine whether parenteral relaxin improves skin tightness, Raynaud's phenomenon, digital morbidity, and digital ulcers in a patient with progressive **systemic sclerosis** (scleroderma). II. Determine whether relaxin decreases collagen production by fibroblasts in vivo and cultured from skin biopsies.

Phase(s): Phase II

Study Type: Interventional

Contact(s): see Web site below

Web Site: http://clinicaltrials.gov/ct/show/NCT00004380

- **Phase III Randomized, Double-Blind, Placebo-Controlled Study of Oral Iloprost for Raynaud's Phenomenon Secondary to Systemic Sclerosis**

  Condition(s): Systemic Sclerosis; Raynaud Disease

  Study Status: This study is completed.

  Sponsor(s): National Center for Research Resources (NCRR); University of Pittsburgh

  Purpose - Excerpt: Objectives: I. Evaluate the safety and efficacy of oral iloprost, a prostacyclin analog, in patients with Raynaud's phenomenon secondary to **systemic sclerosis.**

  Phase(s): Phase III

  Study Type: Interventional

  Contact(s): see Web site below

  Web Site: http://clinicaltrials.gov/ct/show/NCT00004786

- **Study of Silicone-Associated Connective Tissue Diseases**

  Condition(s): Autoimmune Diseases; Connective Tissue Diseases; Scleroderma, Circumscribed; Scleroderma, Systemic

  Study Status: This study is completed.

  Sponsor(s): National Institute of Arthritis and Musculoskeletal and Skin Diseases (NIAMS)

  Purpose - Excerpt: This study will examine the possible relationship between silicone implants or injections and the connective tissue diseases **scleroderma** and myositis. It will explore whether certain factors in the blood or the immune system or other factors are involved in the development of these diseases following silicone implantation or injection. Men and women 18 years of age and older who meet the following criteria may be eligible for this study: Group 1-Patients who have had silicone implants or injections and who later developed **scleroderma** or myositis Group 2-Patients with **scleroderma** or myositis who have not had silicone implants or injections Group 3-Healthy volunteers who have had silicone implants or injections and did not develop symptoms or other medical features of connective tissue disorders. Participants will have a thorough history and physical examination, blood and urine tests, chest X-ray and lung function tests. In addition, patients will complete a questionnaire about their procedure (including information such as the types of implanted devices and injections, reason for the procedure, post-operative complications, other illnesses or medical conditions present before and after the procedure, etc.).

  Study Type: Observational

  Contact(s): see Web site below

  Web Site: http://clinicaltrials.gov/ct/show/NCT00001330

Keeping Current on Clinical Trials

The U.S. National Institutes of Health, through the National Library of Medicine, has developed ClinicalTrials.gov to provide current information about clinical research across the broadest number of diseases and conditions.

The site was launched in February 2000 and currently contains approximately 5,700 clinical studies in over 59,000 locations worldwide, with most studies being conducted in the United States. ClinicalTrials.gov receives about 2 million hits per month and hosts approximately 5,400 visitors daily. To access this database, simply go to the Web site at **http://www.clinicaltrials.gov/** and search by "scleroderma" (or synonyms).

While ClinicalTrials.gov is the most comprehensive listing of NIH-supported clinical trials available, not all trials are in the database. The database is updated regularly, so clinical trials are continually being added. The following is a list of specialty databases affiliated with the National Institutes of Health that offer additional information on trials:

- For clinical studies at the Warren Grant Magnuson Clinical Center located in Bethesda, Maryland, visit their Web site: **http://clinicalstudies.info.nih.gov/**

- For clinical studies conducted at the Bayview Campus in Baltimore, Maryland, visit their Web site: **http://www.jhbmc.jhu.edu/studies/index.html**

- For cancer trials, visit the National Cancer Institute: **http://cancertrials.nci.nih.gov/**

- For eye-related trials, visit and search the Web page of the National Eye Institute: **http://www.nei.nih.gov/neitrials/index.htm**

- For heart, lung and blood trials, visit the Web page of the National Heart, Lung and Blood Institute: **http://www.nhlbi.nih.gov/studies/index.htm**

- For trials on aging, visit and search the Web site of the National Institute on Aging: **http://www.grc.nia.nih.gov/studies/index.htm**

- For rare diseases, visit and search the Web site sponsored by the Office of Rare Diseases: **http://ord.aspensys.com/asp/resources/rsch_trials.asp**

- For alcoholism, visit the National Institute on Alcohol Abuse and Alcoholism: **http://www.niaaa.nih.gov/intramural/Web_dicbr_hp/particip.htm**

- For trials on infectious, immune, and allergic diseases, visit the site of the National Institute of Allergy and Infectious Diseases: **http://www.niaid.nih.gov/clintrials/**

- For trials on arthritis, musculoskeletal and skin diseases, visit newly revised site of the National Institute of Arthritis and Musculoskeletal and Skin Diseases of the National Institutes of Health: **http://www.niams.nih.gov/hi/studies/index.htm**

- For hearing-related trials, visit the National Institute on Deafness and Other Communication Disorders: **http://www.nidcd.nih.gov/health/clinical/index.htm**

- For trials on diseases of the digestive system and kidneys, and diabetes, visit the National Institute of Diabetes and Digestive and Kidney Diseases: **http://www.niddk.nih.gov/patient/patient.htm**

- For drug abuse trials, visit and search the Web site sponsored by the National Institute on Drug Abuse: **http://www.nida.nih.gov/CTN/Index.htm**

- For trials on mental disorders, visit and search the Web site of the National Institute of Mental Health: **http://www.nimh.nih.gov/studies/index.cfm**

- For trials on neurological disorders and stroke, visit and search the Web site sponsored by the National Institute of Neurological Disorders and Stroke of the NIH: **http://www.ninds.nih.gov/funding/funding_opportunities.htm#Clinical_Trials**

CHAPTER 6. PATENTS ON SCLERODERMA

Overview

Patents can be physical innovations (e.g. chemicals, pharmaceuticals, medical equipment) or processes (e.g. treatments or diagnostic procedures). The United States Patent and Trademark Office defines a patent as a grant of a property right to the inventor, issued by the Patent and Trademark Office.[9] Patents, therefore, are intellectual property. For the United States, the term of a new patent is 20 years from the date when the patent application was filed. If the inventor wishes to receive economic benefits, it is likely that the invention will become commercially available within 20 years of the initial filing. It is important to understand, therefore, that an inventor's patent does not indicate that a product or service is or will be commercially available. The patent implies only that the inventor has "the right to exclude others from making, using, offering for sale, or selling" the invention in the United States. While this relates to U.S. patents, similar rules govern foreign patents.

In this chapter, we show you how to locate information on patents and their inventors. If you find a patent that is particularly interesting to you, contact the inventor or the assignee for further information. **IMPORTANT NOTE:** When following the search strategy described below, you may discover <u>non-medical patents</u> that use the generic term "scleroderma" (or a synonym) in their titles. To accurately reflect the results that you might find while conducting research on scleroderma, <u>we have not necessarily excluded non-medical patents</u> in this bibliography.

Patents on Scleroderma

By performing a patent search focusing on scleroderma, you can obtain information such as the title of the invention, the names of the inventor(s), the assignee(s) or the company that owns or controls the patent, a short abstract that summarizes the patent, and a few excerpts from the description of the patent. The abstract of a patent tends to be more technical in nature, while the description is often written for the public. Full patent descriptions contain much more information than is presented here (e.g. claims, references, figures, diagrams, etc.). We will tell you how to obtain this information later in the chapter. The following is an

---

[9]Adapted from the United States Patent and Trademark Office:
http://www.uspto.gov/web/offices/pac/doc/general/whatis.htm.

example of the type of information that you can expect to obtain from a patent search on scleroderma:

- **3,5,6-substituted derivatives of 1,2-O-isopropylidene-.alpha.,D-glucofuranose and intermediates for preparing these derivatives**

Inventor(s): Arora; Sudershan K. (Westchester, IL), Ronsen; Bruce (River Forest, IL), Thomas; Albert V. (Niles, IL)

Assignee(s): 501 Greenwich Pharmaceuticals Incorporated (ft. Washington, Pa)

Patent Number: 5,010,058

Date filed: June 22, 1989

Abstract: Derivatives of 1,2-O-isopropylidene-.alpha.,D-glucofuranose and intermediates for preparing these derivatives are described. These derivatives are useful for treating animals and mammals with inflammatory and/or autoimmune disorders such as autoimmune deficiency syndrome, psoriasis, atopic dermatitus, rheumatoid arthritis, osteoarthritis, **scleroderma** and systemic lupus erythematosus.

Excerpt(s): This invention relates to 3,5,6-substituted derivatives of 1,2-O-isopropylidene-.alpha.,D-glucofuranose compounds and intermediates for preparing these derivatives. More particularly, this invention relates to derivatives of 1,2:3,5-Di-O- and 1,2:5,6-Di-O-isopropylidene-6-deoxy-.alpha.,D-glucofuranose. It also relates to furanosides obtained when 1,2-O-isopropylidene residues are reacted with methanol or other aliphatic alcohols of up to seven carbon atoms, both branching and containing double bonds. It further encompasses glucofuranose and related hexofuranose compounds wherein chirality is changed at positions 3 and 5. The derivatives of this invention have anti-proliferation and anti-inflammatory activity and are useful for treating animals and mammals with inflammatory and/or autoimmune disorders such as autoimmune deficiency syndrome, psoriasis, atopic dermatitis, rheumatoid arthritis, osteoarthritis, **scleroderma** and systemic lupus erythematosus. Blocked acetals of hexoses exist as solids or liquids at room temperature. Various blocking methods are described in U.S. Pat. Nos. 2,715,121 and 4,056,322, the disclosures of which are incorporated by reference herein in their entireties. For example, in instances where an aldehyde or ketone is reacted with the hydroxyl groups on adjacent or neighboring sugar carbon atoms, the hexose may be blocked in a plurality of positions, such as, e.g., the 1,2- and/or 5,6- positions. In the 1,2:5,6-blocked hexoses the ring forms between carbons 1 and 4, leaving carbon 3 free to etherize and in the 1,2:3,5-blocked hexoses, the ring forms between carbons 1 and 4, leaving carbon 6 free to etherize. Thus, 1,2:5,6-blocked hexoses may form 3-O ethers, and 1,2:3,5-blocked hexoses may form 6-O ethers. After the desired blocking of the monosaccharide is obtained, the unblocked position of the monosaccharide can be etherized. The 3- and 6-substituted furanoses thus obtained are generally known to have anti-inflammatory activity. Specific therapeutic compounds such as amiprilose hydrochloride, 1,2-O-Isopropylidene-3-O-3('N,N'-dimethylamino-n-propyl)-.alpha.,D-glucofu ranose (i.e. THERAFECTIN.RTM.), have been known for some time. This compound has demonstrated utility in managing the signs and symptoms of rheumatoid arthritis while exhibiting little toxicity. It is generally known that furanose compounds have activity as immuno-modulators, and therefore, may have a therapeutic effect on other autoimmune disorders such as psoriasis, eczema or lupus. For certain of these indications, high doses of these monosaccharides, such as THERAFECTIN.RTM., are needed to produce effective results. Consequently, they are difficult to prescribe orally. As therapy for those conditions is often midterm or longterm, there is a need to develop potent, non-toxic compounds which can be orally administered to promote patient compliance.

Web site: http://www.delphion.com/details?pn=US05010058__

- **Antigens associated with polymyositis and with dermatomyositis**

Inventor(s): Ge; Qun (Oklahoma City, OK), Targoff; Ira N. (Oklahoma City, OK)

Assignee(s): Board of Regents of the University of Oklahoma (norman, Ok), Oklahoma Medical Research Foundation (oklahoma City, Ok)

Patent Number: 6,610,823

Date filed: September 9, 1992

Abstract: Isolated DNA molecules encoding at least one epitope of the Mi-2 antigen and at least one epitope of the PM-Scl antigen are provided. The DNA may be used as probes to obtain related DNA. Proteins expressed from the DNA may be used in assays for the diagnosis of dermatomyositis and polymyositis, particularly polymyositis-scleroderma overlap disorders. The expressed proteins may also be used for purification of the associated autoantigens.

Excerpt(s): This relates to human antigens that can be used for the diagnosis of myositis and myositis-overlap syndromes that have an autoimmune pathogenesis and more particularly relates to the Mi-2 and PM-Scl antigens. Autoimmune disorders arise when the immune system reacts against its own tissues. Autoimmune diseases are often classified on the basis of whether a single organ or tissue is involved or whether multiple organs or tissues are involved. Generalized or systemic autoimmune diseases, such as systemic lupus erythematosus (SLE), characterized by the involvement of multiple organs and tissues, are often associated with the presence of autoantibodies to fundamental cellular components. Other autoimmune diseases are characterized by autoantibodies to antigens associated with a single organ or tissue. Systemic autoimmune diseases are typically characterized by the presence of autoantibodies. Some of the autoantibodies associated with the particular disease may be disease specific and others may be common to many autoimmune diseases. For example, SLE, which is a prototypical immune disorder, is characterized by the presence of autoantibodies that are detectable in other autoimmune disease, such as anti-single-strand DNA antibodies, anti-histones antibodies, and anti-ribonuclear particle (RNP) antibodies, and also by the presence of autoantibodies that are SLE-specific, such as the anti-double-stranded DNA antibodies. Other systemic autoimmune disorders, such as rheumatoid arthritis and idiopathic inflammatory myopathies, are also characterized by the presence of autoantibodies in the sera of patients that react with fundamental nuclear and cytoplasmic intracellular components. As with SLE, some of these autoantibodies are associated with other autoimmune disorders and some are specifically associated with autoimmune myositis.

Web site: http://www.delphion.com/details?pn=US06610823__

- **Chemical compounds having ion channel blocking activity for the treatment of immune dysfunction**

  Inventor(s):.O slashed.dum; Niels (K.o slashed.benhavn, DK), Christophersen; Palle (Ballerup, DK), J.o slashed.rgensen; Tino D. (Solr.o slashed.d Strand, DK), Jensen; Bo S. (K.o slashed.benhavn S, DK), Olsen; S.o slashed.ren-Peter (Klampenborg, DK), Str.o slashed.b.ae butted.k; Dorte (Farum, DK)

  Assignee(s): Neurosearch A/s (ballerup, Dk)

  Patent Number: 6,545,028

  Date filed: April 14, 2000

  Abstract: This invention relates to treatment or alleviation of a disease, condition or disorder selected from inflammatory bowel disease, Chron's disease, colitis ulcerosa, Coeliac disease, dermatitis herpetiformis, dermatomyositis, enteritis allergia, erytherma nodosum leprosum, ileitis regionalis, psoriasis, purpura, scleritis or **scleroderma** by administering to a living body certain imidazole, triazole, or 1,4-dihydropyridine derivatives.

  Excerpt(s): The present invention relates to chemical compounds having inhibitory activity on an intermediate conductance Ca^{2+} activated potassium channel (IK_{Ca}), and the use of such compounds for the treatment or alleviation of diseases or conditions relating to immune dysfunction. Moreover, the invention relates to a method of screening a chemical compound for inhibitory activity on an intermediate conductance Ca^{2+} activated potassium channel (IK_{Ca}). Ion channels are transmembrane proteins, which catalyse the transport of inorganic ions across cell membranes. The ion channels participate in processes as diverse as the generation and timing of action potentials, synaptic transmissions, secretion of hormones, contraction of muscles, etc.

  Web site: http://www.delphion.com/details?pn=US06545028__

- **Collagen metabolism ameliorant and its use**

  Inventor(s): Inoue; Shintaro (Odawara, JP), Miyamoto; Itaru (Chigasaki, JP), Nakata; Masanori (Odawara, JP), Sotomura; Mikio (Odawara, JP), Taira; Junsei (Hadano, JP)

  Assignee(s): Kanebo, Ltd. (tokyo, Jp)

  Patent Number: 5,332,758

  Date filed: January 13, 1993

  Abstract: This invention relates to a collagen metabolism ameliorant containing N-methyl-L-serine as an active ingredient, more particularly, a collagen metabolism ameliorant efficacious against collagen hypometabolism caused by aging or diseases accompanied with an abnormal cumulation of collagen, such as hepatic and pulmonary fibroses, keloid, hypertrophic scar, **scleroderma,** fibrosis in the scalp, or the like.

  Excerpt(s): The present invention relates to a collagen metabolism ameliorant containing N-methyl-L-serine (hereinafter referred to as "MSE") as an active ingredient, more particularly, a collagen metabolism ameliorant efficacious against collagen hypometabolism caused by aging or diseases accompanied with an abnormal accumulation of collagen, such as hepatic and pulmonary fibroses, keloid, hypertrophic scar, **scleroderma,** fibrosis in the scalp, or the like. Furthermore, this invention relates to hair growth stimulants and skin aging inhibitors containing such a collagen metabolism ameliorant. The term "collagen metabolism amelioration" herein referred to is meant by normalization of a condition such that synthesis of collagen has abnormally progressed due to the loss of balance between synthesis and decomposition of collagen, or reactivation of such a condition as collagen hypometabolism. Further, the term "collagen metabolism" is meant by a phenomenon such that collagen is being renewed at a constant rate as the collagen is undergoing synthesis and decomposition, namely, a metabolic turnover.

Web site: http://www.delphion.com/details?pn=US05332758__

- **Derivatives of.alpha.,D-glucofuranose or.alpha.,D-allofuranose and intermediates for preparing these derivatives**

Inventor(s): Arora; Sudershan K. (Westchester, IL), Ronsen; Bruce (River Forest, IL), Thomas; Albert V. (Niles, IL)

Assignee(s): Greenwich Pharmaceuticals Inc. (ft. Washington, Pa)

Patent Number: 4,996,195

Date filed: January 9, 1989

Abstract: Derivatives of -.alpha.,D-glucofuranose.alpha.,D-allanfuranose and intermediates for preparing these derivatives are described. These derivatives are useful for treating animals and mammals with inflammatory and/or autoimmune disorders such as psoriasis, atopic dermatitus, rheumatoid arthritis, osterarthritis, **scleroderma** and systemic lupus erythematosus.

Excerpt(s): This invention relates to derivatives of.alpha.,D-glucofuranose and.alpha., D-allofuranose compounds and intermediates for preparing these derivatives. More particularly, this invention relates to 1,2 and 1,2:3,5-O-isopropylidene-.alpha.,D-glucofuranose derivatives or.alpha.,D-allofuranose. The derivatives of this invention are useful for treating animals and mammals with inflammatory and/or autoimmune disorders such as psoriasis, atopic dermatitis, rheumatoid arthritis, osteoarthritis, **scleroderma** and systemic lupus erythematosus. After the desired blocking of the monosaccharide is obtained, the unblocked position of the monosaccharide can be etherized. Ethereal substituted hexose monosaccharides, such as 1,2:5,6-Di-O-isopropylidene 3-0-3('N',N'-dimethylamino-n-propyl)-.alpha.,D-glucofuranose (i.e. THERAFECTIN.RTM.), amiprilose hydrochloride are known and have demonstrated utility in managing the signs and symptoms of rheumatoid arthritis. These compounds have activity more generally as immuno-modulators, and therefore have a therapeutic effect on other autoimmune disorders such as psoriasis, eczema or lupus. For certain indications, high doses of these monosaccharides, such as THERAFECTIN.RTM., are needed to produce effective results. These compound, however, can be topically applied. It is therefore an object of the present invention to provide an.alpha.,D-glucofuranose or.alpha.,D-allofuranose compound that exhibits greater potency than THERAFECTIN.RTM. when orally administered.

Web site: http://www.delphion.com/details?pn=US04996195__

- **Diagnosis of scleroderma and related diseases**

Inventor(s): Nelson; J. Lee (Seattle, WA)

Assignee(s): Fred Hutchinson Cancer Research Center (seattle, Wa)

Patent Number: 5,759,766

Date filed: July 19, 1996

Abstract: Allogeneic cells are removed from an individual predisposed to or suffering from **scleroderma** or related diseases, thereby treating the disease and inhibiting or preventing its recurrence. Allogeneic cells are identified in the individual and treatment tailored to remove such cells, in vivo or ex vivo, from the individual by cell separation or cytotoxic agents.

Excerpt(s): This application claims the benefit of U.S. provisional application Ser. No. 60/001,315, filed Jul. 21, 1995. Women are more frequently affected by autoimmune diseases (Rose et al., Immunol. Today 14:426-430 (1993)) than men, including both rheumatologic and non-rheumatologic autoimmune disorders. Female to male ratios of greater than 5 to 1 have been reported, for example, for **scleroderma**, systemic lupus erythematosus, Sjogren's syndrome, Hashimoto's thyroiditis, and primary biliary cirrhosis (Silman, Ann. Rheum. Dis. 50(4):887-893 (1991); Hochberg, Arthritis Rheum. 28:80-86 (1985); Kelly et al., Brit. J. Rheumatol. 30:437-442 (1991); Furszyfer et al., Mayo Clin. Proc. 45:586-596 (1970); and Danielsson et al., Heptology 11:458-464 (1990)). Numerous studies have investigated sex hormones and autoimmunity, particularly in animal models of autoimmune disease, and some have demonstrated immunomodulatory effects of sex steroids (Grossman, Science 227:257-261 (1985); and Lahita, Ann. NY Acad. Sci. 658:278-287 (1993)). Perhaps as a result of these studies, the female predilection for autoimmune disease has sometimes been attributed to female/male differences in sex hormones. However, convincing correlations of studies in animal models with human autoimmune diseases have been limited and at least three additional observations argue against this assumption. These include the age-specific incidence patterns of different autoimmune diseases in women, contrasting effects of exogenous sex steroid administration, and contrasting effects of pregnancy. If sex hormone levels explained the female predominance of autoimmunity, peak age-specific incidence would be expected to occur when sex hormone levels are highest. The peak incidence of systemic lupus erythematosus, at 25 to 34 years in black females (Hochberg, Arthritis Rheum. 28:80-86 (1985)), is consistent with this expectation. However, this age-specific incidence pattern is not the rule. For women with rheumatoid arthritis the incidence of disease continues to rise with age at least into the 8th decade of life (Hochberg, Sem. Arthritis Rheum. 19:294-302 (1990)), thus lacking a correlation with the time when female sex hormone levels are high. Similarly the peak incidence of Hashimoto's thyroiditis in women occurs in postmenopausal years at 50-59 (Furszyfer et al., Mayo Clin. Proc. 45:586-596 (1970)). A bimodal distribution is observed for women with polymyositis with peaks at 10-14 and 45-64 years (Medsger et al., Am. J. Med. 48:715-723 (1970)). The observation that exogenously administered sex steroids do not have similar effects on different autoimmune diseases or susceptibility to disease (Wingrave et al., Lancet 1:569-571 (1978); McHugh et al., Scott and Bird (eds), Oxford Univ. Press., Oxford, p. 81-113 (1990); and Grimes et al., Am J. Obstet Gynecol. 153:179-186 (1985)) also argues against the assumption that differences in sex hormone levels explain the general female predisposition to autoimmunity. Lastly, although sex steroid levels increase during pregnancy, pregnancy has dissimilar effects on different autoimmune diseases both with respect to modulation of existing disease (McHugh et al., supra; and Hench, Proc. Staff Meeting Mayo Clin. 13:161-167 (1938)), and also with respect to susceptibility to development of autoimmune disease (Grimes et al., Am J. Obstet Gynecol. 153:179-186 (1985); and Spector et al., Arthritis Rheum. 33:782-789 (1990)). Thus it is difficult to envision a mechanism by which female/male differences in sex hormone levels provide a unifying explanation for the female predilection to autoimmune disease.

Web site: http://www.delphion.com/details?pn=US05759766__

- **Diagnostic method, test kit, drug and therapeutic treatment for autoimmune diseases**

Inventor(s): Salonen; Eeva-Marjatta (Tunturikatu 15 B 46, FIN-00100 Helsinki, FI)

Assignee(s): None Reported

Patent Number: 5,700,641

Date filed: March 1, 1995

Abstract: Synthesized telomeric sequences bind to and can be used for detecting anti-DNA antibodies in serum. Autoimmune diseases such as Lupus Erythematosus, Rheumatoid Arthritis, and **Scleroderma,** can be detected by detecting an elevated level of anti-DNA antibodies using telomeric sequences. Test kits for such detection are provided including immobilized telomeric sequences capable of binding anti-DNA antibodies. Pharmaceutical compositions for inhibiting or reducing the activity of anti-DNA antibodies contain an effective amount of telomeric sequences effective in inhibiting the antibodies specific to the patient treated.

Excerpt(s): The present invention relates to a method for detecting anti-DNA antibodies in samples obtained from living organisms, especially in mammalian serum, and more particularly to a diagnostic method for detecting anti-DNA-antibodies in serum from human beings and animals. The invention also relates to test kits for performing the said method and to a drug and a therapy for patients suffering from diseases involving the presence of anti-DNA-antibodies, specifically auto-immune disorders such as Lupus Erythematosus. Lupus erythematosus is an autoimmune disorder (antibodies are produced against self antigens), in which the body's immune system, for unknown reasons, attacks the connective tissue as though it were foreign, causing inflammation. Of the multitude of autoreactive antibodies that spontaneously arise during the disease, high levels of circulating autoantibodies to DNA are the best evidence of the pathogenesis. In Systemic Lupus Erythematosus (SLE) there is almost invariable presence in the blood of antibodies directed against one or more components of cell nuclei. Certain manifestations in SLE seem to be associated with the presence of different antinuclear antibodies and genetic markers, which have suggested that SLE may be a family of diseases ›Mills, J. A., Medical Progress 33, 1871-1879 (1994)!.

Web site: http://www.delphion.com/details?pn=US05700641__

- **Diagnostic methods for screening patients for scleroderma**

Inventor(s): Doxsey; Stephen J. (Worcester, MA)

Assignee(s): University of Massachusetts (boston, Ma)

Patent Number: 5,861,260

Date filed: November 5, 1996

Abstract: Disclosed are diagnostic methods for screening a patient for sclerotic disease. One diagnostic method includes obtaining a biological sample from the patient; obtaining a substantially pure CP140 polypeptide fragment; contacting the sample with the CP140 polypeptide; and detecting patient autoantibody:CP140 complexes as an indication of the presence of sclerotic disease in the patient. Other methods of screening patients for **scleroderma** are also described.

Excerpt(s): The invention relates to cell biology, autoimmune disorders, and diagnosis of **scleroderma**. Scleroderma, or **systemic sclerosis,** is characterized by deposition of fibrous connective tissue in the skin, and often in many other organ systems. It may be accompanied by vascular lesions, especially in the skin, lungs, and kidneys. The course of this disease is variable, but it is usually slowly progressive. **Scleroderma** may be limited in scope and compatible with a normal life span. Systemic involvement, however, can be fatal. Scleroderma is classified as diffuse or limited, on the basis of the extent of skin and internal organ involvement. The diffuse form is characterized by thickening and fibrosis of skin over the proximal extremities and trunk. The heart, lungs, kidneys, and gastrointestinal tract below the esophagus are often involved. Limited **scleroderma** is characterized by cutaneous involvement of the hands and face. Visceral involvement occurs less commonly. The limited form has a better prognosis than the diffuse form, except when pulmonary hypertension is present.

Web site: http://www.delphion.com/details?pn=US05861260__

- **Disubstituted and deoxydisubstituted derivatives of.alpha.-d-lyxofuranosides having anti-inflammatory and anti-proliferative activity**

Inventor(s): Arora; Sudershan K. (Lansdale, PA), Schied; Peter J. (Southampton, PA)

Assignee(s): Medicarb Inc. (southampton, Pa)

Patent Number: 5,367,062

Date filed: August 21, 1992

Abstract: Derivatives of disubstituted and deoxydisubstituted.alpha.-D-lyxofuranosides and intermediates for preparing these derivatives are described. These compounds exhibit significant antiinflammatory and anti-proliferative activity and are useful for treating inflammatory and/or autoimmune disorders such as psoriasis, asthma, atopic dermatitis, rheumatoid arthritis, osteoarthritis, **scleroderma,** systemic lupus erythematosus, and cancer (particularly melanoma and colon cancer).

Excerpt(s): The present invention relates to novel disubstituted or deoxydisubstituted.alpha.-D-lyxofuranosides, their synthesis, and intermediates for preparing these compounds. More specifically, the present invention relates to alkyl, alkoxyalkyl, or aralkyl 2,3-0-(1-methlethylidene)   -.alpha.-D-lyxofuranosides unsubstituted or substituted at the 5-position. This invention further relates to the replacement of oxygen at 5-position of lyxofuranosides by N or S to form 5-deoxy-5-amino substituted or 5-deoxy-5-thio substituted lyxofuranosides. These compounds show significant anti-inflammatory and anti-proliferative activity and are useful for treating warm blooded animals and mammals with rheumatoid arthritis, osteoarthritis, **scleroderma,** systemic lupus erythematosus, autoimmune deficiency syndrome, atopic dermatitis, cancer (particularly colon and melanoma), and psoriasis. Thus, this invention also relates to the pharmaceutical compositions containing lyxofuranoside compounds and methods of treating inflammatory and/or autoimmune disorders. The most reactive functional group in D-lyxose is the anomeric hydroxyl group. A glycoside is formed when the hydrogen atom of an anomeric hydroxyl group is replaced by a substituted or unsubstituted carbon atom. Typically, glycosides are formed either for group protection or as part of the synthesis of a larger molecule. The Fischer Method is particularly effective for synthesizing glycosides from unprotected reducing sugars and low molecular weight alcohols. After the glycosides are formed, various blocking methods are used to block or protect one or more of the hydroxyl group(s) thus leaving one or two hydroxyls free to derivatize. Isopropylidene and benzylidene groups are the most commonly used protective groups in carbohydrate chemistry. These groups are introduced into a molecule under similar conditions; however, the location of the protection can be quite different. The reason for this difference is directly related to the stability of each protected molecule. Since protection normally occurs under conditions which allow reversibility, reaction proceeds until equilibrium is reached. The distribution of products at equilibrium is determined by their relative thermodynamic stabilities. In other words, these reactions are thermodynamically controlled. Benzylidene groups prefer to be part of six-membered ring acetals, while the ketals resulting from acetonation generally are 5-membered rings. The difference is attributed to the effect of the methyl and phenyl substituents on the stability of the particular ring systems. These blocking methods are described in U.S. Pat. Nos. 2,715,121, 4,056,322, 4,735,934, 4,996,195, and 5,010,054 the disclosure of which are incorporated herein by reference. Other blocking methods are described in J. Carbohydr. Chem., 4, 227 (1985); 3, 331 (1984); Methods in Carbohydr. Chem., 1, 191 (1962); 1, 107 (1962); Can. J. Chem., 62, 2728 (1984); 47, 1195, 1455 (1969); 48, 1754 (1970). The therapeutic activity of hexoses and their derivatives are also disclosed in several of the above references. A well known derivative of.alpha.-D glucose having beneficial therapeutic properties is Amiprilose. HCl, 1,2-0-isopropylidene-3-0-3'-(N',N'-dimethylaminopropyl)-.alpha.-D-glucofur anose. This compound, which is in late Phase III clinical trials, is known to have anti-inflammatory activity and demonstrated utility in managing the signs and symptoms of rheumatoid arthritis.

Web site: http://www.delphion.com/details?pn=US05367062__

- **H.sub.3 -receptor agonists as therapeutic agents**

Inventor(s): Theoharides; Theoharis C. (14 Parkman St., #2, Brookline, MA 02146)

Assignee(s): None Reported

Patent Number: 5,821,259

Date filed: September 6, 1995

Abstract: The invention provides a method for preventing and alleviating the harmful biological effects of secretion of chemicals from mast cells in the organism of mammals which leads to clinical conditions namely allergy, asthma, arthritis, dermatitis, interstitial cystitis, inflammatory and irritable bowel disease, migraines, multiple sclerosis, **scleroderma** or **systemic sclerosis**, ulcerative disease of the gastro-intestinal tract and urticaria, among others. The method consists in administering to said mammals and especially to human beings an amount, effective against said conditions, of an H.sub.3 receptor agonist which has inhibitory activity of neurohormonal activation of mast cell secretion.

Excerpt(s): The present invention relates to the use of histamine-3 (H.sub.3)-agonists as therapeutic agents with inhibitory activity of neurohormonal activation of mast cell secretion. It also relates to the use of pharmaceutical compositions containing such agonists as active ingredients. More particularly, the present invention pertains to a method of preventing or alleviating in mammals a disease characterized by an abnormally high number of mast cells, increased activation of mast cells or large amounts of mediators secreted therefrom by administering an H.sub.3 -agonist with inhibitory activity of neurohormonal activation of mast cell secretion. Histamine is a molecule found in many tissues where it can bind to specific receptors and lead to particular biologic actions. The histamine-1 (H.sub.1) receptor is found on vessels, and its activation leads to dilation and oedema; histamine-2 (H.sub.2) receptors are found on exocrine glands, such as the parietal cells in the stomach, where their activation leads to gastric acid secretion and ulcers. Recently, an H.sub.3 receptor was identified (Schwartz, J-C. Arrang, J. M., Garbarg, M. and Korner, M. Properties and roles of the three subclasses of histamine receptors in brain. J. Exp. Biol. 124:203-224, 1986) and seems to be involved in regulation of perivascular nerve activity (Ishikawa, S. and Sperelakis, N. A novel class (H.sub.3) of histamine receptors on perivascular nerve terminals. Nature 327:158-160, 1987). Prior art findings relate to the possible action of H.sub.3 -agonists to inhibit histamine release (Theoharides, T. C. Histamine.sub.2 (H.sub.2)-receptor antagonists in the treatment of urticaria. Drugs 37:345-355, 1989), to decrease bronchoconstriction (Ichinose, M. and Barnes, P. J. Histamine H3-receptors modulate nonadrenergic noncholinergic neural bronchoconstriction in guinea pig in vitro. Euro. J. Pharmacol. 174:49-55, 1989), or to increase the resistance of bronchial blood vessels and lower their permeability so that hemorrhagic phenomena due to vascular fragility will not occur (Ichinose, M., Belvisi, M. G. and Barnes, P. J. Histamine H3-receptors inhibit neurogenic microvascular leakage in airways. J. Appl. Physiol. 68:21-25, 1990). However, none of these findings lead one to the claims of this invention and a recent review of H.sub.3 -agonists does not mention any such claims as potential therapeutic prospects (Timmerman, H. Histamine H.sub.3 ligands: just pharmacological tools or potential therapeutic agents? J. Med. Chem. 33:4-11, 1990).

Web site: http://www.delphion.com/details?pn=US05821259__

- **Identification of a novel retrovirus associated with primary biliary cirrhosis and autoimmune disorders**

Inventor(s): Mason; Andrew L. (New Orleans, LA), Neuberger; James (Worcester, GB), Xu; Lizhe (Metairie, LA)

Assignee(s): Alton Ochsner Medical Foundation (new Orleans, La)

Patent Number: 6,468,737

Date filed: June 1, 2000

Abstract: The present invention relates, first, to the discovery, identification, and characterization of novel nucleic acid molecules, that are associated with PBC, Sjogren's syndrome, scleroderma, SLE, autoimmune thyroiditis and various other connective tissue disorders. The novel nucleotide sequences of the present invention are retroviral in origin and are indicative of a PBC retrovirus which bears a strong correlation with PBC. The present invention is based, in part, on the Applicant's data which is the first evidence to suggest that PBC patient's tissue may harbor a transmissible agent. The association of a retroviral infectious agent with PBC was first demonstrated by Applicants in vitro by co-culture of periportal lymph nodes derived from patients at time of transplantation and healthy biliary epithelium cells. The Applicant's discoveries as described herein, report the characterization of PBC-associated infectious agent as retroviral as demonstrated by electron microscopy and immunoblot reactivity. In addition, Applicants have characterized novel nucleotide sequences which are associated with the PBC-associated retrovirus.

Excerpt(s): The present invention relates first, to the identification of a novel human retrovirus and the novel nucleotide sequences encoding a retroviral long terminal repeat and reverse transcriptase nucleotides associated with the existence of primary biliary cirrhosis (PBC), and other immune disorders such as Sjogren's syndrome, **scleroderma,** systemic lupus erythematosus (SLE), autoimmune thyroiditis and various other connective tissue disorders, in addition to lymphoma and breast cancer. The present invention further relates to methods for using the PBC retroviral nucleotides for the detection of PBC, Sjogren's syndrome, **scleroderma,** SLE, autoimmune thyroiditis and various other connective tissue disorders in patient samples. The present invention also relates to methods for using and targeting the PBC retroviral long terminal repeat and reverse transcriptase nucleotides in gene therapy protocols for the treatment of PBC, Sjogren's syndrome, **scleroderma,** SLE, autoimmune thyroiditis and various other connective tissue disorders in patients in need of such treatment. The present invention also relates to methods of treating or inhibiting PBC retroviral infection with antiviral agents, such as cytokines, inhibitors of reverse transcriptase, inhibitors of viral capping, and inhibitors of viral protease. The present invention further relates to diagnostic protocols and kits for the detection of PBC, Sjogren's syndrome, **scleroderma,** SLE, autoimmune thyroiditis and various other connective tissue disorders in tissue samples. Primary biliary cirrhosis (PBC) is a progressive pluriglandular disease affecting the liver, pancreas, salivary and lachrymal glands (Neuberger, 1997, Lancet 850:875-79; Epstein et al., 1980, Lancet 1:1166-68). The hepatic disease is characterized by a florid bile duct lesion with lymphocytic infiltration and granulomatous destruction of 30 to 80.mu.m sized interlobular bile ducts (Rubin et al., 1965, Am. J. Pathol. 46:387-407). There is no curative therapy, apart from liver transplantation, and patients usually develop cirrhosis (Neuberger et al., 1997, Lancet 250:875-879). It is estimated to account for approximately 2% of patients dying from cirrhosis in Europe and 10% of patients that requiring orthotopic liver transplantation in North America (Neuberger et al., 1997, Lancet 250:875-879). The autoimmune phenomena associated with PBC have been well characterized. Over 95% of PBC patients have antibodies that bind and inhibit the dihydrolipoamide acetyltransferase enzymatic function of the E2 subunit of the pyruvate dehydrogenase complex (PDC) (Gershwin et al., 1992, Molecular biology of the 2-oxo-acid dehydrogenase complexes and anti-microbial antibodies. Philadelphia W. B. Saunders) These AMA have a higher affinity to the dehydrogenase E2 enzymes of mammals as compared to invertebrates and react to the E2 sub-units of other highly conserved inner membrane mitochondrial proteins of the oxoglutarate dehydrogenase complex, and branched chain 2-oxoacid dehydrogenase complex, and also the E1.alpha. and E1.beta. sub-units of PDC. For patients with liver disease, reactivity to the E2 mitochondrial enzymes is specific to PBC but these AMA have been observed in individuals with Sjogren's syndrome and SLE as well (Van-de-Water et al., 1989, New Eng. J. Med. 320: 1377-80). The reason why PBC patients have an antigen driven immune response to human PDC-E2 may be partially explained by the findings of immunohistochemical studies. Using monoclonal and combinatorial AMA, PDC-E2 or antigens resembling PDC-E2 have been observed on the surface of cultured PBC biliary epithelium cells (Joplin et al., 1992, Lancet 339: 93-94), biliary epithelium and lymph node macrophages in PBC patient's tissues (Joplin et al., 1991, Hepatology 14: 442-447, Van-de-Water et al., 1993, J. Clin. Invest. 91: 2654-64), and salivary glands of patients with PBC and Sjogrens syndrome (Tsuneyama et al., 1994, Hepatology 20: 893-898). In essence, the tissues affected by the pluriglandular disease process are the same as those with the abnormal distribution of PDC-E2 antigens on epithelial cell surface.

Web site: http://www.delphion.com/details?pn=US06468737__

- **Local delivery of dipyridamole for the treatment of proliferative diseases**

    Inventor(s): Kauffman; Raymond F. (11420 Saint Andrews La., Carmel, IN 46032), Singh; Jai P. (13774 Hill Crest Ct., Carmel, IN 46032)

    Assignee(s): None Reported

    Patent Number: 5,270,047

    Date filed: November 21, 1991

    Abstract: A method of inhibiting cell proliferation in mammals which comprises the local delivery of an inhibitory amount of dipyridamole. Inhibiting cell proliferation is useful for the treatment of proliferaive diseases such as vascular restonesis, **scleroderma**, psoriasis, and rheumatoid arthritis. This method includes the local delivery of dipyridamole to the proliferative site by various techniques including local delivery catheters, site specific carriers, implants, direct injection, or direct application.

    Excerpt(s): Proliferative diseases such as vascular restenosis, **scleroderma**, psoriasis, and rheumatoid arthritis share the fundamental mechanism of excessive proliferation of cells in a specific tissue or organ. In each of these diseases, the excessive proliferation of cells contributes significantly to the pathogenesis of the disease. For example, the excessive proliferation of vascular smooth muscle cells contributes to the reocclusion of coronary arteries following percutaneous transluminal coronary angioplasty (PTCA), atherectomy, laser angioplasty and arterial bypass graft surgery. See "Intimal Proliferation of Smooth Muscle Cells as an Explanation for Recurrent Coronary Artery Stenosis after Percutaneous Transluminal Coronary Angioplasty," Austin et al., Journal of the American College of Cardiology 8:369-375 (August 1985). Vascular restenosis remains a major long term complication following surgical intervention of blocked arteries by percutaneous transluminal coronary angioplasty (PTCA), atherectomy, laser angioplasty and arterial bypass graft surgery. In about 35% of the patients who undergo PTCA, reocclusion occurs within three to six months after the procedure. The current strategies for treating vascular restenosis include mechanical intervention by devices such as stents or pharmacologic therapies including heparin, low molecular weight heparin, coumarin, aspirin, fish oil, calcium antagonist, steroids, and prostacyclin. These strategies have failed to curb the reocclusion rate and have been ineffective for the treatment and prevention of vascular restenosis. See "Prevention of Restenosis after Percutaneous Transluminal Coronary Angioplasty: The Search for a `Magic Bullet`," Hermans et al., American Heart Journal 122:171-187 (July 1991).

    Web site: http://www.delphion.com/details?pn=US05270047__

- **Methods and compositions for treating Raynaud's Phenomenon and scleroderma**

    Inventor(s): Chotani; Maqsood (Columbus, OH), Flavahan; Nicholas (Columbus, OH), Flavahan; Sheila (Columbus, OH), Mitra; Srabani (Worthington, OH), Su; Baogen (Columbus, OH)

    Assignee(s): The Ohio State University Research Foundation (columbus, Oh)

    Patent Number: 6,444,681

    Date filed: June 9, 2000

Abstract: A method for treating conditions or diseases associated with deleterious vasoconstriction of the small arteries and arterioles of one or more organs or parts of a patient's body. In one embodiment, the method comprises administering a therapeutically effective amount of an antagonist to the.alpha.sub.2C -adrenergic receptor (.alpha.sub.2C -AR) to a patient with Raynaud's Phenomenon. Such method is used to ameliorate the cold-induced or stress-induced vasoreactive response that is associated with Raynaud's Phenomenon. The.alpha.sub.2C -AR antagonist is administered to the subject either prior to or after exposure of the patient to the cold or to stressIn another embodiment, the method is used to reduce the extent of deleterious vasoconstriction that occurs in the small arteries, arterioles, and microcirculation of the lungs, heart, kidneys, skin, or gastrointestinal tract of a patient, particularly a **scleroderma** patient. The method comprises administering a therapeutically effective amount of an.alpha.sub.2C -AR antagonist to a patient who is in need of the same. Such treatment serves to maintain or restore, at least in part, blood flow through the small arteries, arterioles, and microcirculation of the lungs, heart, kidneys, skin, and/or gastrointestinal tract in a such patient. The present invention also relates to a pharmaceutical compositions comprising an.alpha.sub.2C -AR antagonist and a pharmaceutically acceptable carrier.

Excerpt(s): Raynaud's Phenomenon is one example of a disease that involves deleterious vasoconstriction of the small arteries and/or arterioles of one or more organs of a subject's body. Raynaud's Phenomenon is an abnormal vasoreactive response to cold or emotional stress of the small arteries and arterioles in the subject's digits. Individuals who suffer from Raynaud's Phenomenon experience episodic, sharp, demarcated, cutaneous pallor and cyanosis of their digits. These symptoms result from spasm or closure of the digital arteries. The condition is painful and debilitating. Under severe conditions, it can even lead to digital ulcers or amputation of the affected digit. Another, more problematic disease that is associated with a deleterious vasoconstriction of the small arteries and arterioles in one or more organs of a subject's body is **Scleroderma**. **Scleroderma** is a devastating disease of unknown etiology or origin that is associated with severe morbidity and mortality. Vascular dysfunction is an important early defect in **Scleroderma** (SSc). Raynaud's phenomenon is one of the earliest manifestations of SSc, occurring in approximately 95% of patients. In addition to the digital arteries, reversible vasospasm also occurs in the terminal arterial supply of the kidney, heart, lung, and gastrointestinal tract of patients with **scleroderma.** Such vasospastic activity causes ischemia, reperfusion injury and increased oxidant stress of the affected organs and is thought to thereby contribute to endothelial injury and the vascular and extravascular lesions that subsequently occur in this disease. The vascular lesions are found in the small arteries, arterioles (50-500.mu. in diameter) and the microcirculation of the affected organ and are characterized by concentric intimal thickening and adventitial fibrosis of the small arteries and arterioles. The loss of function and structure of the affected blood vessels leads to ischemia of the organ supplied by these vessels, organ failure, and death. At present there is no cure and no effective therapy for the diseases that involve deleterious vasoconstriction of the small arteries and arterioles, including **scleroderma.** In addition, there is no therapy that is specifically targeted to Raynaud's phenomenon. Current therapy for this condition is limited to broad spectrum vasodilator therapy which affects every blood vessel of the treated individual and, thus, causes significant side effects, such as dizziness, nausea, and severe headaches, vasodilator therapy could also exacerbate the problem by directing blood away from the affected organ.

Web site: http://www.delphion.com/details?pn=US06444681__

- **Methods and polycyclic aromatic compound containing compositions for treating T-cell-mediated diseases**

Inventor(s): Lavie; Gad (Tenafly, NJ), Meruelo; Daniel (Scarborough, NY)

Assignee(s): New York University (new York, Ny)

Patent Number: 5,514,714

Date filed: March 30, 1993

Abstract: T cell-mediated diseases in mammals are treated using compositions comprising a polycyclic aromatic compound, preferably hypericin or pseudohypericin, and related compounds, including isomers, analogs, derivatives, salts, or ion pairs of hypericin or pseudohypericin. The above composition may be administered in combination with an immunosuppressive agent. Pharmaceutical compositions useful for treating a T cell-mediated disease comprise the above polycyclic aromatic compound, alone or in combination with an immunosuppressive agent. The compositions and methods are useful in treating diseases which include multiple sclerosis, myasthenia gravis, **scleroderma**, polymyositis, graft-versus-host disease, graft rejection, Graves disease, Addison's disease, autoimmune uveoretinitis, autoimmune thyroiditis, pemphigus vulgaris and rheumatoid arthritis. Psoriasis and systemic lups erythematosus. Also provided are methods for diminishing the expression of CD4 Molecules on the surface of a T lymphocyte, and for inducing multidrug resistance in a cell, comprising incubating the cell with an effective concentration of a polycyclic aromatic compound.

Excerpt(s): This invention pertains to the administration of polycyclic aromatic compounds for the treatment of T cell-mediated diseases in mammals and compositions useful for treating T cell-mediated diseases. T cell-mediated diseases have been characterized by the induction of cytotoxic T-lymphocytes expressing the CD8 antigen on their cell surface and/or helper T cells expressing the CD4 antigen on their cell surface. These diseases, non-limiting examples being graft-versus-host diseaser graft rejection, and autoimmune disorders, such as multiple sclerosis, rheumatoid arthritis, Graves diseases Addison's diseases polymyositis, insulin dependent diabetes, primary biliary cirrhosis, systemic Lupus erythematosus, psoriasis, **scleroderma,** represent a large number of host immune system disorders. Graft-versus-host disease may occur when cells of the immune system such as stem cells or lymphocytes are transplanted into an allogeneic host, such as one genetically different at the major histocompatibility complex, which encodes cell surface antigens that give rise to strong immunological reactions. Transplants of cells of the immune system are made for treating certain forms of leukemia, aplastic anemia, and various immunodeficiency diseases. In order to prevent rejection of the foreign cells, the host is typically immunosuppressed, as with irradiation and/or immunosuppressive drugs. The transplanted immunocompetent cells recognize the host as foreign and mount an immune response directed against the host. In humans, the clinical manifestations of this graft-versus-host disease include fever, rash, anorexia, nausea, vomiting and watery or bloody diarrhea, weight loss and death.

Web site: http://www.delphion.com/details?pn=US05514714__

- **Monoclonal antibodies to nucleolar protein**

Inventor(s): Aris; John (New York, NY), Blobel; Gunter (New York, NY)

Assignee(s): The Rockefeller University (new York, Ny)

Patent Number: 5,811,247

Date filed: February 28, 1994

Abstract: The invention relates to a hybridoma cell line which produces a monoclonal antibody which cross reacts with both yeast and human fibrillarin. Diagnostic kits are also described. These are useful in diagnosing diseases such as **scleroderma.**

Excerpt(s): We have produced monoclonal antibodies against purified nuclei from the yeast Saccharomyces cerevisiae and have characterized three different antibodies that recognize a protein with an apparent molecular weight of 38,000 termed p38. See in this regard, J. Cell. Biol. 107:17-31 (1988) which is hereby incorporated by reference. Subcellular fractionation shows that virtually all of p38 occurs in the nuclear fraction. High concentrations of salt (1M) or urea (6M) effectively solubilized p38 from a nuclear envelope fraction prepared by digestion of nuclei with DNase. Indirect immunofluorescence demonstrates a crescent shaped distribution of p38 at the inner periphery of the nucleus, with p38 extending between dividing pairs of cells during mitosis. Postembedding immunogold electron microscopy shows decoration of the densely stained "crescent" region of the yeast nucleus, confirming the localization of p38 to the nucleolus. One of the monoclonals, D77, cross reacts on immunoblots with a single protein of molecular weight 37,000 from purified rat liver nuclei. Indirect immunofluorescence localizes this protein to the nucleolus, and shows that it is dispersed throughout the cell during mitosis. The yeast and rat liver nucleolar proteins behave similarly when electrophoresed in two dimensions, and appear to have basic pI (i.e., isoelectric point) values. Analysis of immunological cross-reactivity using D77, and antibodies specific for nucleolar proteins from other sources, suggests that the rat liver protein is fibrillarin, and demonstrates that p38 shares epitopes with fibrillarin, as well as with other vertebrate nucleolar proteins. The nucleolus of Saccharomyces cerevisiae differs from the more familiar vertebrate cell nucleolus in several aspects of its morphology and functional organization. The yeast nucleolus typically has the appearance of a single crescent-shaped region, when viewed by phase contrast (Gordon, C. N., (1977) J. Cell Sci. 24:81-93; Molenaar, I., et al. (1970) Exp. Cell Res. 60:148-156; and Sillevis Smitt, W. W., et al. (1973) Exp. Cell Res. 80:313-321). The crescent-shaped region may occupy a significant portion of the nucleus, and its location is not central but rather juxtaposed to the inner membrane of the nuclear envelope. Electron microscopy reveals a crescent-shaped region that is more densely stained than the area occupied by chromatin, which has a uniform appearance and does not appear to be separated into euchromatic and heterochromatic domains (Gordon, C. N., (1977) Supra; Molenaar, I., et al. (1970) Supra; and Sillevis Smitt, W. W., et al. (1973) Supra). Thus, the region has been commonly termed the "dense crescent" (Carter, B. L. A., (1978) Adv. Microb. Physiol. 17:243-302; Gordon, C. N., (1977) Supra; and Sillevis Smitt, W. W., et al. (1973) Supra). The dense staining of the yeast nucleolus is uniform and does not show the heterogeneous staining that characterizes the subdivisions of the vertebrate nucleolus, which are known as the granular, fibrillar, and fibrillar center components (Fakan, S., et al. (1986) Biol. Cell. 56:189-206; Goessens, G., (1984) Int. Rev. Cytol. 87:107-158; and Hadjiolov, A. A. (1985) Cell Biol. Monogr. 12:1-268). The yeast nucleolus has a simple functional organization. The tandemly repeated ribosomal RNA genes are clustered at the terminus of a single chromosome, number XII, instead of distributed onto multiple chromosomes (Bollon, A. P. (1982) in The Cell Nucleus. rDNA. Part A. Vol. 10. H. Busch and L. Rothblun eds. Academic Press, New York 67-125 and Kuroiwa, T., et al. (1986) Exp. Cell Res. 165:199-206). The organization of the approximately 120 copies (per haploid) of tandemly repeating units of rDNA into the nucleolus organizer region (NOR) is unlike that in higher cells because of the failure of a synaptonemal complex to form in the yeast NOR during meiosis (Moens, P. B., et al. (1985) Chromosoma (Berl.) 91:113-120). On the other hand, the yeast nucleolus resembles the nucleolus of higher eucaryotes in terms of one of its main functions, the synthesis of rRNA molecules and the assembly of preribosomal particles (Carter, B. L. A. (1978) Supra; and Warner, J. R. (1982), in The Molecular Biology of the Yeast Saccharomyces, Metabolism and Gene Expression, J. N. Strathern, E. W. Jones and J. R. Broach, Cold Spring Harbor Laboratory, Cold Spring Harbor, N.Y. 529-560). Both 37S and 28S ribosomal precursor RNAs are highly enriched in the dense crescent (Sillevis Smitt, W. W., et al. (1973) Supra). Pulse labeling with uracil and high-resolution autoradiography show that label is predominantly incorporated into 37S RNA, and results in a majority of grains over the dense crescent. In terms of structure, the yeast nucleolus contains a fibrillar meshwork similar to that in higher cell nucleoli but embedded in an electron-dense background (Molenaar, I., et al. (1970) Exp. Cell Res. 60:148-156).

Web site: http://www.delphion.com/details?pn=US05811247___

- **Mutant proteins of human DNA topoisomerase I**

  Inventor(s): Kurita; Noriko (Osaka, JP), Wagatsuma; Masako (Tokyo, JP)

  Assignee(s): Nippon Hoechst Marion Roussel Limited (tokyo, Jp)

  Patent Number: 5,849,503

  Date filed: November 26, 1996

  Abstract: Mutant proteins of human DNA topoisomerase I having an amino acid sequence in which tyrosine at the 592nd position of human DNA topoisomerase I is lacking or replaced with phenylalanine and which contains at least 30 amino acids in succession of the amino acid sequence subsequent to the 542nd amino acid of human DNA topoisomerase I. Above described mutant proteins react with anti-Scl-70, antibody in the sera of autoimmune disease patients of diffuse **scleroderma** and can be produced by genetic engineering using E. coli, and therefore they are useful as a diagnostic agent of **scleroderma**.

  Excerpt(s): This invention relates to novel mutant proteins of human DNA topoisomerase I. These mutant proteins are preferably produced by genetic engineering and useful for a diagnosis of autoimmune diseases and for analysis of topological interconversion of genes. The autoantibodies against various nuclear antigens are detected in the sera of patients with autoimmune diseases, and it is possible to diagnose autoimmune diseases by detecting these autoantibodies. It is known that, among these autoantibodies, the autoantibodies against a nuclear antigen, Scl-70 having a molecular weight of 70 kD, are detected in sera of many patients with an autoimmune disease named diffuse **scleroderma**. In recent years it has been demonstrated that Scl-70 is a 70 kD-molecular-weight protein of the C-terminal fragment of DNA topoisomerase I (J. H. Sero et al., 1986, Science, Vol. 231, pp. 737-740). DNA topoisomerases catalyze the breaking and rejoining of DNA strands in a way that allows the strands to pass through one another, thus altering the topology of DNA. There exist two kinds of DNA topoisomerases, Type I and Type II. Type I cleaves a single chain DNA while Type II cleaves a double-chain DNA.

Web site: http://www.delphion.com/details?pn=US05849503__

- **Nucleic acid sequence which codes for and expresses human fibrillarin and uses thereof**

Inventor(s): Aris; John (New York, NY), Blobel; Gunter (New York, NY)

Assignee(s): The Rockefeller University (new York, Ny)

Patent Number: 5,310,892

Date filed: December 10, 1990

Abstract: Substantially pure nucleic acid sequences coding for human fibrillarin have been identified and isolated. The isolated material is used to generate the protein in vitro, which is then used to identify autoimmune antibodies in patients suffering from **scleroderma.**

Excerpt(s): This invention refers to recombinant DNA technology and its application to immune diagnosis. More particularly, it refers to the isolation of nucleic acid molecules which code for or express a protein associated with the autoimmune disease **scleroderma,** and the protein product of transcription and translation of the nucleic acid, human fibrillarin. One of the features of the immune system currently under study is the process by which the immune system "fails", and generates antibodies against so-called "self" antigens in the subject. This phenomenon leads to the development of the so-called autoimmune diseases which include arthritis, rheumatism, some forms of diabetes and the disease under discussion herein, **scleroderma.** In the autoimmune diseases studied, one generally finds that the disease can be correlated to an immune response against a normal protein produced by the organism, a particular cell type, etc. The mechanism by which this takes place is under intensive investigation, but for now, most efforts center on the diagnosis of the conditions.

Web site: http://www.delphion.com/details?pn=US05310892__

- **Oral appliance for burn patients**

Inventor(s): Buckner; Horst E. (R.R. No. 1, Iowa City, IA 52240)

Assignee(s): None Reported

Patent Number: 3,938,508

Date filed: July 26, 1974

Abstract: An oral appliance for persons who have suffered facial burns to prevent shrinkage of the tissues around the mouth and lips during the healing process (microstomia). The appliance is adjustable to fit the patient's mouth and can be enlarged to progressively widen the opening of the mouth if shrinkage has already occurred. It may be employed to prevent shrinkage of the mouth and the lips by other causes (scleroderma, etc.).

Excerpt(s): Each year thousands of persons suffer burns as the result of accidents. Unfortunately, many of these individuals suffer extensive facial burns which result in scarring. During the healing process, the tissues around the mouth and the lips shrink. This shrinkage can permanently reduce the size of the mouth opening resulting in problems in eating, dental care, and speech as well as appearance. Presently, correction of microstomia requires surgical treatment. But the result may be functionally and cosmetically less than perfect, and the microstomia may recur. It is known that scars from burns can be remodelled by pressure. However, there is no known technique for retarding or preventing shrinkage of the tissues around the mouth and the lips. Because of the number of burn patients who suffer this deformity, there is a need for any technique or device which can help these persons, particularly if the technique or device is simple and inexpensive. The invention employs a technique and device which will maintain the size of the opening of the mouth during the healing process in a simple painless manner. The device constructed according to the principles of the invention is preferably made in two different sizes, each of which is adjustable to fit the patient. Because of its adjustability, the device can also be used to progressively widen the oral opening if shrinkage has already occurred. The device of the invention is very simple consisting of two end members contoured to fit the lips at the sides of the opening of the mouth, the end members being connected by two bars which are movable to each other and which can be maintained in a desired relative position thus providing for adjustment of the distance between the two end members. The device is very simple and inexpensive to manufacture and is very simple to use so that the patient himself can use the device without assistance. End member 10 has rigidly affixed to it a convexly curved bar 22 which has affixed to it at its opposite end an abutment member 24 that extends forwardly and substantially transversely to the curved bar 22. Abutment member 24 has an opening 26 extending transversely through it near its forward end which opening extends in a direction somewhat parallel to the bar 22. The opening 26 has slidably received therein a second curved bar 28 which has one end rigidly affixed to end member 12 and has at its opposite end an abutment member 30 which extends rearwardly and substantially transversely to the curved bar 28. Abutment member 30 has an opening 32 extending transversely near its rearward end which opening slidably receives the curved bar 22. Thus, although each of the curved bars 22 and 28 are rigidly affixed to the end members, and end members 10 and 12 are movable generally toward and away from each other as the curved bars 22 and 28 slide respectively in the openings 26 and 32 in the abutment members 24 and 30.

Web site: http://www.delphion.com/details?pn=US03938508__

- **S-nitroso derivatives of ACE inhibitors and the use thereof**

Inventor(s): Cooke; John (Needham Heights, MA), Loscalzo; Joseph (Dedham, MA)

Assignee(s): Brigham and Women's Hospital (boston, Ma)

Patent Number: 5,025,001

Date filed: March 24, 1989

Abstract: The invention relates to novel S-nitroso derivatives of ACE inhibitors and to pharmaceutical compositions comprising the S-nitrosothiol derivatives of the invention together with a pharmaceutically acceptable carrier.The invention also relates to methods for treating various pathophysiological conditions including acute myocardial infarction, left ventricular dysfunction without overt heart failure, hypertension, pulmonary hypertension, congestive heart failure, angina pectoris, vascular thrombosis, Raynauds syndrome, **scleroderma,** toxemia of pregnancy, acute renal failure, diabetic nephropathy, and renal artery stenosis, and to methods of inhibiting ACE and effecting vasodilation comprising administering the S-nitrosothiol derivatives of the ACE inhibitors of the invention to an animal.

Excerpt(s): This invention relates to new pharmaceutical preparations and the use thereof for the treatment of various pathophysiological diseases including acute myocardial infarction, left ventricular dysfunction without overt heart failure, congestive heart failure, angina pectoris, vascular thrombosis, hypertension, Raynauds syndrome, **scleroderma,** toxemia of pregnancy, acute renal failure, diabetic nephropathy, renal artery stenosis, and pulmonary hypertension. The invention also relates to methods for inhibiting ACE and effecting vasodilation by administering the pharmaceutical preparations of the invention to an animal. A variety of vasodilators currently exist for the treatment of hypertensive states, angina pectoris, and congestive heart failure. These agents may be classified according to their primary mechanism of action. Two important groups of these agents are the angiotensin converting enzyme inhibitors (useful in hypertension and congestive heart failure, but not angina) and nitrates (useful in angina and congestive heart failure, but less effective in hypertension). Neither of these groups are believed to be clinically important as antiplatelet agents. Angiotensin converting enzyme (ACE) is capable of converting angiotensin I to angiotensin II by removal of the carboxy terminal His-Leu. Angiotensin II is formed by the action of the enzyme renin and endopeptidase found in the kidney, other tissues, and plasma. Blood pressure is affected by various peptides found in the blood including angiotensin II. Angiotensin II is reported to be a powerful pressor agent found at elevated concentrations in the blood of patients with renal hypertension.

Web site: http://www.delphion.com/details?pn=US05025001__

- **Stabilization and purification of interferon with propylene glycol, resulting in a non-toxic product**

Inventor(s): Carter; William A. (HEM Research, 5451 Randolph Rd., Rockville, MD 20852), Silver; Gerald (HEM Research, 5451 Randolph Rd., Rockville, MD 20852)

Assignee(s): None Reported

Patent Number: 4,483,849

Date filed: January 7, 1983

Abstract: A new process for stabilizing purified human interferon is described, using propylene glycol. Propylene glycol also aids in the interferon purification procedure. Older methods used stabilizing agents which are toxic, antigenic or irritating. The new process will make available significantly more interferon of clinical purity for use in patients with cancer, viral illnesses and other diseases as yet undesignated (e.g. multiple sclerosis, amyotropic lateral sclerosis, **scleroderma,** etc.).

Excerpt(s): The purification and stabilization of human interferon has become increasingly important as its use as an antiviral and anticancer agent grows. The most powerful technique for purifying interferon from media of interferon-producing cells involves binding of the protein to a hydrophobic ligand carrying primary amino groups, such as Cibarcron Blue F3G-A, and its subsequent elution by solutions containing ethylene glycol (Jankowski, et al., 1976, Biochemistry 15:5182-5187; Knight and Fahey, 1981, J. Biol. Chem. 256:3609-3611). A slight modification of the procedure starting from "serum-free" media was patented by Knight U.S. patent application No. 84,632, filed Oct. 12, 1979) but in our hands the advantage in purity is more than offset by yields which are diminished 4-10 fold and, more importantly, by the need to use ethylene glycol. Ethylene glycol is toxic to human beings. The lethal dose in humans is about 1.4 ml/kg or 100 ml (Merck Index, pp. 3736, 9th Edition). Lower doses can cause central nervous system depression, vomiting, drowsiness, respiratory failure, coma, convulsions, renal damage which may proceed to anuria, uremia and death. Consequently, the presence of ethylene glycol in preparations of interferon severely limits the clinical use of such interferon preparations, particularly for chronic, long-term, drug administration. These features have importance because larger volumes require more extensive concentration steps, increasing the probability of encountering serious contamination problems and severe losses in bioactivity and potency. Lower yields reduce the economy of the purification procedure and increase purification difficulties which inevitably result from needing larger amounts of starting material, handling larger volumes, etc. Interferon is probably the most costly human medicinal thus far discovered and, accordingly any steps which increase its cost-effective manufacture are to be greatly coveted and esteemed in value.

Web site: http://www.delphion.com/details?pn=US04483849__

- **Tetracyclines including non-antimicrobial chemically-modified tetracyclines inhibit excessive glycosylation of different types of collagen and other proteins during diabetes**

Inventor(s): Golub; Lorne M. (Smithtown, NY), McNamara; Thomas F. (Port Jefferson, NY), Ramamurthy; Nungavarum S. (Smithtown, NY), Ryan; Maria E. (Port Jefferson Station, NY)

Assignee(s): The Research Foundation of State University of New York (albany, Ny)

Patent Number: 5,532,227

Date filed: December 21, 1994

Abstract: A method for treating mammals suffering from excessive extracellular protein glycosylation which is associated with diabetes, **scleroderma** and progeria by administering to the mammal a tetracycline which effectively inhibits excessive protein glycosylation.

Excerpt(s): The present invention relates to a method of treating mammals suffering from conditions associated with an excessive amount of protein glycosylation, by administering to the mammal an amount and/or type of a tetracycline that is not effectively antimicrobial but which effectively inhibits excessive protein glycosylation. All somatic proteins with exposed amino groups are subject to extracellular non-enzymatic glycosylation. Several proteins including collagens (e.g., Type I and Type IV collagen), lens crystallins, laminin, albumin, fibrin and low-density lipoproteins are known to be glycosylated in various disease states. For example, excessive glycosylation of the diabetic basement membrane contributes to the complication of kidney disease or nephropathy. In diabetes mellitus excessive glycosylation of collagen results in an excessive amount of collagen crosslinking. This pathological complication of excessive collagen glycosylation and the resulting excessive collagen crosslinking during diabetes mellitus is discussed in detail below. Other conditions associated with an excessive amount of collagen glycosylation and resulting collagen crosslinking include **scleroderma** and progeria. Diabetes mellitus (diabetes) is a complex disease that affects several hundred million people world wide. Diabetes is characterized by an elevated level of glucose in the blood. Glucose cannot enter the body's cells to be utilized and therefore remains in the blood in high concentrations. When the blood glucose level exceeds the reabsorptive capacity of the renal tubules, glucose is excreted in the urine. Diabetes produces a number of debilitating and life-threatening complications.

Web site: http://www.delphion.com/details?pn=US05532227__

- **Topical application of thioglycolic acid in the treatment of dermatological conditions**

  Inventor(s): Sheffner; Aaron L. (18 Trombley Dr., Livingston, NJ 07039)

  Assignee(s): None Reported

  Patent Number: 4,195,095

  Date filed: August 14, 1978

  Abstract: A preparation containing as an active ingredient 0.1 to 10% by weight of thioglycolic acid and the salts, esters, and acid amides thereof, is employed in the treatment of fatty cysts, dandruff, **scleroderma** and other dermatological disorders.

  Excerpt(s): This invention relates to compositions useful in the treatment of acne and other dermatological disorders. More specifically the present invention relates to a pharmaceutical composition containing minor, effective amounts of thioglycolic acid and the salts, esters and acid amides thereof, which composition can be applied topically to soften the skin and render it more permeable, particularly to secretions from the sebaceous glands. The skin covers the surface of the body and consists of two main layers, the eipdermis and the subjacent connective tissue layer--the corium, or dermis. The epidermis is a stratified squamous epithelium, the external layer of which keratinizes, or cornifies. The hairs are slender keratinous threads which develop from the matrix cells of the follicular epithelium. Each hair arises in a tubular invagination of the epidermis, the hair follicle, the walls of which are composed of epithelial and connective tissue. One or more sebaceous glands are connected with each hair. Through a short duct they empty their excretion product into the follicular canal in the upper third of its length. In sebaceous glands the secretions result from the destruction of the epithelial cells. These cells break down yielding the oily secretion of the gland, and also a small number of cornified cells. The pathological changes common to acne vulgaris consist of a follicular hyperkeratosis and a hypersecretion of sebum. The result of this process is the comedo, or "blackhead", which is composed at its outer end of concentric layers of horny cells, dried sebum, acne bacillus and staphylococci, and at its inner end mainly of sebum. The outer end of the comedo is dark-colored from oxidation of the sebum as well as from dirt. The pressure of the comedo causes some atrophy of the epithelium of the follicle. Sometimes the hyperkeratosis of the mouths of the follicles closes them completely, so that small sebaceous cysts are formed rather than comedones.

  Web site: http://www.delphion.com/details?pn=US04195095__

Patent Applications on Scleroderma

As of December 2000, U.S. patent applications are open to public viewing.[10] Applications are patent requests which have yet to be granted. (The process to achieve a patent can take several years.) The following patent applications have been filed since December 2000 relating to scleroderma:

---

[10] This has been a common practice outside the United States prior to December 2000.

- **Attenuation of fibroblast proliferation**

  Inventor(s): Cauchon, Elizabeth; (Ile Perrot, CA), Denholm, Elizabeth M.; (Pointe Claire, CA), Silver, Paul J.; (Spring City, PA)

  Correspondence: Patrea L. Pabst; Arnall Golden & Gregory, Llp; 2800 One Atlantic Center; 1201 West Peachtree Street; Atlanta; GA; 30309-3450; US

  Patent Application Number: 20020102249

  Date filed: December 1, 2000

  Abstract: Highly purified and specific glycosaminoglycan degrading enzymes, chondroitinase B and chondroitinase AC, are used to treat fibroproliferative diseases. The enzymatic removal of chondroitin sulfate B (dermatan sulfate), and to a lesser extent, chondroitin sulfate A or C, from cell surfaces effectively decreases growth factor receptors on the cells and thereby decreases the cell proliferative response to such growth factors. In addition, removal of chondroitin sulfates reduces secretion of collagen, one of the major extracellular matrix components. Through the combined inhibition of fibroblast proliferation and collagen synthesis, treatment with chondroitinase B or chondroitinase AC decreases the size of fibrous tissue found in psoriasis, **scleroderma**, keloids, pulmonary fibrosis and surgical adhesions.

  Excerpt(s): The present invention is a method and composition using chondroitinase B and chondroitinase AC, glycosaminoglycan degrading enzymes, to inhibit the formation of fibrotic tissue. This application claims priority to U.S. Ser. No. 60/168,518, filed Dec. 2, 1999. Proteoglycans on the cell surface and in the extracellular matrix contain variable glycosaminoglycan chains, which include heparan sulfate and chondroitin sulfates A, B, or C. While some proteoglycans contain only one type of glycosaminoglycan, others contain a mixture of heparan and chondroitin sulfates (Jackson et. al., Physiol. Rev. 71:481-530,1991). Extracellular proteoglycans form a structural framework for cells and tissues, and together with cell-associated proteoglycans, have major functions in regulating cell adhesion, migration, and proliferation. The functions of proteoglycans and their component parts have been extensively studied, with much of the emphasis on the roles of heparin and heparan sulfate on cell metabolism (Kjellen, L., and Lindahl, U. (1991) Ann. Rev. Biochem. 60:443-475; Vlodavsky, et al. (1995) Thrombosis Haemostasis 74:534-540; Yayon, et al. (1991) Cell 64:841-848)). Much less is known about the biological activities of proteoglycans containing chondroitin sulfate glycosaminoglycans, and in particular, their effects on cell proliferation.

  Web site: http://appft1.uspto.gov/netahtml/PTO/search-bool.html

- **Copper lowering treatment of inflammatory and fibrotic diseases**

  Inventor(s): Brewer, George J.; (Ann Arbor, MI)

  Correspondence: Thomas J. Bordner; Medlen & Carroll, Llp; Suite 350; 101 Howard Street; San Francisco; CA; 94105; US

  Patent Application Number: 20040009237

  Date filed: May 23, 2003

  Abstract: The present invention relates generally to the field of prophylaxis and therapy for inflammatory and/or fibrotic diseases which include responses to injuries. In particular, the present invention is related to agents that can bind or complex copper such as thiomolybdate, and to the use of these agents in the prevention and treatment of inflammatory and/or fibrotic diseases. Exemplary thiomolybdates include mono-, di-, tri- and tetrathiomolybdate; these agents are administered to patients to prevent and/or treat inflammatory and/or fibrotic diseases, such as pulmonary disease including pulmonary fibrosis and acute respiratory distress syndrome, liver disease including liver cirrhosis and hepatitis C, kidney disease including renal interstitial fibrosis, **scleroderma,** cystic fibrosis, pancreatic fibrosis, keloid, secondary fibrosis in the gastrointestinal tract, hypertrophic bum scars, myocardial fibrosis, Alzheimer's disease, retinal detachment inflammation and/or fibrosis resulting after surgery, and graft versus host and host versus graft rejections.

Excerpt(s): The present invention claims priority to U.S. No. 60/382,993 filed on May 24, 2002, the disclosure of which is herein incorporated by reference in its entirety. The present invention relates generally to the field of prophylaxis and therapy for inflammatory and fibrotic diseases. In particular, the present invention is related to agents that can bind or complex copper, and to the use of these agents in the prevention and treatment of inflammatory and fibrotic diseases. Many diseases begin with inflammation, which if excessive, may overwhelm and kill the patient, or if the patient survives, often leads to a disabling fibrosis, which ultimately may also kill the patient.

Web site: http://appft1.uspto.gov/netahtml/PTO/search-bool.html

- **Herbal composition for treating various disorders including psoriasis, a process for preparation thereof and method for treatment of such disorders**

Inventor(s): Arora, Sudershan Kumar; (Maharashtra, IN), Gupta, Lavleen Kumar; (Maharashtra, IN), Sanganabhatla, Narender; (Maharashtra, IN), Saraf, Dinesh Balakrishna; (Maharashtra, IN), Srivastava, Vandita; (Maharashtra, IN)

Correspondence: Ladas & Parry; 26 West 61 Street; New York; NY; 10023; US

Patent Application Number: 20030194456

Date filed: January 10, 2003

Abstract: The invention provides a novel herbal composition containing the extracts of the leaves and/or stem of Argemone mexicana plant, optionally containing the extracts of the fruits of Cuminum cyminum, which exhibits useful in vitro, in vivo and interesting immunological and pharmacological activities; a process for preparation thereof; and a method of treatment of psoriasis and related immunological and biological disorders by administration of the said novel herbal composition. The useful in vitro, in vivo and interesting immunological and pharmacological activities exhibited by the extracts and fractions of the leaves and/or stem of Argemone mexicana plant include immunosuppression, lymphoproliferation inhibition, cytokine modulation such as IL-2 inhibition, IFNgamma inhibition, IL-10 induction, keratinocyte proliferation inhibition, keratolytic activity, endothelial cell proliferation inhibition, inhibition of cell adhesion molecule expression such as ICAM-1, MEST inhibition, and enzymes inhibition such as p60src Tyrosine kinase, which are known to be involved in anti-psoriatic activity. The novel herbal composition(s) is useful in the treatment of various disorders, such as psoriasis including plaque psoriasis, gutatte psoriasis, pustular psoriasis and psoriasis of the nails; dermatitis and **scleroderma;** eczema; inflammatory disorders and other autoimmune diseases like psoriatic arthritis, rheumatoid arthritis, Crohn's disease, multiple sclerosis, irritable bowel disease, ankylosing spondilitis, systemic lupus erythremetosus and Sjogren's syndrome; allergies like asthma and chronic obstructive pulmonary disease and is safe, well-tolerated, non-toxic, with minimal and reversible adverse reactions or side effects, and most importantly, with minimal relapse or recurrence of the disease following completion of a treatment regimen. The invention also describes the presence of phosphodiesterase (III, IV and V) inhibition and 5-Lipoxygenase inhibition in the aqueous, ethanolic or aqueous-ethanolic extracts of fruits of Cuminum cyminum plant.

Excerpt(s): The present invention relates to a herbal composition comprising aqueous, ethanolic or aqueous-ethanolic extracts obtained from leaves and/or stem of Argemone mexicana plant, containing a mixture of alkaloids, flavonoids, organic acids, amino acids, sugars/glycosides and salts, optionally in combination with an aqueous, ethanolic or aqueous-ethanolic extract obtained from the fruits of Cuminum cyminum plant, which exhibit useful in vitro and in vivo immunological and pharmacological activities, hitherto not known and which provide significant reduction in the rate of PASI score with better tolerability within the range of normal permissible limit. The present invention also relates to a herbal composition comprising fractions of the aqueous, ethanolic and aqueous-ethanolic extracts obtained from leaves and/or stem of Argemone mexicana plant, containing a mixture of alkaloids, flavonoids, organic acids, amino acids, sugars/glycosides and salts, which exhibit useful in vitro and in vivo immunological and pharmacological activities, hitherto not known.

Web site: http://appft1.uspto.gov/netahtml/PTO/search-bool.html

- **Mammalian relaxin receptors**

  Inventor(s): Hsu, Sheau Yu; (Mountain View, CA), Hsueh, Aaron J.W.; (Stanford, CA)

  Correspondence: Bozicevic, Field & Francis Llp; 200 Middlefield RD; Suite 200; Menlo Park; CA; 94025; US

  Patent Application Number: 20030088884

  Date filed: August 15, 2002

  Abstract: High affinity relaxin receptors, polypeptide compositions related thereto, as well as nucleotide compositions encoding the same, are provided. These proteins, herein termed LGR7 and LGR8, are orphan leucine-repeat-containi- ng, G protein-coupled receptors. These receptors have a wide and a unique tissue expression pattern. The receptors, particularly soluble fragments thereof, are useful as therapeutic agents capable of inhibiting the action of relaxin and InsL3. The receptors and fragments thereof also find use in the screening and design of relaxin agonists and antagonists. Conditions treatable with relaxin agonists or antagonists include prevention or induction of labor, treatment of endometriosis, treatment of skin conditions such as **scleroderma** that require collagen or extracellular matrix remodelling. Additionally, relaxin has been implicated in the dilation of blood vessels' smooth muscle cells directly and through release of nitric oxide and atrial natriuretic peptide. Relaxin has also been used in the treatment of severe chronic pain, particularly pain arising from stretching, swelling, or dislocation of tissues.

  Excerpt(s): Relaxin is a pregnancy hormone discovered in 1926 (Hisaw (1926) Proc. Soc. Exp. Biol. Med. 23: 661-663), based on its ability to relax the public ligament in guinea pig. Mature human relaxin is a hormonal peptide of approximately 6000 daltons known to be responsible for remodelling the reproductive tract before parturition, thus facilitating the birth process. A concise review of relaxin was provided by Sherwood, D. in The Physiology of Reproduction, Chapter 16, "Relaxin", Knobil, E. and Neill, J., et al. (eds.), (Raven Press Ltd., New York), pp. 585-673 (1988). Relaxin has local autocrine and/or paracrine roles that contribute to connective tissue remodeling at the maternal-fetal interface during late pregnancy and at parturition, including an increase in the expression of the genes, proteins, and enzyme activities of the matrix metalloproteinases interstitial collagenase (MMP-1), stromelysin (MMP-3), and gelatinase B (MMP-9). Two human gene forms of relaxin have been identified, (H1) and (H2) (Hudson et al. (1983) Nature 301:628-631; Hudson et al. (1984) EMBO Journal 3:2333-2339; U.S. Pat. Nos. 4,758,516 and 4,871,670). Only the H2 form is expressed in corpus luteum. The primary translation product of H2 relaxin is a preprorelaxin consisting of a 24 amino acid signal sequence followed by a B chain of about 29 amino acids, a connecting peptide of 104-107 amino acids, and an A chain of about 24 amino acids. Although relaxin itself has been well-characterized for a number of years, it's receptor has remained elusive. To date, binding studies have had to rely on crude cellular extracts, which indicated that a specific binding molecule was present, but gave no clue as to its molecular identity. Relaxin binding sites have been reported in the reproductive tract (Kohsaka et al. (1998) Biol Reprod 59(4):991-9), as well as other tissues, including cardiac and other smooth muscle, and specific nuclei in the brain (Tan et al. (1999) Br J Pharmacol 127(1):91-8).

Web site: http://appft1.uspto.gov/netahtml/PTO/search-bool.html

- **METHOD FOR TREATMENT OF FIBROSIS RELATED DISEASES BY THE ADMINISTRATION OF PROSTACYCLIN DERIVATIVES**

Inventor(s): BLACK, CAROL M.; (LONDON, GB), CARMICHAEL, DAVID F.; (PACIFICA, CA), MARTIN, GEORGE R.; (PALO ALTO, CA), STRATTON, RICHARD; (LONDON, GB)

Correspondence: Legal Department; Fibrogen Inc; 225 Gateway Blvd; South San Francisco; CA; 94080

Patent Application Number: 20010006979

Date filed: July 8, 1999

Abstract: The present invention is directed to methods for treating fibrosis related diseases and disorders, particularly **scleroderma** by treating a patient in need with a pharmaceutically efficacious amount of a prostacyclin derivative. The most preferred prostacyclin derivatives are cicaprost and iloprost.

Excerpt(s): This application is a continuation-in-part of U.S. Provisional Application Ser. No.: 60/092,044, filed, Jul. 8, 1998. Fibrosis Related Diseases And Disorders. The deposition of excess connective tissue is found in a variety of diseases and disorders. These diseases and disorders has been designated as "fibrosis-related" disorders and are implicated in over 56% of the deaths in the United States and a comparable percentage worldwide. Fibrosis-related disorders include, excessive scarring, fibrosis of the internal organs (e.g. liver cirrhosis), and **scleroderma**. Scleroderma is a connective tissue disease characterized by the deposition of excess collagen in skin and internal organs. Various estimates of the incidence of this disease worldwide suggest that approximately four- to twelve-million patients are afflicted with some form of **scleroderma** (Medsger & Masi, 1971, Ann. Intern. Med. 74:714-721), although hospital based studies may underestimate the true incidence of the condition by failing to record mild cases of the disorder that are treated for by general practioners.

Web site: http://appft1.uspto.gov/netahtml/PTO/search-bool.html

- **Method of treating the symptoms of scleroderma**

  Inventor(s): Ross, Jesse; (Great Neck, NY)

  Correspondence: Myron Amer, P.C.; Suite 310; 114 Old Country Road; Mineola; NY; 11501; US

  Patent Application Number: 20020169356

  Date filed: May 14, 2001

  Abstract: Using to a first and second advantage for **scleroderma** a known treatment of a high frequency electromagnetic field, the first advantage being that the rest period between the pulses is approximately twenty-four times as great as the duration of each pulse, so that any heat that might be accumulated in the patient during the occurrence of the pulse has many times longer for its dissipation, thereby providing a treatment which is not harmful to the patient, and now a second advantage that it can be applied to an exact location of the patient, wherein the site of the **scleroderma** which can visually determined is correlated to the exact site of the applied treatment.

  Excerpt(s): The present invention relates generally to a new treatment to relieve the symptoms of **scleroderma,** which will provide noteworthy quality of life benefits without deleterious consequences. Scleroderma, a condition preventing a normal lifestyle, is a chronic hardening and thickening of tissue, which may be a finding in several different diseases, occurring in a localized area and frequently confined to the skin and subcutaneous tissue, although it can occur in organ tissue. The cause of **scleroderma** is unknown, and there is no cure; but treatments can ease symptoms. These treatments include, for localized **scleroderma,** skin protection measures such as cold-water room humidifiers, superfatted soaps, and lubricants and moisturizers to help prevent dry skin. Topical corticosteroids may also help.

  Web site: http://appft1.uspto.gov/netahtml/PTO/search-bool.html

- **Method of treatment and pharmaceutical composition**

  Inventor(s): Gasparo, Marc de; (Es Planches, CH), Webb, Randy Lee; (Flemington, NJ)

  Correspondence: Thomas Hoxie; Novartis Corporation; Patent And Trademark Dept; 564 Morris Avenue; Summit; NJ; 079011027

  Patent Application Number: 20010049384

  Date filed: January 9, 2001

  Abstract: The invention relates to a method for the treatment or prevention of a condition or disease selected from the group consisting of hypertension, (acute and chronic) congestive heart failure, left ventricular dysfunction and hypertrophic cardiomyopathy, myocardial infarction and its sequelae, supraventricular and ventricular arrhythmias, atrial fibrillation or atrial flutter, atherosclerosis, angina (whether stable or ustable), renal insufficiency (diabetic and non-diabetic), heart failure, angina pectoris, diabetessecondary aldosteronism, primary and secondary pulmonary hyperaldosteronism, primary and pulmonary hypertension, renal failure conditions, such as diabetic nephropathy,glomerulonephritis, **scleroderma,** glomerular sclerosis, proteinuria of primary renal disease, and also renal vascular hypertension, diabetic retinopathy, the management of other vascular disorders, such as migraine, Raynaud's disease, luminal hyperplasia, cognitive dysfunction (such as Alzheimer's), and stroke, comprising administering a therapeutically effective amount of combination of (i) the

AT.sub.1-antagonists valsartan or a pharmaceutically acceptable salt thereof and (ii) a Calcium channel blocker or a pharmaceutically acceptable salt thereof and a pharmaceutically acceptable carrier to a mammal in need of such treatment and to corresponding pharmaceutical combination composition.

Excerpt(s): (iii) a pharmaceutically acceptable carrier. Valsartan is disclosed in EP 0443983 A. A CCB useful in said combination is preferably selected from the group consisting of amlodipine, diltiazem, felodipine, fendiline, flunarizine, gallopamil, isradipine, lacidipine, mibefradil, nicardipine, nifedipine, niguldipine, niludipine, nimodipine, nisoldipine, nitrendipine, nivaldipine, ryosidine, tiapamil and verapamil, and in each case, a pharmaceutically acceptable salt thereof. All these drugs are therapeutically used as CCBs, e.g. as anti-hypertensive, anti-angina pectoris or anti-arrhythmic drugs.

Web site: http://appft1.uspto.gov/netahtml/PTO/search-bool.html

• **Methods for treatment of scleroderma**

Inventor(s): Alila, Hector W.; (North Wales, PA), Earle, Keith A.; (North Wales, PA), Thompson, W. Joseph; (Doylestown, PA), Whitehead, Clark M.; (Warminster, PA)

Correspondence: Robert W. Stevenson; Cell Pathways, INC.; 702 Electronic Drive; Horsham; PA; 19044; US

Patent Application Number: 20030073711

Date filed: August 23, 2001

Abstract: Substituted condensation products of N-benzyl-3-indenylacetamides with heterocyclic aldehydes and other such inhibitors are useful for the treatment of **scleroderma.**

Excerpt(s): This invention relates to the treatment **scleroderma.** The cause of **scleroderma** is unknown. Some cases of **scleroderma** have been linked to chemical exposures. Genetics and viruses might also be factors in the development of **scleroderma.** At present, there are no proven treatments or cure for any forms of **scleroderma;** that is, no drugs have been shown to have an impact on the fibrosis which is the hallmark of this disease.

Web site: http://appft1.uspto.gov/netahtml/PTO/search-bool.html

• **Methods of treatment and pharmaceutical composition**

Inventor(s): Ksander, Gary Michael; (Amherst, NH), Webb, Randy Lee; (Flemington, NJ)

Correspondence: Thomas Hoxie; Novartis, Corporate Intellectual Property; One Health Plaza 430/2; East Hanover; NJ; 07936-1080; US

Patent Application Number: 20030144215

Date filed: January 14, 2003

Abstract: The invention relates a pharmaceutical composition comprising a combination of:(i) the AT 1-antagonist valsartan or a pharmaceutically acceptable salt thereof; and(ii) a NEP inhibitor or a pharmaceutically acceptable salt thereof and optionally a pharmaceutically acceptable carrier and to a method for the treatment or prevention of a condition or diseaseselected from the group consisting of hypertension, heart failure, such as (acute and chronic) congestive heart failure, left ventricular dysfunction and hypertrophic cardiomyopathy, diabetic cardiac myopathy, supraventricular and ventricular arrhythmias, atrial fibrillation, atrial flutter, detrimental vascular remodeling, myocardial infarction and its sequelae, atherosclerosis, angina (whether unstable or stable), renal insufficiency (diabetic and non-diabetic), heart failure, angina pectoris, diabetes, secondary aldosteronism, primary and secondary pulmonary hypertension, renal failure conditions, such as diabetic nephropathy, glomerulonephritis, **scleroderma**, glomerular sclerosis, proteinuria of primary renal disease, and also renal vascular hypertension, diabetic retinopathy, the management of other vascular disorders, such as migraine, peripheral vascular disease, Raynaud's disease, luminal hyperplasia, cognitive dysfunction, such as Alzheimer's, glaucoma and stroke, comprising administering a therapeutically effective amount of the pharmaceutical composition to a mammal in need thereof.

Excerpt(s): The renin angiotensin system is a complex hormonal system comprised of a large molecular weight precursor, angiotensinogen, two processing enzymes, renin and angiotensin converting enzyme (ACE), and the vasoactive mediator angiotensin II (Ang II). See J. Cardiovasc. Pharmacol., Vol. 15, Suppl. B, pp. S1-S5 (1990). The enzyme renin catalyzes the cleavage of angiotensinogen into the decapeptide angiotensin I, which has minimal biological activity on its own and is converted into the active octapeptide Ang II by ACE. Ang II has multiple biological actions on the cardiovascular system, including vasoconstriction, activation of the sympathetic nervous system, stimulation of aldosterone production, anti-natriuresis, stimulation of vascular growth and stimulation of cardiac growth. Ang II functions as a pressor hormone and is involved the pathophysiology of several forms of hypertension. The vasoconstrictive effects of angiotensin II are produced by its action on the non-striated smooth muscle cells, the stimulation of the formation of the adrenergenic hormones epinephrine and norepinephrine, as well as the increase of the activity of the sympathetic nervous system as a result of the formation of norepinephrine. Ang II also has an influence on electrolyte balance, produces, e.g., anti-natriuretic and anti-diuretic effects in the kidney and thereby promotes the release of, on the one hand, the vasopressin peptide from the pituitary gland and, on the other hand, of aldosterone from the adrenal glomerulosa. All these influences play an important part in the regulation of blood pressure, in increasing both circulating volume and peripheral resistance. Ang II is also involved in cell growth and migration and in extracellular matrix formation. Ang II interacts with specific receptors on the surface of the target cell. It has been possible to identify receptor subtypes that are termed, e.g., AT 1- and AT 2-receptors. In recent times great efforts have been made to identify substances that bind to the AT 1-receptor. Such active ingredients are often termed Ang II antagonists. Because of the inhibition of the AT 1-receptor such antagonists can be used, e.g., as anti-hypertensives or for the treatment of congestive heart failure, among other indications. Ang II antagonists are therefore understood to be those active ingredients which bind to the AT 1-receptor subtype.

Web site: http://appft1.uspto.gov/netahtml/PTO/search-bool.html

- **Methods to treat autoimmune and inflammatory conditions**

Inventor(s): Shepard, H. Michael; (Encinitas, CA)

Correspondence: Mccutchen, Doyle, Brown & Enersen Llp; Suite 1800; Three Embarcadero Center; San Francisco; CA; 94111; US

Patent Application Number: 20020151519

Date filed: January 18, 2002

Abstract: This invention provides methods for treating inflammatory or autoimmune diseases by contacting the affected cell or tissue with a therapeutic compound as described herein. Such pathologies include, but are not limited to rheumatoid arthritis, systemic lupus erythmatosus, psoriatic arthritis, reactive arthritis, Crohn's disease, ulcerative colitis and **scleroderma.** Therapeutic compounds useful in the methods of this invention are selected from the group consisting of a 1,5-substituted pyrimidine derivative or analog and substituted furano-pyrimidone analog.

Excerpt(s): This application claims priority under 35 U.S.C.sctn. 119(e) of U.S. Provisional Application No. 60/262,849, filed Jan. 19, 2001, the contents of which are hereby incorporated by reference into the present disclosure. The present invention is in the field of medicinal chemistry and relates to other areas such as pharmacology and immunology. In particular, it provides methods to treat autoimmune disorders and inflammatory conditions. The function of tumor suppressor genes is a major focus of recent attempts to develop innovative therapeutics for the treatment cancer. The products of tumor suppressor gene expression are generally characterized as negative regulators of cell proliferation (Knudson, A. G. (1993), Weinberg, R. A. (1995)). Thus, therapeutic approaches to date include gene therapies to restore inactive or missing tumor suppressor function in cancer cells to re-establish normal cellular function or induce apoptosis (Clayman, G. L. (2000), Knudson, A. G. (1993)).

Web site: http://appft1.uspto.gov/netahtml/PTO/search-bool.html

- **Methods, compositions and kits relating to chitinases and chitinase-like molecules and inflammatory disease**

Inventor(s): Elias, Jack A.; (Woodbridge, CT), Zhu, Zhou; (Woodbridge, CT)

Correspondence: Morgan, Lewis & Bockius Llp; 1701 Market Street; Philadelphia; PA; 19103-2921; US

Patent Application Number: 20030049261

Date filed: July 23, 2002

Abstract: The present invention includes compositions and methods for the treatment of inflammatory disease (e.g., asthma, COPD, inflammatory bowel disease, atopic dermatitis, atopy, allergy, allergic rhinitis, **scleroderma,** and the like), relating to inhibiting a chitinase-like molecule. The invention further includes methods to identify new compounds for the treatment of inflammatory disease, including, but not limited to, asthma, COPD and the like. This is because the present invention demonstrates, for the first time, that expression of IL-13, and of a chitinase-like molecule, mediates and/or is associated with inflammatory disease and that inhibiting the chitinase-like molecule treats and even prevents, the disease. Thus, the invention relates to the novel discovery that inhibiting a chitinase-like molecule treats and prevents an inflammatory disease.

Excerpt(s): This application is entitled to priority pursuant to 35 U.S.C.sctn.119(e) to U.S. Provisional Patent Application No. 60/307,432, which was filed on Jul. 24, 2001. The prevalence of asthma has been steadily increasing for the past two decades, with an estimated 17 million cases in the United States alone. Once believed to be primarily a dysfunction in the contractile mechanisms of airway smooth muscles, recent studies have indicated the role of the immune system and inflammation in asthma and other pulmonary diseases. Asthma is now characterized as a complex inflammatory disease attributed to the inappropriate stimulation of the immune system. In some cases, the inflammation is triggered by airborne antigens. In others, exogenous triggers cannot be defined (intrinsic asthma). The immune cells and mediators implicated in asthmatic inflammation include IgE, mast cells, eosinophils, T cells, interleukin-4 (IL-4), IL-5, IL-9, IL-13 and other cytokines (Bradding et al., 1994, Am. J. Respir. Cell Mol. Biol. 10:471-480; Bradding et al., 1997, Airway Wall Remodeling in Asthma, CRC Press, Boca Raton, Fla.; Nicolaides et al., 1997, Proc. Natl. Acad. Sci. USA 94:13175-13180; Wills-Karp, 1998, Science 282:2258-2260; Hamid et al., 1991, J. Clin. Invest. 87:1541-1546; Kotsimbos et al., 1996, Proc. Assoc. Am. Physicians 108:368-373). Of these immune cells and mediators, the role of T-helper type 2 (Th2) cells and cytokines is proving to be increasingly important, as they are believed to be responsible for initiation and maintenance of airway inflammation, as well as vital to B cell regulation, eosinophil function, mucus responses, and stimulation of airway remodeling (Elias et al., 1999, J. Clin. Invest. 104:1001-1006; Ray et al., 1999, J. Clin. Invest. 104:985-993).

Web site: http://appft1.uspto.gov/netahtml/PTO/search-bool.html

• Regulation of human substance p-like g protein-coupled receptor

Inventor(s): Ramakrishnan, Shyam; (Brighton, MA)

Correspondence: Banner & Witcoff; 1001 G Street N W; Suite 1100; Washington; DC; 20001; US

Patent Application Number: 20030104435

Date filed: September 11, 2002

Abstract: Reagents which regulate human substance P G protein-coupled receptor (SP-GPCR) protein and reagents which bind to human SP-GPCR gene products can play a role in preventing, ameliorating, or correcting dysfunctions or diseases including, but not limited to, urinary incontinence, inflammatory diseases (e.g., arthritis, psoriasis, asthma and inflammatory bowel disease), anxiety, depression or dysthymic disorders, cluster headache, colitis, psychosis, pain, allergies such as eczema and rhinitis, chronic obstructive airways disease, hypersensitivity disorders such as poison ivy, vasospastic diseases such as angina, migraine and Reynaud's disease, fibrosing and collagen diseases such as scleroderma and eosinophilic fascioliasis, reflex sympathetic dystrophy such as shoulder/hand syndrome, addiction disorders such as alcoholism, stress related somatic disorders, peripheral neuropathy, neuralgia, neuropathological disorders such as Alzheimer's disease, AIDS related dementia, diabetic neuropathy and multiple sclerosis, disorders related to immune enhancement or suppression such as systemic lupus erythematosus, and rheumatic diseases such as fibrositis.

Excerpt(s): The invention relates to the area of G-protein coupled receptors. More particularly, it relates to the area of human substance P-like G protein-coupled receptor and its regulation. Many medically significant biological processes are mediated by signal transduction pathways that involve G-proteins (Lefkowitz, Nature 351, 353-354, 1991). The family of G-protein coupled receptors (GPCR) includes receptors for hormones, neurotransmitters, growth factors, and viruses. Specific examples of GPCRs include receptors for such diverse agents as dopamine, calcitonin, adrenergic hormones, endothelin, cAMP, adenosine, acetylcholine, serotonin, histamine, thrombin, kinin, follicle stimulating hormone, opsins, endothelial differentiation gene-1, rhodopsins, odorants, cytomegalovirus, G-proteins themselves, effector proteins such as phospholipase C, adenyl cyclase, and phosphodiesterase, and actuator proteins such as protein kinase A and protein kinase C. GPCRs possess seven conserved membrane-spanning domains connecting at least eight divergent hydrophilic loops. GPCRs (also known as 7TM receptors) have been characterized as including these seven conserved hydrophobic stretches of about 20 to 30 amino acids, connecting at least eight divergent hydrophilic loops. Most GPCRs have single conserved cysteine residues in each of the first two extracellular loops, which form disulfide bonds that are believed to stabilize functional protein structure. The seven transmembrane regions are designated as TM1, TM2, TM3, TM4, TM5, TM6, and TM7. TM3 has been implicated in signal transduction.

Web site: http://appft1.uspto.gov/netahtml/PTO/search-bool.html

- **Treatment of inflammatory diseases including psoriasis**

Inventor(s): Dedhar, Shoukat; (Richmond, CA), Fazli, Ladan; (North Vancouver, CA), Hannigan, Greg; (Toronto, CA), Hunt, David W.C.; (Surrey, CA), Tao, Jing-Song; (Vancouver, CA)

Correspondence: Pamela J. Sherwood; Bozicevic, Field And Francis Llp; Suite 200; 200 Middlefield Road; Menlo Park; CA; 94025; US

Patent Application Number: 20020155179

Date filed: November 30, 2001

Abstract: Inhibitors of integrin-linked kinase (ILK) are used in the treatment of inflammatory disease, including cutaneous inflammatory diseases, such as psoriasis, **scleroderma**, systemic lupus erythematosus and atopic dermatitis.

Excerpt(s): This application is a continuation-in-part of U.S. patent application Ser. No. 09/390,425, filed Sep. 3, 1999, which is a continuation of U.S. patent application Ser. No. 09/035,706, filed Mar. 5, 1998, now issued as U.S. Patent No. 6,001,622, which is a continuation-in-part of U.S. patent application Ser. No. 08/955,841 filed Oct. 21, 1997, now issued as U.S. Patent No. 6,013,782, which is a continuation-in-part of U.S. patent application Ser. No. 08/752,345, filed Nov. 19, 1996, now abandoned, which claims priority to provisional patent application no. 60/009,074, filed Dec. 21, 1995. The invention relates to the use of inhibitors of integrin-linked kinase (ILK) in the treatment of inflammatory diseases and autoimmune conditions such as psoriasis in which the immune system directly contributes to disease pathogenesis. Psoriasis is a chronic skin disease, characterized by scaling and inflammation. Psoriasis affects 1.5 to 2 percent of the United States population, or almost 5 million people. It occurs in all age groups and about equally in men and women. People with psoriasis suffer discomfort, restricted motion of joints, and emotional distress. When psoriasis develops, patches of skin thicken, redden, and become covered with silvery scales, referred to as plaques. Psoriasis most often occurs on the elbows, knees, scalp, lower back, face, palms, and soles of the feet. The disease also may affect the fingernails, toenails, and the soft tissues inside the mouth and genitalia. About 10 percent of people with psoriasis have joint inflammation that produces symptoms of arthritis.

Web site: http://appft1.uspto.gov/netahtml/PTO/search-bool.html

- **Vaccines for the treatment of autoimmune disease**

  Inventor(s): Mocci, Simonetta; (Belmont, CA), Solvason, Nannette; (Palo Alto, CA)

  Correspondence: Townsend And Townsend And Crew, Llp; Two Embarcadero Center; Eighth Floor; San Francisco; CA; 94111-3834; US

  Patent Application Number: 20030104012

  Date filed: May 13, 2002

  Abstract: The present invention provides pharmaceutical compositions comprising M. vaccae cells for treatment of autoimmune diseases such as diabetes, multiple sclerosis, rheumatoid arthritis, and **scleroderma.** The compositions may comprise either killed cells or delipidated and deglycolipidated cells.

  Excerpt(s): This application claims priority to U.S. Ser. No. 06/290,498, filed May 11, 2001 and is related to U.S. Ser. No. 60/147,626, filed Aug. 6, 1999, and U.S. Ser. No. 09/632,893, filed Aug. 7, 2000, all of which are incorporated herein by reference. The present invention relates to compositions and methods for treating autoimmune diseases. The compositions comprise as an active ingredient Mycobacteria vaccae. A number of pathological responses involving unwanted immune responses are known. For instance, autoimmune disease is a particularly important class of deleterious immune response. In autoimmune diseases, self-tolerance is lost and the immune system attacks "self" tissue as if it were a foreign target. More than 30 autoimmune diseases are presently known, including rheumatoid arthritis (RA), insulin-dependent diabetes mellitus (IDDM), multiple sclerosis (MS), myasthenia gravis (MG), systemic lupus erythematosis (SLE), and **scleroderma.**

  Web site: http://appft1.uspto.gov/netahtml/PTO/search-bool.html

Keeping Current

In order to stay informed about patents and patent applications dealing with scleroderma, you can access the U.S. Patent Office archive via the Internet at the following Web address: **http://www.uspto.gov/patft/index.html**. You will see two broad options: (1) Issued Patent, and (2) Published Applications. To see a list of issued patents, perform the following steps: Under "Issued Patents," click "Quick Search." Then, type "scleroderma" (or synonyms) into the "Term 1" box. After clicking on the search button, scroll down to see the various patents which have been granted to date on scleroderma.

You can also use this procedure to view pending patent applications concerning scleroderma. Simply go back to **http://www.uspto.gov/patft/index.html**. Select "Quick Search" under "Published Applications." Then proceed with the steps listed above.

CHAPTER 7. BOOKS ON SCLERODERMA

Overview

This chapter provides bibliographic book references relating to scleroderma. In addition to online booksellers such as **www.amazon.com** and **www.bn.com**, excellent sources for book titles on scleroderma include the Combined Health Information Database and the National Library of Medicine. Your local medical library also may have these titles available for loan.

Book Summaries: Federal Agencies

The Combined Health Information Database collects various book abstracts from a variety of healthcare institutions and federal agencies. To access these summaries, go directly to the following hyperlink: **http://chid.nih.gov/detail/detail.html**. You will need to use the "Detailed Search" option. To find book summaries, use the drop boxes at the bottom of the search page where "You may refine your search by." Select the dates and language you prefer. For the format option, select "Monograph/Book." Now type "scleroderma" (or synonyms) into the "For these words:" box. You should check back periodically with this database which is updated every three months. The following is a typical result when searching for books on scleroderma:

- **Systemic Sclerosis**

  Source: Baltimore, MD: Williams and Wilkins. 1996. 679 p.

  Contact: Available from Williams and Wilkins, Special Sales Department. (800) 358-3583.

  Summary: This textbook for health professionals provides them with up-to-date information on systemic sclerosis (SSc). Part one presents information on the history, epidemiology, demographics, genetic aspects, classification, prognosis, and differential diagnosis of SSc. Localized **scleroderma** is described, and the role of environmental factors in scleroderma and pseudoscleroderma is examined. Part two explores the pathogenesis of **scleroderma**, focusing on cellular aspects, vascular involvement, serologic correlates, environmental aspects, immune aspects, and animal models of systemic sclerosis. Part three discusses pulmonary, cardiac, peripheral vascular, skin, musculoskeletal, renal, nervous system, and gastrointestinal involvement in SSc. In addition, the association between Sjogren's syndrome and SSc is examined, and the sexual and psychosocial aspects of SSc are explored. Part four addresses issues related to designing trials of therapeutic interventions in SSc and describes the use of disease modifying drugs, unproven remedies, surgery, and occupational and physical therapy in treating SSc. Part five examines ancillary and supportive care for SSc patients and lists available resources. Appendices list resources for devices and modalities, **Scleroderma** Foundation Offices, and products and services. Numerous references, numerous figures, numerous tables, and 15 color plates.

Book Summaries: Online Booksellers

Commercial Internet-based booksellers, such as Amazon.com and Barnes&Noble.com, offer summaries which have been supplied by each title's publisher. Some summaries also include customer reviews. Your local bookseller may have access to in-house and commercial databases that index all published books (e.g. Books in Print®). **IMPORTANT NOTE:** Online booksellers typically produce search results for medical and non-medical books. When searching for "scleroderma" at online booksellers' Web sites, you may discover non-medical books that use the generic term "scleroderma" (or a synonym) in their titles. The following is indicative of the results you might find when searching for "scleroderma" (sorted alphabetically by title; follow the hyperlink to view more details at Amazon.com):

- **An Intimate Account: My Twenty-Five Year Battle Before and After the Diagnosis of Scleroderma and Periarthritis** by Victoria E. Murray Pruitt; ISBN: 0533130921; http://www.amazon.com/exec/obidos/ASIN/0533130921/icongroupinterna

- **Connective Tissue Diseases: Holistic Therapy Options--Sjoegren¿s Syndrome; Systemic Sclerosis - Scleroderma; Systemic Lupus Erythematosus; Discoid Lupus Erythematosus; Secondary and Primary Raynaud¿s phenomenon; Raynaud¿s Disease; Polymyositis ¿ Dermatomyositis** by Hannelore Helbing-Sheafe; ISBN: 1591099803; http://www.amazon.com/exec/obidos/ASIN/1591099803/icongroupinterna

- **Connective Tissue Diseases: Lupus, Scleroderma and Rheumatoid Arthritis** by Susan Brown (Editor), Robert P. Sundel (Editor); ISBN: 187977206X; http://www.amazon.com/exec/obidos/ASIN/187977206X/icongroupinterna

- **JABLONSKA SCLERODERMA AND PSEUDOSCLERO** by JABLONSKA *SCLE; ISBN: 0470151153; http://www.amazon.com/exec/obidos/ASIN/0470151153/icongroupinterna

- **Progressive Systemic Sclerosis (Current Topics in Rheumatology)** by Carol M. Black, Allen R. Myers (Editor); ISBN: 0912143088; http://www.amazon.com/exec/obidos/ASIN/0912143088/icongroupinterna

- **Scleroderma (Progressive Systemic Sclerosis)** by Alfred John Barnett; ISBN: 0398029555; http://www.amazon.com/exec/obidos/ASIN/0398029555/icongroupinterna

- **Scleroderma and pseudoscleroderma** by Stefania Jab±onska; ISBN: 0879331402; http://www.amazon.com/exec/obidos/ASIN/0879331402/icongroupinterna

- **Scleroderma: A New Role For Patients and Families** by Michael Brown; ISBN: 0971752400; http://www.amazon.com/exec/obidos/ASIN/0971752400/icongroupinterna

- **Scleroderma: Caring for Your Hands & Face** by Jeanne L. Melvin, Bradley O. Pomeroy (Illustrator); ISBN: 1569000069;
  http://www.amazon.com/exec/obidos/ASIN/1569000069/icongroupinterna

- **Scleroderma: The Proven Therapy That Can Save Your Life** by Henry Scammell; ISBN: 1590770234;
  http://www.amazon.com/exec/obidos/ASIN/1590770234/icongroupinterna

- **Successful Living with Scleroderma** by Robert H. Phillips; ISBN: 1888614102;
  http://www.amazon.com/exec/obidos/ASIN/1888614102/icongroupinterna

- **Systemic Sclerosis** by Philip J. Clements (Editor), et al; ISBN: 0781737443;
  http://www.amazon.com/exec/obidos/ASIN/0781737443/icongroupinterna

- **Systemic sclerosis: current research**; ISBN: 084227202X;
  http://www.amazon.com/exec/obidos/ASIN/084227202X/icongroupinterna

- **Systemic Sclerosis: Scleroderma** by Malcolm I. Jayson (Editor), et al; ISBN: 0471908460;
  http://www.amazon.com/exec/obidos/ASIN/0471908460/icongroupinterna

- **The First Year -- Scleroderma : An Essential Guide for the Newly Diagnosed** by Karen Gottesman (Author); ISBN: 1569244391;
  http://www.amazon.com/exec/obidos/ASIN/1569244391/icongroupinterna

- **The Official Patient's Sourcebook on Scleroderma** by James N. Parker, Icon Health Publications; ISBN: 0597829896;
  http://www.amazon.com/exec/obidos/ASIN/0597829896/icongroupinterna

- **The Scleroderma Book: A Guide for Patients and Families** by Maureen D. Mayes; ISBN: 0195115074;
  http://www.amazon.com/exec/obidos/ASIN/0195115074/icongroupinterna

- **Voices of Scleroderma, Vol. 1** by Judith R. Thompson, Shelley Ensz; ISBN: 0972462309;
  http://www.amazon.com/exec/obidos/ASIN/0972462309/icongroupinterna

Chapters on Scleroderma

In order to find chapters that specifically relate to scleroderma, an excellent source of abstracts is the Combined Health Information Database. You will need to limit your search to book chapters and scleroderma using the "Detailed Search" option. Go to the following hyperlink: **http://chid.nih.gov/detail/detail.html**. To find book chapters, use the drop boxes at the bottom of the search page where "You may refine your search by." Select the dates and language you prefer, and the format option "Book Chapter." Type "scleroderma" (or synonyms) into the "For these words:" box. The following is a typical result when searching for book chapters on scleroderma:

- **History of Scleroderma**

  Source: in Clements, P.J.; Furst, D.E., Eds. Systemic Sclerosis. Baltimore, MD: Williams and Wilkins. 1996. p. 3-22.

  Contact: Available from Williams and Wilkins, Special Sales Department. (800) 358-3583.

  Summary: This chapter for health professionals presents an overview of the history of scleroderma. Possible early cases of scleroderma are identified. Descriptions of scleroderma in the nineteenth century are highlighted. Subdivisions of types of scleroderma are discussed, focusing on systemic sclerosis (SSc) and morphea.

Subdivisions of SSc are examined. Descriptions of the involvement of the skin, joints, blood vessels, alimentary tract, lungs, heart, and kidneys are presented. The concept of scleroderma as a systemic disease is discussed. Research on the nature of scleroderma is highlighted, focusing on investigations of scleroderma as a connective tissue disease, a vascular disease, and an autoimmune disease. Views on the causes of scleroderma are presented. In addition, types of therapies that have been used to treat scleroderma are described. 121 references.

- **Morphea and Scleroderma**

Source: in Bork, K., et al. Diseases of the Oral Mucosa and the Lips. Orlando, FL: W.B. Saunders Company. 1993. p. 204-210.

Contact: Available from W.B. Saunders Company. Order Fulfillment, 6277 Sea Harbor Drive, Orlando, FL 32887-4430. (800) 545-2522 (individuals) or (800) 782-4479 (schools); Fax (800) 874-6418 or (407) 352-3445; http://www.wbsaunders.com. PRICE: $99.00 plus shipping and handling. ISBN: 0721640397.

Summary: This chapter, from a textbook on diseases of the oral mucosa and the lips, discusses morphea and scleroderma, two distinct clinical disorders with an almost identical histologic appearance. Morphea is generally localized and limited to the skin. Scleroderma or progressive systemic sclerosis (PSS) is a wide-spread systemic, often fatal disorder involving the lungs, heart, kidneys, and many other organs. In the skin, both disorders show marked dermal thickening. The chapter also discusses facial hemiatrophy. For each topic, the authors describe the clinical features and present brief therapeutic recommendations. Full-color photographs illustrate the chapter; references are provided for some sections. 15 figures. 26 references. (AA-M).

CHAPTER 8. MULTIMEDIA ON SCLERODERMA

Overview

In this chapter, we show you how to keep current on multimedia sources of information on scleroderma. We start with sources that have been summarized by federal agencies, and then show you how to find bibliographic information catalogued by the National Library of Medicine.

Video Recordings

An excellent source of multimedia information on scleroderma is the Combined Health Information Database. You will need to limit your search to "Videorecording" and "scleroderma" using the "Detailed Search" option. Go directly to the following hyperlink: **http://chid.nih.gov/detail/detail.html**. To find video productions, use the drop boxes at the bottom of the search page where "You may refine your search by." Select the dates and language you prefer, and the format option "Videorecording (videotape, videocassette, etc.)." Type "scleroderma" (or synonyms) into the "For these words:" box. The following is a typical result when searching for video recordings on scleroderma:

- **What You Should Know About Xerostomia (Dry Mouth)**

  Source: Fairburn, GA: National Oral Cancer Awareness (NOCAP). 199x. (videocassette).

  Contact: Available from American Dental Hygienists' Association (ADHA). 444 North Michigan Avenue, Suite 3400, Chicago, IL 60611. (800) 243-2342 (press 2) or (312) 440-8900. Fax (312) 467-1806. Website: www.adha.org. PRICE: $18.00. Item Number 3917 COM.

  Summary: This videocassette program describes the problem of xerostomia (dry mouth). The introduction stresses that the health impact of saliva goes far beyond the mouth and includes eating, talking, tooth maintenance, and tasting. The program then features a person with xerostomia describing how it feels to have problems with dry mouth. A brief description of the chemical makeup of salivary and the anatomy of the salivary glands follow. The next section discusses the potential causes of xerostomia, including radiation therapy, especially for cancer of the head and neck; drug effects, particularly from antihistamines, tranquilizers, and some blood pressure medications;

anxiety or depression, even without drug therapy; dehydration; and systemic diseases, including Sjogren's syndrome, lupus, cystic fibrosis, rheumatoid arthritis, and **scleroderma.** The narrator stresses that aging itself is not necessarily the cause of xerostomia. Complications of xerostomia include dry lips, burning mouth or tongue, constant thirst, difficulty talking or swallowing, impaired taste, dental caries (cavities), candidiasis (a fungal infection), and problems related to dehydration. Viewers are encouraged to work closely with health care providers to obtain an accurate diagnosis and employ strategies to cope with xerostomia. Treatment encompasses three options: eliminating the cause of the xerostomia, if possible; stimulating the salivary glands with sugar-free chewing gum, oral moisturizers, or the prescription drug pilocarpine; and using other measures to get relief, including saliva substitutes, frequent sips of water, room humidifiers (especially during winter), and lip balm. The program concludes with a reminder that xerostomia results in the need for increased attention to dental hygiene, including increased dental visits, limiting sugar intake, the use of fluoride, and the prevention of candidiasis. The program encourages viewers to learn about xerostomia, seek help, and improve the quality of their lives.

- **Health Care Professionals' Guide to Xerostomia**

Source: Bethesda, MD: Sjogren's Syndrome Foundation, Inc. 1997. (videocassette).

Contact: Available from Sjogren's Syndrome Foundation, Inc. 8120 Woodmont Avenue, Suite 530, Bethesda MD 20814-1437. (301) 718-0300 or (800) 475-6473. Fax (301) 718-0322. Website: www.sjogrens.org. PRICE: $29.00.

Summary: This videotape program reviews xerostomia (dry mouth). The program begins with an overview of the anatomy and physiology of the salivary glands, followed by a discussion of the three functional roles of saliva: digestion (and taste facilitation), lubrication, and protection (including antimicrobial and pH mechanisms). The narrator notes that saliva is also being used more and more as a diagnostic tool to measure systemic health. The program begins with a physician narrating, then includes interviews with two middle age women who have xerostomia; the interviews focus on the impact xerostomia has on quality of life and on the difficulties of obtaining an accurate diagnosis. The program then details the three causes of xerostomia: medical therapies (including drug side effects, radiation therapy, and surgery or trauma of the salivary glands), systemic disorders (including Sjogren's syndrome, HIV, rheumatoid arthritis, systemic lupus erythematosus, **scleroderma,** graft versus host disease, sarcoidosis, amyloidosis, cystic fibrosis, and neural disease affecting the salivary glands), and dehydration. The program emphasizes that xerostomia is not a natural consequence of the aging process. The program then reviews the clinical signs and oral complications of xerostomia; each is illustrated with a color photograph. Other topics include problems associated with xerostomia, the need for a multidisciplinary team approach to patients with salivary gland dysfunction, diagnostic tests used, treatment options (including chewing activity, oral moisturizing agents, and oral pilocarpine hydrochloride), determining residual salivary gland function, and the behavioral and lifestyle changes that can help patients cope with xerostomia.

CHAPTER 9. PERIODICALS AND NEWS ON SCLERODERMA

Overview

In this chapter, we suggest a number of news sources and present various periodicals that cover scleroderma.

News Services and Press Releases

One of the simplest ways of tracking press releases on scleroderma is to search the news wires. In the following sample of sources, we will briefly describe how to access each service. These services only post recent news intended for public viewing.

PR Newswire

To access the PR Newswire archive, simply go to **http://www.prnewswire.com/**. Select your country. Type "scleroderma" (or synonyms) into the search box. You will automatically receive information on relevant news releases posted within the last 30 days. The search results are shown by order of relevance.

Reuters Health

The Reuters' Medical News and Health eLine databases can be very useful in exploring news archives relating to scleroderma. While some of the listed articles are free to view, others are available for purchase for a nominal fee. To access this archive, go to **http://www.reutershealth.com/en/index.html** and search by "scleroderma" (or synonyms). The following was recently listed in this archive for scleroderma:

- **Actelion says Tracleer also prevents scleroderma ulcers**
  Source: Reuters Medical News
  Date: October 29, 2002

- **Genetic predisposition to high TGF production seen in systemic sclerosis**
  Source: Reuters Medical News
  Date: August 09, 2002

- **Combination regimen effective against systemic sclerosis lung disease**
  Source: Reuters Medical News
  Date: March 07, 2002

- **Scleroderma family registry launched in US**
  Source: Reuters Health eLine
  Date: June 26, 2001

- **Early organ involvement linked to poor outcome in systemic sclerosis**
  Source: Reuters Medical News
  Date: December 26, 2000

- **Greater skin thickness predicts early mortality in patients with systemic sclerosis**
  Source: Reuters Medical News
  Date: December 22, 2000

- **GI involvement common in children with scleroderma and MCTD**
  Source: Reuters Medical News
  Date: December 20, 2000

- **Drug combats scleroderma in lab tests**
  Source: Reuters Health eLine
  Date: November 07, 2000

- **Cellular microchimerism linked to systemic sclerosis**
  Source: Reuters Medical News
  Date: June 22, 2000

- **Relaxin improves skin symptoms of scleroderma**
  Source: Reuters Medical News
  Date: June 06, 2000

- **Pregnancy hormone promising for scleroderma**
  Source: Reuters Health eLine
  Date: June 06, 2000

- **Collgard scleroderma drug gets orphan drug designation**
  Source: Reuters Medical News
  Date: March 13, 2000

- **Fetal Antimaternal Graft-Vs-Host Reaction Has Role In Scleroderma**
  Source: Reuters Medical News
  Date: April 23, 1998

- **Fetal Cells May Trigger Scleroderma**
  Source: Reuters Health eLine
  Date: April 22, 1998

- **Maternal-Fetal Microchimerism May Be Involved In Scleroderma**
  Source: Reuters Medical News
  Date: February 20, 1998

- **Fetal Cells May Cause Scleroderma**
  Source: Reuters Health eLine
  Date: February 20, 1998

- **Low-Dose Ultraviolet Light Effective Against Localized Scleroderma**
  Source: Reuters Medical News
  Date: February 03, 1998

- **Intestinal Perforations Common In Patients With Scleroderma**
  Source: Reuters Medical News
  Date: April 04, 1997

- **Abnormal Metal Status May Underlie Scleroderma Etiology**
  Source: Reuters Medical News
  Date: January 16, 1997

- **Early Clues To Scleroderma**
  Source: Reuters Health eLine
  Date: January 14, 1997

- **[] - Connective Therapeutics Initiates Phase II Scleroderma Trial**
  Source: Reuters Medical News
  Date: June 24, 1996

- **Scleroderma Symptoms Develop In Three Patients Treated With Docetaxel**
  Source: Reuters Medical News
  Date: July 04, 1995

The NIH

Within MEDLINEplus, the NIH has made an agreement with the New York Times Syndicate, the AP News Service, and Reuters to deliver news that can be browsed by the public. Search news releases at **http://www.nlm.nih.gov/medlineplus/alphanews_a.html**. MEDLINEplus allows you to browse across an alphabetical index. Or you can search by date at the following Web page: **http://www.nlm.nih.gov/medlineplus/newsbydate.html**. Often, news items are indexed by MEDLINEplus within its search engine.

Business Wire

Business Wire is similar to PR Newswire. To access this archive, simply go to **http://www.businesswire.com/**. You can scan the news by industry category or company name.

Market Wire

Market Wire is more focused on technology than the other wires. To browse the latest press releases by topic, such as alternative medicine, biotechnology, fitness, healthcare, legal, nutrition, and pharmaceuticals, access Market Wire's Medical/Health channel at **http://www.marketwire.com/mw/release_index?channel=MedicalHealth**. Or simply go to Market Wire's home page at **http://www.marketwire.com/mw/home**, type "scleroderma" (or synonyms) into the search box, and click on "Search News." As this service is technology oriented, you may wish to use it when searching for press releases covering diagnostic procedures or tests.

Search Engines

Medical news is also available in the news sections of commercial Internet search engines. See the health news page at Yahoo (**http://dir.yahoo.com/Health/News_and_Media/**), or you can use this Web site's general news search page at **http://news.yahoo.com/**. Type in "scleroderma" (or synonyms). If you know the name of a company that is relevant to scleroderma, you can go to any stock trading Web site (such as **http://www.etrade.com/**) and search for the company name there. News items across various news sources are reported on indicated hyperlinks. Google offers a similar service at **http://news.google.com/**.

BBC

Covering news from a more European perspective, the British Broadcasting Corporation (BBC) allows the public free access to their news archive located at **http://www.bbc.co.uk/**. Search by "scleroderma" (or synonyms).

Newsletter Articles

Use the Combined Health Information Database, and limit your search criteria to "newsletter articles." Again, you will need to use the "Detailed Search" option. Go directly to the following hyperlink: **http://chid.nih.gov/detail/detail.html**. Go to the bottom of the search page where "You may refine your search by." Select the dates and language that you prefer. For the format option, select "Newsletter Article." Type "scleroderma" (or synonyms) into the "For these words:" box. You should check back periodically with this database as it is updated every three months. The following is a typical result when searching for newsletter articles on scleroderma:

- **Scleroderma and Sexuality**

    Source: The Beacon. 5(1):1,3,15,19-21; Winter 1997.

    Contact: Available from Scleroderma Foundation. 12 Kent Way, Suite 101, Byfield, MA 01922. (800) 722-4673 or (978) 463-5843. Fax (978) 463-5809. E-mail: sfinfo@scleroderma.org. Website: www.scleroderma.org.

    Summary: This newsletter article for health professionals and individuals with scleroderma presents available medical information on the effect of scleroderma symptoms on sexuality. Symptoms of scleroderma that can potentially affect sexuality are discussed, focusing on skin changes; calcinosis; joint pain and stiffness; muscle weakness; fixation of the fingers in a bent position; esophageal dysfunction; Raynaud's phenomenon; and lung, cardiac, and renal abnormalities. Specific problems for both women and men are highlighted. Suggestions for alleviating the negative effects of scleroderma on sexuality are offered, including altering the physical environment to enhance comfort during sexual activity, improving communication between sexual partners, making adjustments to accommodate hand deformities, and re-evaluating medications. In addition, the article highlights the intimate relationship problems confronting individuals with scleroderma and stresses the need for sexuality educators and therapists to help individuals with scleroderma improve the sexual aspect of their life.

- **Update on Scleroderma Kidney**

    Source: The Beacon. 5(4):1,8-9. Fall 1997.

Contact: Available from Scleroderma Foundation. 12 Kent Way, Suite 101, Byfield, MA 01922. (800) 722-4673 or (978) 463-5843. Fax (978) 463-5809. E-mail: sfinfo@scleroderma.org. Website: www.scleroderma.org.

Summary: This newsletter article for individuals with scleroderma presents updated information on scleroderma kidney. It reviews the function of the normal kidney, explains the consequences of kidney failure, and describes the impact of scleroderma on kidney function. Although scleroderma kidney was the worst complication of scleroderma 25 years ago, significant advances in treatment have occurred, including the development of new blood pressure medications and the use of dialysis and transplantation. Despite these advances, researchers need to find a medication that will control blood pressure, allow healing of the lining of the blood vessels of the kidney, and reverse the blood flow problems within the kidney. 2 figures.

- **Pulmonary Arterial Hypertension in Scleroderma: A New Treatment**

Source: Scleroderma Voice. Number 2: 9-10,23. 2002.

Contact: Available from Scleroderma Foundation. 12 Kent Way, Suite 101, Byfield, MA 01922. (800) 722-HOPE or (978) 463-5843. Fax (978) 463-5809. E-mail: sfinfo@scleroderma.org. Website: www.scleroderma.org.

Summary: This newsletter article provides health professionals and people who have scleroderma with information on the diagnosis and treatment of pulmonary arterial hypertension (PAH). This serious condition occurs when the blood vessels that supply the lungs constrict, making it more difficult for blood to get through to the lungs. As time passes, scarring makes the vessels stiffer and thicker. The extra stress on the heart causes it to enlarge and become less flexible. As a result, less and less blood flows out of the heart, through the lungs, and into the body. PAH can occur by itself or in association with another disease. Scleroderma is the most common disease associated with PAH. It is more common in patients with limited scleroderma. The exact cause of PAH is unknown. However, many factors may have a role in the process of blood vessel thickening and stiffening, including the elevation of a substance in the body called endothelin, a potent vasoconstrictor. Symptoms of PAH include shortness of breath during exercise and at rest, chest pain, dizziness, and fainting. Diagnosis of PAH related to scleroderma is based on the results of a series of tests given to determine the specific cause of shortness of breath, including pulmonary function tests, chest x rays, high resolution computed tomography scans, scans for blood clots, and bronchoscopy. Doppler echocardiogram is the best screening tool for PAH. A right heart catheterization can confirm a diagnosis. Medications that relax and open up blood vessels are the mainstay of treatment for PAH; they include calcium channel blockers such as nifedifine or diltiazem, water pills, blood thinners, and drugs that block endothelin such as bosentan. Bosentan is the first oral medication approved by the Food and Drug Administration to block endothelin receptors. The drug is generally well tolerated, and it may have additional treatment applications in patients with scleroderma. 5 references.

- **Practical Tips for Living With Scleroderma**

Source: Scleroderma Voice. p. 21-22. Winter 2000-2001.

Contact: Available from Scleroderma Foundation. 12 Kent Way, Suite 101, Byfield, MA 01922. (800) 722-HOPE or (978) 463-5843. Fax (978) 463-5809. E-mail: sfinfo@scleroderma.org. Website: www.scleroderma.org.

Summary: This newsletter article provides people who have scleroderma with information on practical tips for living with the disease. The article offers suggestions for grasping items with the fingers, coping with problems associated with eating and drinking, sitting comfortably, keeping the hands warm, bathing, sleeping, and dressing. General advice includes avoiding loose rugs or mats that can slip and cause falls and placing keys in a special attachment that can provide a better grip for holding and turning.

Academic Periodicals covering Scleroderma

Numerous periodicals are currently indexed within the National Library of Medicine's PubMed database that are known to publish articles relating to scleroderma. In addition to these sources, you can search for articles covering scleroderma that have been published by any of the periodicals listed in previous chapters. To find the latest studies published, go to **http://www.ncbi.nlm.nih.gov/pubmed**, type the name of the periodical into the search box, and click "Go."

If you want complete details about the historical contents of a journal, you can also visit the following Web site: **http://www.ncbi.nlm.nih.gov/entrez/jrbrowser.cgi**. Here, type in the name of the journal or its abbreviation, and you will receive an index of published articles. At **http://locatorplus.gov/**, you can retrieve more indexing information on medical periodicals (e.g. the name of the publisher). Select the button "Search LOCATORplus." Then type in the name of the journal and select the advanced search option "Journal Title Search."

CHAPTER 10. RESEARCHING MEDICATIONS

Overview

While a number of hard copy or CD-ROM resources are available for researching medications, a more flexible method is to use Internet-based databases. Broadly speaking, there are two sources of information on approved medications: public sources and private sources. We will emphasize free-to-use public sources.

U.S. Pharmacopeia

Because of historical investments by various organizations and the emergence of the Internet, it has become rather simple to learn about the medications recommended for scleroderma. One such source is the United States Pharmacopeia. In 1820, eleven physicians met in Washington, D.C. to establish the first compendium of standard drugs for the United States. They called this compendium the U.S. Pharmacopeia (USP). Today, the USP is a non-profit organization consisting of 800 volunteer scientists, eleven elected officials, and 400 representatives of state associations and colleges of medicine and pharmacy. The USP is located in Rockville, Maryland, and its home page is located at **http://www.usp.org/**. The USP currently provides standards for over 3,700 medications. The resulting USP DI® Advice for the Patient® can be accessed through the National Library of Medicine of the National Institutes of Health. The database is partially derived from lists of federally approved medications in the Food and Drug Administration's (FDA) Drug Approvals database, located at **http://www.fda.gov/cder/da/da.htm**.

While the FDA database is rather large and difficult to navigate, the Phamacopeia is both user-friendly and free to use. It covers more than 9,000 prescription and over-the-counter medications. To access this database, simply type the following hyperlink into your Web browser: **http://www.nlm.nih.gov/medlineplus/druginformation.html**. To view examples of a given medication (brand names, category, description, preparation, proper use, precautions, side effects, etc.), simply follow the hyperlinks indicated within the United States Pharmacopeia (USP).

Below, we have compiled a list of medications associated with scleroderma. If you would like more information on a particular medication, the provided hyperlinks will direct you to ample documentation (e.g. typical dosage, side effects, drug-interaction risks, etc.). The following drugs have been mentioned in the Pharmacopeia and other sources as being potentially applicable to scleroderma:

Aminobenzoate Potassium

- **Systemic - U.S. Brands:** Potaba
  http://www.nlm.nih.gov/medlineplus/druginfo/uspdi/202025.html

Angiotensin-Converting Enzyme (Ace) Inhibitors

- **Systemic - U.S. Brands:** Accupril; Aceon; Altace; Capoten; Lotensin; Mavik; Monopril; Prinivil; Univasc; Vasotec 4; Zestril
  http://www.nlm.nih.gov/medlineplus/druginfo/uspdi/202044.html

Bleomycin

- **Systemic - U.S. Brands:** Blenoxane
  http://www.nlm.nih.gov/medlineplus/druginfo/uspdi/202093.html

Clindamycin

- **Systemic - U.S. Brands:** Cleocin
  http://www.nlm.nih.gov/medlineplus/druginfo/uspdi/202145.html
- **Topical - U.S. Brands:** Clinda-Derm
  http://www.nlm.nih.gov/medlineplus/druginfo/uspdi/202146.html
- **Vaginal - U.S. Brands:** Cleocin
  http://www.nlm.nih.gov/medlineplus/druginfo/uspdi/202700.html

Dimethyl Sulfoxide

- **Mucosal - U.S. Brands:** Rimso-50
  http://www.nlm.nih.gov/medlineplus/druginfo/uspdi/202196.html

Epoprostenol

- **Systemic - U.S. Brands:** Flolan
  http://www.nlm.nih.gov/medlineplus/druginfo/uspdi/203429.html

Erythromycin

- **Ophthalmic - U.S. Brands:** Ilotycin
  http://www.nlm.nih.gov/medlineplus/druginfo/uspdi/202220.html

Silver Sulfadiazine

- **Topical - U.S. Brands:** Silvadene; SSD; Thermazene
  http://www.nlm.nih.gov/medlineplus/druginfo/uspdi/202521.html

Commercial Databases

In addition to the medications listed in the USP above, a number of commercial sites are available by subscription to physicians and their institutions. Or, you may be able to access these sources from your local medical library.

Mosby's Drug Consult™

Mosby's Drug Consult™ database (also available on CD-ROM and book format) covers 45,000 drug products including generics and international brands. It provides prescribing information, drug interactions, and patient information. Subscription information is available at the following hyperlink: **http://www.mosbysdrugconsult.com/.**

PDR*health*

The PDR*health* database is a free-to-use, drug information search engine that has been written for the public in layman's terms. It contains FDA-approved drug information adapted from the Physicians' Desk Reference (PDR) database. PDR*health* can be searched by brand name, generic name, or indication. It features multiple drug interactions reports. Search PDR*health* at **http://www.pdrhealth.com/drug_info/index.html.**

Other Web Sites

Drugs.com (**www.drugs.com**) reproduces the information in the Pharmacopeia as well as commercial information. You may also want to consider the Web site of the Medical Letter, Inc. (**http://www.medletter.com/**) which allows users to download articles on various drugs and therapeutics for a nominal fee.

Researching Orphan Drugs

Although the list of orphan drugs is revised on a daily basis, you can quickly research orphan drugs that might be applicable to scleroderma by using the database managed by the National Organization for Rare Disorders, Inc. (NORD), at **http://www.rarediseases.org/.** Scroll down the page, and on the left toolbar, click on "Orphan Drug Designation Database." On this page (**http://www.rarediseases.org/search/noddsearch.html**), type "scleroderma" (or synonyms) into the search box, and click "Submit Query." When you receive your results, note that not all of the drugs may be relevant, as some may have been withdrawn from orphan status. Write down or print out the name of each drug and the relevant contact information. From there, visit the Pharmacopeia Web site and type the name of each orphan drug into the search box at **http://www.nlm.nih.gov/medlineplus/druginformation.html.** You may need to contact the sponsor or NORD for further information.

NORD conducts "early access programs for investigational new drugs (IND) under the Food and Drug Administration's (FDA's) approval 'Treatment INDs' programs which allow for a limited number of individuals to receive investigational drugs before FDA marketing approval." If the orphan product about which you are seeking information is approved for marketing, information on side effects can be found on the product's label. If the product is not approved, you may need to contact the sponsor.

The following is a list of orphan drugs currently listed in the NORD Orphan Drug Designation Database for scleroderma:

- **Halofuginone (trade name: Stenorol)**
  http://www.rarediseases.org/nord/search/nodd_full?code=1021

- **human anti-transforming growth factor beta 1 monoc (trade name: NONE Assigned)**
  http://www.rarediseases.org/nord/search/nodd_full?code=1243

- **human anti-transforming growth factor beta 1 monoc**
  http://www.rarediseases.org/nord/search/nodd_full?code=1271

- **8-methoxsalen (trade name: Uvadex)**
  http://www.rarediseases.org/nord/search/nodd_full?code=505

If you have any questions about a medical treatment, the FDA may have an office near you. Look for their number in the blue pages of the phone book. You can also contact the FDA through its toll-free number, 1-888-INFO-FDA (1-888-463-6332), or on the World Wide Web at **www.fda.gov**.

APPENDICES

APPENDIX A. PHYSICIAN RESOURCES

Overview

In this chapter, we focus on databases and Internet-based guidelines and information resources created or written for a professional audience.

NIH Guidelines

Commonly referred to as "clinical" or "professional" guidelines, the National Institutes of Health publish physician guidelines for the most common diseases. Publications are available at the following by relevant Institute[11]:

- Office of the Director (OD); guidelines consolidated across agencies available at **http://www.nih.gov/health/consumer/conkey.htm**

- National Institute of General Medical Sciences (NIGMS); fact sheets available at **http://www.nigms.nih.gov/news/facts/**

- National Library of Medicine (NLM); extensive encyclopedia (A.D.A.M., Inc.) with guidelines: **http://www.nlm.nih.gov/medlineplus/healthtopics.html**

- National Cancer Institute (NCI); guidelines available at **http://www.cancer.gov/cancerinfo/list.aspx?viewid=5f35036e-5497-4d86-8c2c-714a9f7c8d25**

- National Eye Institute (NEI); guidelines available at **http://www.nei.nih.gov/order/index.htm**

- National Heart, Lung, and Blood Institute (NHLBI); guidelines available at **http://www.nhlbi.nih.gov/guidelines/index.htm**

- National Human Genome Research Institute (NHGRI); research available at **http://www.genome.gov/page.cfm?pageID=10000375**

- National Institute on Aging (NIA); guidelines available at **http://www.nia.nih.gov/health/**

---

[11] These publications are typically written by one or more of the various NIH Institutes.

- National Institute on Alcohol Abuse and Alcoholism (NIAAA); guidelines available at http://www.niaaa.nih.gov/publications/publications.htm

- National Institute of Allergy and Infectious Diseases (NIAID); guidelines available at http://www.niaid.nih.gov/publications/

- National Institute of Arthritis and Musculoskeletal and Skin Diseases (NIAMS); fact sheets and guidelines available at http://www.niams.nih.gov/hi/index.htm

- National Institute of Child Health and Human Development (NICHD); guidelines available at http://www.nichd.nih.gov/publications/pubskey.cfm

- National Institute on Deafness and Other Communication Disorders (NIDCD); fact sheets and guidelines at http://www.nidcd.nih.gov/health/

- National Institute of Dental and Craniofacial Research (NIDCR); guidelines available at http://www.nidr.nih.gov/health/

- National Institute of Diabetes and Digestive and Kidney Diseases (NIDDK); guidelines available at http://www.niddk.nih.gov/health/health.htm

- National Institute on Drug Abuse (NIDA); guidelines available at http://www.nida.nih.gov/DrugAbuse.html

- National Institute of Environmental Health Sciences (NIEHS); environmental health information available at http://www.niehs.nih.gov/external/facts.htm

- National Institute of Mental Health (NIMH); guidelines available at http://www.nimh.nih.gov/practitioners/index.cfm

- National Institute of Neurological Disorders and Stroke (NINDS); neurological disorder information pages available at http://www.ninds.nih.gov/health_and_medical/disorder_index.htm

- National Institute of Nursing Research (NINR); publications on selected illnesses at http://www.nih.gov/ninr/news-info/publications.html

- National Institute of Biomedical Imaging and Bioengineering; general information at http://grants.nih.gov/grants/becon/becon_info.htm

- Center for Information Technology (CIT); referrals to other agencies based on keyword searches available at http://kb.nih.gov/www_query_main.asp

- National Center for Complementary and Alternative Medicine (NCCAM); health information available at http://nccam.nih.gov/health/

- National Center for Research Resources (NCRR); various information directories available at http://www.ncrr.nih.gov/publications.asp

- Office of Rare Diseases; various fact sheets available at http://rarediseases.info.nih.gov/html/resources/rep_pubs.html

- Centers for Disease Control and Prevention; various fact sheets on infectious diseases available at http://www.cdc.gov/publications.htm

NIH Databases

In addition to the various Institutes of Health that publish professional guidelines, the NIH has designed a number of databases for professionals.[12] Physician-oriented resources provide a wide variety of information related to the biomedical and health sciences, both past and present. The format of these resources varies. Searchable databases, bibliographic citations, full-text articles (when available), archival collections, and images are all available. The following are referenced by the National Library of Medicine:[13]

- **Bioethics:** Access to published literature on the ethical, legal, and public policy issues surrounding healthcare and biomedical research. This information is provided in conjunction with the Kennedy Institute of Ethics located at Georgetown University, Washington, D.C.: **http://www.nlm.nih.gov/databases/databases_bioethics.html**

- **HIV/AIDS Resources:** Describes various links and databases dedicated to HIV/AIDS research: **http://www.nlm.nih.gov/pubs/factsheets/aidsinfs.html**

- **NLM Online Exhibitions:** Describes "Exhibitions in the History of Medicine": **http://www.nlm.nih.gov/exhibition/exhibition.html**. Additional resources for historical scholarship in medicine: **http://www.nlm.nih.gov/hmd/hmd.html**

- **Biotechnology Information:** Access to public databases. The National Center for Biotechnology Information conducts research in computational biology, develops software tools for analyzing genome data, and disseminates biomedical information for the better understanding of molecular processes affecting human health and disease: **http://www.ncbi.nlm.nih.gov/**

- **Population Information:** The National Library of Medicine provides access to worldwide coverage of population, family planning, and related health issues, including family planning technology and programs, fertility, and population law and policy: **http://www.nlm.nih.gov/databases/databases_population.html**

- **Cancer Information:** Access to cancer-oriented databases: **http://www.nlm.nih.gov/databases/databases_cancer.html**

- **Profiles in Science:** Offering the archival collections of prominent twentieth-century biomedical scientists to the public through modern digital technology: **http://www.profiles.nlm.nih.gov/**

- **Chemical Information:** Provides links to various chemical databases and references: **http://sis.nlm.nih.gov/Chem/ChemMain.html**

- **Clinical Alerts:** Reports the release of findings from the NIH-funded clinical trials where such release could significantly affect morbidity and mortality: **http://www.nlm.nih.gov/databases/alerts/clinical_alerts.html**

- **Space Life Sciences:** Provides links and information to space-based research (including NASA): **http://www.nlm.nih.gov/databases/databases_space.html**

- **MEDLINE:** Bibliographic database covering the fields of medicine, nursing, dentistry, veterinary medicine, the healthcare system, and the pre-clinical sciences: **http://www.nlm.nih.gov/databases/databases_medline.html**

---

[12] Remember, for the general public, the National Library of Medicine recommends the databases referenced in MEDLINE*plus* (**http://medlineplus.gov/** or **http://www.nlm.nih.gov/medlineplus/databases.html**).

[13] See **http://www.nlm.nih.gov/databases/databases.html**.

- **Toxicology and Environmental Health Information (TOXNET):** Databases covering toxicology and environmental health: **http://sis.nlm.nih.gov/Tox/ToxMain.html**

- **Visible Human Interface:** Anatomically detailed, three-dimensional representations of normal male and female human bodies: **http://www.nlm.nih.gov/research/visible/visible_human.html**

The NLM Gateway[14]

The NLM (National Library of Medicine) Gateway is a Web-based system that lets users search simultaneously in multiple retrieval systems at the U.S. National Library of Medicine (NLM). It allows users of NLM services to initiate searches from one Web interface, providing one-stop searching for many of NLM's information resources or databases.[15] To use the NLM Gateway, simply go to the search site at **http://gateway.nlm.nih.gov/gw/Cmd**. Type "scleroderma" (or synonyms) into the search box and click "Search." The results will be presented in a tabular form, indicating the number of references in each database category.

Results Summary

Category	Items Found
Journal Articles	13761
Books / Periodicals / Audio Visual	93
Consumer Health	600
Meeting Abstracts	1
Other Collections	84
Total	14539

HSTAT[16]

HSTAT is a free, Web-based resource that provides access to full-text documents used in healthcare decision-making.[17] These documents include clinical practice guidelines, quick-reference guides for clinicians, consumer health brochures, evidence reports and technology assessments from the Agency for Healthcare Research and Quality (AHRQ), as well as AHRQ's Put Prevention Into Practice.[18] Simply search by "scleroderma" (or synonyms) at the following Web site: **http://text.nlm.nih.gov**.

---

[14] Adapted from NLM: **http://gateway.nlm.nih.gov/gw/Cmd?Overview.x**.

[15] The NLM Gateway is currently being developed by the Lister Hill National Center for Biomedical Communications (LHNCBC) at the National Library of Medicine (NLM) of the National Institutes of Health (NIH).

[16] Adapted from HSTAT: **http://www.nlm.nih.gov/pubs/factsheets/hstat.html**.

[17] The HSTAT URL is **http://hstat.nlm.nih.gov/**.

[18] Other important documents in HSTAT include: the National Institutes of Health (NIH) Consensus Conference Reports and Technology Assessment Reports; the HIV/AIDS Treatment Information Service (ATIS) resource documents; the Substance Abuse and Mental Health Services Administration's Center for Substance Abuse Treatment (SAMHSA/CSAT) Treatment Improvement Protocols (TIP) and Center for Substance Abuse Prevention (SAMHSA/CSAP) Prevention Enhancement Protocols System (PEPS); the Public Health Service (PHS) Preventive Services Task Force's *Guide to Clinical Preventive Services*; the independent, nonfederal Task Force on Community Services' *Guide to Community Preventive Services*; and the Health Technology Advisory Committee (HTAC) of the Minnesota Health Care Commission (MHCC) health technology evaluations.

Coffee Break: Tutorials for Biologists[19]

Coffee Break is a general healthcare site that takes a scientific view of the news and covers recent breakthroughs in biology that may one day assist physicians in developing treatments. Here you will find a collection of short reports on recent biological discoveries. Each report incorporates interactive tutorials that demonstrate how bioinformatics tools are used as a part of the research process. Currently, all Coffee Breaks are written by NCBI staff.[20] Each report is about 400 words and is usually based on a discovery reported in one or more articles from recently published, peer-reviewed literature.[21] This site has new articles every few weeks, so it can be considered an online magazine of sorts. It is intended for general background information. You can access the Coffee Break Web site at the following hyperlink: **http://www.ncbi.nlm.nih.gov/Coffeebreak/**.

Other Commercial Databases

In addition to resources maintained by official agencies, other databases exist that are commercial ventures addressing medical professionals. Here are some examples that may interest you:

- **CliniWeb International:** Index and table of contents to selected clinical information on the Internet; see **http://www.ohsu.edu/cliniweb/**.

- **Medical World Search:** Searches full text from thousands of selected medical sites on the Internet; see **http://www.mwsearch.com/**.

The Genome Project and Scleroderma

In the following section, we will discuss databases and references which relate to the Genome Project and scleroderma.

Online Mendelian Inheritance in Man (OMIM)

The Online Mendelian Inheritance in Man (OMIM) database is a catalog of human genes and genetic disorders authored and edited by Dr. Victor A. McKusick and his colleagues at Johns Hopkins and elsewhere. OMIM was developed for the World Wide Web by the National Center for Biotechnology Information (NCBI).[22] The database contains textual information, pictures, and reference information. It also contains copious links to NCBI's Entrez database of MEDLINE articles and sequence information.

---

[19] Adapted from **http://www.ncbi.nlm.nih.gov/Coffeebreak/Archive/FAQ.html**.

[20] The figure that accompanies each article is frequently supplied by an expert external to NCBI, in which case the source of the figure is cited. The result is an interactive tutorial that tells a biological story.

[21] After a brief introduction that sets the work described into a broader context, the report focuses on how a molecular understanding can provide explanations of observed biology and lead to therapies for diseases. Each vignette is accompanied by a figure and hypertext links that lead to a series of pages that interactively show how NCBI tools and resources are used in the research process.

[22] Adapted from **http://www.ncbi.nlm.nih.gov/**. Established in 1988 as a national resource for molecular biology information, NCBI creates public databases, conducts research in computational biology, develops software tools for analyzing genome data, and disseminates biomedical information--all for the better understanding of molecular processes affecting human health and disease.

To search the database, go to **http://www.ncbi.nlm.nih.gov/Omim/searchomim.html**. Type "scleroderma" (or synonyms) into the search box, and click "Submit Search." If too many results appear, you can narrow the search by adding the word "clinical." Each report will have additional links to related research and databases. In particular, the option "Database Links" will search across technical databases that offer an abundance of information. The following is an example of the results you can obtain from the OMIM for scleroderma:

- **Polymyositis/scleroderma Autoantigen 1**
  Web site: http://www.ncbi.nlm.nih.gov/htbin-post/Omim/dispmim?606180

- **Polymyositis/scleroderma Autoantigen 2**
  Web site: http://www.ncbi.nlm.nih.gov/htbin-post/Omim/dispmim?605960

- **Scleroderma, Familial Progressive**
  Web site: http://www.ncbi.nlm.nih.gov/htbin-post/Omim/dispmim?181750

- **Sjogren Syndrome/scleroderma Autoantigen 1**
  Web site: http://www.ncbi.nlm.nih.gov/htbin-post/Omim/dispmim?606044

Genes and Disease (NCBI - Map)

The Genes and Disease database is produced by the National Center for Biotechnology Information of the National Library of Medicine at the National Institutes of Health. This Web site categorizes each disorder by system of the body. Go to **http://www.ncbi.nlm.nih.gov/disease/**, and browse the system pages to have a full view of important conditions linked to human genes. Since this site is regularly updated, you may wish to revisit it from time to time. The following systems and associated disorders are addressed:

- **Cancer:** Uncontrolled cell division.
  Examples: Breast and ovarian cancer, Burkitt lymphoma, chronic myeloid leukemia, colon cancer, lung cancer, malignant melanoma, multiple endocrine neoplasia, neurofibromatosis, p53 tumor suppressor, pancreatic cancer, prostate cancer, Ras oncogene, RB: retinoblastoma, von Hippel-Lindau syndrome.
  Web site: **http://www.ncbi.nlm.nih.gov/disease/Cancer.html**

- **Immune System:** Fights invaders.
  Examples: Asthma, autoimmune polyglandular syndrome, Crohn's disease, DiGeorge syndrome, familial Mediterranean fever, immunodeficiency with Hyper-IgM, severe combined immunodeficiency.
  Web site: **http://www.ncbi.nlm.nih.gov/disease/Immune.html**

- **Metabolism:** Food and energy.
  Examples: Adreno-leukodystrophy, atherosclerosis, Best disease, Gaucher disease, glucose galactose malabsorption, gyrate atrophy, juvenile-onset diabetes, obesity, paroxysmal nocturnal hemoglobinuria, phenylketonuria, Refsum disease, Tangier disease, Tay-Sachs disease.
  Web site: **http://www.ncbi.nlm.nih.gov/disease/Metabolism.html**

- **Muscle and Bone:** Movement and growth.
  Examples: Duchenne muscular dystrophy, Ellis-van Creveld syndrome, Marfan syndrome, myotonic dystrophy, spinal muscular atrophy.
  Web site: **http://www.ncbi.nlm.nih.gov/disease/Muscle.html**

- **Nervous System:** Mind and body.
  Examples: Alzheimer disease, amyotrophic lateral sclerosis, Angelman syndrome, Charcot-Marie-Tooth disease, epilepsy, essential tremor, fragile X syndrome, Friedreich's ataxia, Huntington disease, Niemann-Pick disease, Parkinson disease, Prader-Willi syndrome, Rett syndrome, spinocerebellar atrophy, Williams syndrome.
  Web site: **http://www.ncbi.nlm.nih.gov/disease/Brain.html**

- **Signals:** Cellular messages.
  Examples: Ataxia telangiectasia, Cockayne syndrome, glaucoma, male-patterned baldness, SRY: sex determination, tuberous sclerosis, Waardenburg syndrome, Werner syndrome.
  Web site: **http://www.ncbi.nlm.nih.gov/disease/Signals.html**

- **Transporters:** Pumps and channels.
  Examples: Cystic fibrosis, deafness, diastrophic dysplasia, Hemophilia A, long-QT syndrome, Menkes syndrome, Pendred syndrome, polycystic kidney disease, sickle cell anemia, Wilson's disease, Zellweger syndrome.
  Web site: **http://www.ncbi.nlm.nih.gov/disease/Transporters.html**

Entrez

Entrez is a search and retrieval system that integrates several linked databases at the National Center for Biotechnology Information (NCBI). These databases include nucleotide sequences, protein sequences, macromolecular structures, whole genomes, and MEDLINE through PubMed. Entrez provides access to the following databases:

- **3D Domains:** Domains from Entrez Structure,
  Web site: **http://www.ncbi.nlm.nih.gov/entrez/query.fcgi?db=geo**

- **Books:** Online books,
  Web site: **http://www.ncbi.nlm.nih.gov/entrez/query.fcgi?db=books**

- **Genome:** Complete genome assemblies,
  Web site: **http://www.ncbi.nlm.nih.gov/entrez/query.fcgi?db=Genome**

- **NCBI's Protein Sequence Information Survey Results:**
  Web site: **http://www.ncbi.nlm.nih.gov/About/proteinsurvey/**

- **Nucleotide Sequence Database (Genbank):**
  Web site: **http://www.ncbi.nlm.nih.gov/entrez/query.fcgi?db=Nucleotide**

- **OMIM:** Online Mendelian Inheritance in Man,
  Web site: **http://www.ncbi.nlm.nih.gov/entrez/query.fcgi?db=OMIM**

- **PopSet:** Population study data sets,
  Web site: **http://www.ncbi.nlm.nih.gov/entrez/query.fcgi?db=Popset**

- **ProbeSet:** Gene Expression Omnibus (GEO),
  Web site: **http://www.ncbi.nlm.nih.gov/entrez/query.fcgi?db=geo**

- **Protein Sequence Database:**
  Web site: **http://www.ncbi.nlm.nih.gov/entrez/query.fcgi?db=Protein**

- **PubMed:** Biomedical literature (PubMed),
  Web site: **http://www.ncbi.nlm.nih.gov/entrez/query.fcgi?db=PubMed**

- **Structure:** Three-dimensional macromolecular structures,
  Web site: **http://www.ncbi.nlm.nih.gov/entrez/query.fcgi?db=Structure**

- **Taxonomy:** Organisms in GenBank,
  Web site: **http://www.ncbi.nlm.nih.gov/entrez/query.fcgi?db=Taxonomy**

To access the Entrez system at the National Center for Biotechnology Information, go to **http://www.ncbi.nlm.nih.gov/entrez/query.fcgi?CMD=search&DB=genome**, and then select the database that you would like to search. The databases available are listed in the drop box next to "Search." Enter "scleroderma" (or synonyms) into the search box and click "Go."

Jablonski's Multiple Congenital Anomaly/Mental Retardation (MCA/MR) Syndromes Database[23]

This online resource has been developed to facilitate the identification and differentiation of syndromic entities. Special attention is given to the type of information that is usually limited or completely omitted in existing reference sources due to space limitations of the printed form.

At **http://www.nlm.nih.gov/mesh/jablonski/syndrome_toc/toc_a.html**, you can search across syndromes using an alphabetical index. Search by keywords at **http://www.nlm.nih.gov/mesh/jablonski/syndrome_db.html**.

The Genome Database[24]

Established at Johns Hopkins University in Baltimore, Maryland in 1990, the Genome Database (GDB) is the official central repository for genomic mapping data resulting from the Human Genome Initiative. In the spring of 1999, the Bioinformatics Supercomputing Centre (BiSC) at the Hospital for Sick Children in Toronto, Ontario assumed the management of GDB. The Human Genome Initiative is a worldwide research effort focusing on structural analysis of human DNA to determine the location and sequence of the estimated 100,000 human genes. In support of this project, GDB stores and curates data generated by researchers worldwide who are engaged in the mapping effort of the Human Genome Project (HGP). GDB's mission is to provide scientists with an encyclopedia of the human genome which is continually revised and updated to reflect the current state of scientific knowledge. Although GDB has historically focused on gene mapping, its focus will broaden as the Genome Project moves from mapping to sequence, and finally, to functional analysis.

To access the GDB, simply go to the following hyperlink: **http://www.gdb.org/**. Search "All Biological Data" by "Keyword." Type "scleroderma" (or synonyms) into the search box, and

---

[23] Adapted from the National Library of Medicine:
http://www.nlm.nih.gov/mesh/jablonski/about_syndrome.html.
[24] Adapted from the Genome Database: **http://gdbwww.gdb.org/gdb/aboutGDB.html - mission**.

review the results. If more than one word is used in the search box, then separate each one with the word "and" or "or" (using "or" might be useful when using synonyms).

APPENDIX B. PATIENT RESOURCES

Overview

Official agencies, as well as federally funded institutions supported by national grants, frequently publish a variety of guidelines written with the patient in mind. These are typically called "Fact Sheets" or "Guidelines." They can take the form of a brochure, information kit, pamphlet, or flyer. Often they are only a few pages in length. Since new guidelines on scleroderma can appear at any moment and be published by a number of sources, the best approach to finding guidelines is to systematically scan the Internet-based services that post them.

Patient Guideline Sources

The remainder of this chapter directs you to sources which either publish or can help you find additional guidelines on topics related to scleroderma. Due to space limitations, these sources are listed in a concise manner. Do not hesitate to consult the following sources by either using the Internet hyperlink provided, or, in cases where the contact information is provided, contacting the publisher or author directly.

The National Institutes of Health

The NIH gateway to patients is located at **http://health.nih.gov/**. From this site, you can search across various sources and institutes, a number of which are summarized below.

Topic Pages: MEDLINEplus

The National Library of Medicine has created a vast and patient-oriented healthcare information portal called MEDLINEplus. Within this Internet-based system are "health topic pages" which list links to available materials relevant to scleroderma. To access this system, log on to **http://www.nlm.nih.gov/medlineplus/healthtopics.html**. From there you can either search using the alphabetical index or browse by broad topic areas. Recently, MEDLINEplus listed the following when searched for "scleroderma":

- Guides on scleroderma

  Scleroderma
  http://www.nlm.nih.gov/medlineplus/scleroderma.html

- Other guides

  Arthritis
  http://www.nlm.nih.gov/medlineplus/arthritis.html

  Autoimmune Diseases
  http://www.nlm.nih.gov/medlineplus/autoimmunediseases.html

  Juvenile Rheumatoid Arthritis
  http://www.nlm.nih.gov/medlineplus/juvenilerheumatoidarthritis.html

  Lupus
  http://www.nlm.nih.gov/medlineplus/lupus.html

  Multiple Sclerosis
  http://www.nlm.nih.gov/medlineplus/multiplesclerosis.html

  Myositis
  http://www.nlm.nih.gov/medlineplus/myositis.html

  Neurologic Diseases
  http://www.nlm.nih.gov/medlineplus/neurologicdiseases.html

  Raynaud's Disease
  http://www.nlm.nih.gov/medlineplus/raynaudsdisease.html

  Tuberous Sclerosis
  http://www.nlm.nih.gov/medlineplus/tuberoussclerosis.html

Within the health topic page dedicated to scleroderma, the following was listed:

- General/Overviews

  Scleroderma
  Source: American College of Rheumatology
  http://www.rheumatology.org/public/factsheets/scler.asp?aud=prs

  Scleroderma
  Source: Arthritis Foundation
  http://www.arthritis.org/conditions/DiseaseCenter/scleroderma.asp

  Scleroderma
  Source: Mayo Foundation for Medical Education and Research
  http://www.mayoclinic.com/invoke.cfm?id=DS00362

- Diagnosis/Symptoms

  Antinuclear Antibody Test
  Source: American Association for Clinical Chemistry
  http://www.labtestsonline.org/understanding/analytes/ana/test.html

Understanding Scleroderma: Diagnosis and Care
Source: Scleroderma Research Foundation
http://www.srfcure.org/sclerod/diagnosis.html

Understanding Scleroderma: Symptoms
Source: Scleroderma Research Foundation
http://www.srfcure.org/sclerod/symptoms.html

- Specific Conditions/Aspects

CREST Syndrome
Source: Mayo Foundation for Medical Education and Research
http://www.mayoclinic.com/invoke.cfm?id=HQ00495

Localized Scleroderma (Morphea)
Source: Scleroderma Foundation
http://www.scleroderma.org/pdf/Medical%2520Brochures/local.PDF

Understanding Scleroderma: Types
Source: Scleroderma Research Foundation
http://www.srfcure.org/sclerod/types.html

- Children

Getting to Know Your Child's Health Care Team
Source: Juvenile Scleroderma Network
http://www.jsdn.org/healthCareTeam.html

Laboratory Tests in Juvenile Scleroderma
Source: Juvenile Scleroderma Network
http://www.jsdn.org/jsdlabtests.html

What Is Juvenile Scleroderma?
Source: Juvenile Scleroderma Network
http://www.jsdn.org/whatis.html

- Organizations

American College of Rheumatology
http://www.rheumatology.org/

Arthritis Foundation
http://www.arthritis.org/

Juvenile Scleroderma Network
http://www.jsdn.org

National Institute of Arthritis and Musculoskeletal and Skin Diseases
http://www.niams.nih.gov/

Scleroderma Research Foundation
http://www.srfcure.org/home/index.html

- Research

  Bosentan Effectively Treats Painful Ulcer Condition
  Source: American College of Rheumatology
  http://www.rheumatology.org/press/am2003/pr14.asp

  Lung Transplants Might Be Effective for People with Scleroderma
  Source: American College of Rheumatology
  http://www.rheumatology.org/press/am2003/pr12.asp

  Scleroderma and Kidney Disease
  Source: Arthritis Foundation
  http://www.arthritis.org/research/researchupdate/03jan_feb/scleroderma.asp

You may also choose to use the search utility provided by MEDLINEplus at the following Web address: **http://www.nlm.nih.gov/medlineplus/**. Simply type a keyword into the search box and click "Search." This utility is similar to the NIH search utility, with the exception that it only includes materials that are linked within the MEDLINEplus system (mostly patient-oriented information). It also has the disadvantage of generating unstructured results. We recommend, therefore, that you use this method only if you have a very targeted search.

The Combined Health Information Database (CHID)

CHID Online is a reference tool that maintains a database directory of thousands of journal articles and patient education guidelines on scleroderma. CHID offers summaries that describe the guidelines available, including contact information and pricing. CHID's general Web site is **http://chid.nih.gov/**. To search this database, go to **http://chid.nih.gov/detail/detail.html**. In particular, you can use the advanced search options to look up pamphlets, reports, brochures, and information kits. The following was recently posted in this archive:

- **Sexuality in Scleroderma**

  Source: Watsonville, CA: United Scleroderma Foundation Inc. 1990. 4 p.

  Contact: Available from United Scleroderma Foundation Inc. P.O. Box 350, Watsonville, CA 95077. (408) 728-2202. PRICE: $0.20.

  Summary: The United Scleroderma Foundation has published a number of brochures intended to give scleroderma patients a better understanding of their illness and to extend encouragement in coping with the difficulties of daily living. This brochure was produced in an effort to aid patients in dealing with scleroderma and sexuality. The authors note that scleroderma is a chronic disease, difficult to diagnose, and requiring understanding, communication, and support as vital factors in patients coping with the disease. Topics include self image; the role of health professionals; sexual functioning and scleroderma; physical concerns related to women; contraception; pregnancy; physical concerns related to men; using condoms; renal problems; Peyronie's disease; and resources for additional help. The addresses of five resource organizations conclude the brochure.

- **Understanding and Managing Scleroderma**

  Source: Peabody, MA: Scleroderma Federation. 1991. 40 p.

Contact: Available from Scleroderma Federation. Peabody Office Building, One Newbury Street, Peabody, MA 01960. (800) 422-1113 or (508) 535-6600. PRICE: $5.00 for individuals; $1.00 for health care professionals.

Summary: This booklet is intended to help persons with scleroderma and their families to better understand what scleroderma is, what effects it may have, and what those with scleroderma can do to help themselves and their physicians in the management of the disease. Specific topics covered include a definition of scleroderma; who develops scleroderma and when; the causes of scleroderma; the different types of scleroderma; diagnosis; symptoms, including Raynaud's phenomenon, pain and stiffness of the joints, skin disorders, sclerodactyly and joint contractures; oral, facial and dental problems of scleroderma, and major organ involvement; managing scleroderma; and advances in research. The brochure concludes with a glossary and a brief description of the Scleroderma Federation, an international nonprofit federation of scleroderma support groups.

- **Scleroderma Handbook**

Source: Santa Barbara, CA: Scleroderma Research Foundation. 199x. 20 p.

Contact: Available from Scleroderma Research Foundation. Pueblo Medical Commons, 2320 Bath Street, Suite 307, Santa Barbara, CA 93105. (800) 441-CURE or (805) 563-9133. Website: www.srfcure.org. PRICE: Single copy free.

Summary: This booklet provides people who have scleroderma, a chronic, degenerative disease that causes overproduction of collagen in the body's connective tissue, with information on its symptoms, diagnosis, treatment, and prognosis. The booklet describes the cutaneous, vascular, and other manifestations of scleroderma; lists the common manifestations represented by the CREST acronym, and outlines general symptoms. The features of several types of scleroderma are described, especially systemic scleroderma and limited forms of scleroderma. Although no one specific test can accurately and definitively determine whether a patient has scleroderma, the nailfold capillary test is a useful clinical tool. Physicians commonly consulted for diagnosis and treatment include a rheumatologist, a dermatologist, and an internist. Other topics discussed are the importance of becoming one's own health advocate and obstacles to and progress in scleroderma research.

- **Handout on Health: Scleroderma**

Source: Bethesda, MD: National Institute of Arthritis and Musculoskeletal and Skin Diseases (NIAMS) Information Clearinghouse. 2001. 48 p.

Contact: Available from National Institute of Arthritis and Musculoskeletal and Skin Diseases (NIAMS) Information Clearinghouse. 1 AMS Circle, Bethesda, MD 20892-3675. (877) 226-4267 toll-free or (301) 495-4484. Fax (301) 718-6366. TTY (301) 565-2966. E-mail: NIAMSInfo@mail.nih.gov. Website: www.niams.nih.gov. PRICE: 1 to 25 free. Order Number: AR-113 HH (booklet), or AR-113L HH (large print fact sheet).

Summary: This booklet uses a question and answer format to provide people who have scleroderma and their family members and friends with information on the types, symptoms, causes, diagnosis, and treatment of this disease. Scleroderma is a symptom of a group of diseases that involve the abnormal growth of connective tissue. It is classified as both a rheumatic disease and a connective tissue disease. The main types are localized scleroderma and systemic sclerosis. Localized scleroderma includes morphea and linear scleroderma. Systemic scleroderma, which is also known as systemic sclerosis, can be broken down into limited or diffuse scleroderma. Although the exact cause is unknown, scientists suspect that scleroderma is caused by several factors, including abnormal immune or inflammatory activity, genetic makeup, environmental triggers, and hormones. Scleroderma affects people of all races and ethnic groups, and it is more common in women. The disease can affect various aspects of life, including appearance and self esteem, self care, family relationships, sexual relations, and pregnancy and childbearing. Diagnosis is based on medical history, physical examination, and laboratory tests. Many conditions can mimic the symptoms of scleroderma, including eosinophilic fasciitis, undifferentiated connective tissue disease, and overlap syndromes. Management may involve many doctors. There is no treatment that controls or stops the underlying problem, so treatment and management focus on relieving symptoms and limiting damage. The booklet discusses the medical and nonmedical treatments for various problems that can occur in systemic scleroderma, including Raynaud's phenomenon; stiff and painful joints; skin problems; dry mouth and dental problems; gastrointestinal, heart, and kidney problems; lung damage; and cosmetic problems. Other topics includes ways people can manage their own health and current research aimed at understanding and treating scleroderma, particularly research supported by the National Institute of Arthritis and Musculoskeletal and Skin Diseases and other components of the National Institutes of Health. The booklet includes a glossary and list of national resources.

- **Scleroderma**

  Source: Atlanta, GA: Arthritis Foundation. 1997. 10 p.

  Contact: Available from Arthritis Foundation. P.O. Box 1616, Alpharetta, GA 30009-1616. (800) 207-8633. Fax (credit card orders only) (770) 442-9742. http://www.arthritis.org. PRICE: Single copy free from local Arthritis Foundation chapter (call 800-283-7800 for closest local chapter); bulk orders may be purchased from address above.

  Summary: This brochure for people with scleroderma uses a question and answer format to provide information on this rare, chronic disease, which affects women much more often than men. Although the cause is unknown, scientists know that a person with scleroderma produces too much collagen, which causes thickening and hardening of the skin and affects the functioning of internal organs. The brochure outlines the ways in which the various forms of scleroderma affect the body and it explains how the disease is diagnosed and treated. Treatment may consist of medication, exercise, joint and skin protection, and stress management. The brochure also provides information on the Arthritis Foundation.

- **Scleroderma Fact Sheet**

  Source: Danvers, MA: Scleroderma Foundation. 199X. 2 p.

  Contact: Available from Scleroderma Foundation. 12 Kent Way, Suite 101, Byfield, MA 01922. (800) 722-4673 or (978) 463-5843. Fax (978) 463-5809. E-mail: sfinfo@scleroderma.org. Website: www.scleroderma.org. PRICE: $0.25.

  Summary: This fact sheet for people with scleroderma presents facts about this chronic, autoimmune connective tissue disease, which is also known as systemic sclerosis. It explains that scleroderma is a highly individualized disease with wide-ranging symptoms that may affect the skin or internal organs, but that as a general rule, scleroderma is not contagious, cancerous, or inherited. It answers questions on the number of people with scleroderma, what causes it, and how it is diagnosed. In addition, the fact sheet provides information on localized scleroderma and systemic sclerosis.

- **Systemic Scleroderma**

  Source: Detroit, MI: American Autoimmune Related Diseases Association, Inc. 1998. 3 p.

  Contact: Available from American Autoimmune Related Diseases Association, Inc. (AARDA). Michigan National Bank Building, 15475 Gratiot Avenue, Detroit, MI 48205. (313) 371-8600. Website: www.aarda.org. PRICE: Single copy free; send self-addressed, stamped envelope.

  Summary: This fact sheet for people with systemic scleroderma discusses the affected population, symptoms, diagnosis, and treatment of this chronic autoimmune disease involving the skin and connective tissue. Localized and systemic forms have been identified. Systemic forms of scleroderma include the CREST syndrome (i.e., Calcinosis, Raynaud's phenomenon, Esophageal dysfunction, Sclerodactyly, and Telangiectasia). Although systemic scleroderma can occur in both men and women, it usually affects women in their thirties and forties. Subtle symptoms, including swelling or thickening of the skin of the fingers, Raynaud's phenomenon, changes in the esophagus, and shortness of breath on exertion and cough, usually exist for years. The disease is diagnosed by observing the patient over time, and treatment in the form of various drugs and exercises is based on the particular manifestations the patient is experiencing. The fact sheet also explains what autoimmunity is, lists other common autoimmune diseases, and outlines the activities of the American Autoimmune Related Diseases Association. 2 references.

- **Scleroderma: The CREST Variant**

  Source: Danvers, MA: Scleroderma Foundation. 1998. 1 p.

  Contact: Available from Scleroderma Foundation. 12 Kent Way, Suite 101, Byfield, MA 01922. (800) 722-4673 or (978) 463-5843. Fax (978) 463-5809. E-mail: sfinfo@scleroderma.org. Website: www.scleroderma.org. PRICE: Single copy $1.00.

  Summary: This fact sheet provides people who have scleroderma with information on the CREST variant of the systemic form of scleroderma. CREST is an acronym that stands for calcinosis, Raynaud's phenomenon, esophageal dysfunction, sclerodactyly, and telangiectasia. The fact sheet describes each of these features. Calcinosis is characterized by deposits of calcium in the skin. Raynaud's phenomenon, which occurs in about 90 percent of patients with scleroderma, involves constriction of the blood vessels in response to cold or to emotional upset and causes a series of color changes in the skin. Improper closing of the lower esophageal sphincter causes a backwash of acid and a burning sensation as food and acid return to the esophagus. Sclerodactyly is characterized by tight shiny skin on the fingers and toes. Affected digits may be difficult to bend or become fixed in a bent position. Telangiectasia involves dilation of small blood vessels near the surface of the skin.

- **Scleroderma: An Overview**

  Source: Danvers, MA: Scleroderma Foundation. 2000. 6 p.

  Contact: Available from Scleroderma Foundation. 12 Kent Way, Suite 101, Byfield, MA 01922. (800) 722-4673 or (978) 463-5843. Fax (978) 463-5809. E-mail: sfinfo@scleroderma.org. Website: www.scleroderma.org. PRICE: Single copy $1.00.

Summary: This pamphlet for people with scleroderma provides an overview of this autoimmune connective tissue disease that affects the skin and internal organs. It presents the features of the systemic and localized forms of scleroderma. In systemic scleroderma, the immune system causes damage to the small blood vessels and the collagen-producing cells located in the skin and throughout the body. Systemic scleroderma is categorized as limited or diffuse, although both forms are associated with internal organ damage. The limited form tends to have less severe organ problems than the diffuse form. The limited form is frequently referred to as the CREST form, which is an acronym that stands for calcinosis, Raynaud's phenomenon, esophageal dysfunction, sclerodactyly, and telangiectasias. Localized scleroderma affects the collagen producing cells in some of the areas of the skin and usually spares the internal organs and blood vessels. The pamphlet also answers questions about who gets scleroderma, whether genetic factors are involved, and how it is treated. It concludes with information on the mission of the Scleroderma Foundation.

- **Coping With Scleroderma**

Source: Danvers, MA: Scleroderma Foundation. 1998. 8 p.

Contact: Available from Scleroderma Foundation. 12 Kent Way, Suite 101, Byfield, MA 01922. (800) 722-4673 or (978) 463-5843. Fax (978) 463-5809. E-mail: sfinfo@scleroderma.org. Website: www.scleroderma.org. PRICE: Single copy $1.00.

Summary: This pamphlet intended for people with scleroderma, focuses on adjusting to the disease. It discusses the emotional stages that people often go through before they acknowledge their changed lives. The initial stages involve waiting for and receiving the diagnosis. Subsequent stages may involve denying the reality of the disease, getting angry and depressed, bargaining, and finally accepting it. The pamphlet provides practical tips for coping with each stage and highlights some of the characteristics of people who have learned to cope with the disease. It concludes with information on the mission of the Scleroderma Foundation.

- **Gastrointestinal Tract in Scleroderma**

Source: Danvers, MA: Scleroderma Foundation. 1999. 6 p.

Contact: Available from Scleroderma Foundation. 12 Kent Way, Suite 101, Byfield, MA 01922. (800) 722-4673 or (978) 463-5843. Fax (978) 463-5809. E-mail: sfinfo@scleroderma.org. Website: www.scleroderma.org. PRICE: Single copy $1.00.

Summary: This pamphlet provides people who have scleroderma with information on its gastrointestinal tract manifestations. The pamphlet focuses on manifestations involving the mouth, esophagus, stomach, and small intestine and large intestines. People who have scleroderma may experience dry mouth, which may lead to impairment of early digestion and occurrence of dental caries and periodontitis. Involvement of the esophagus may cause heartburn, difficulty with swallowing, and aspiration. Stomach involvement occurs in only 10 percent of patients, but it can be associated with bloating, satiety, abdominal pain, nausea, and vomiting. Involvement of the small intestine may cause nausea, vomiting, bloating, diarrhea, and malabsorption, while muscle impairment of the large intestine may result in constipation, bloating, and diarrhea. The pamphlet also includes a glossary of terms. 1 figure.

- **Localized Scleroderma**

Source: Danvers, MA: Scleroderma Foundation. 1999. 8 p.

Contact: Available from Scleroderma Foundation. 12 Kent Way, Suite 101, Byfield, MA 01922. (800) 722-4673 or (978) 463-5843. Fax (978) 463-5809. E-mail: sfinfo@scleroderma.org. Website: www.scleroderma.org. PRICE: Single copy $1.00.

Summary: This pamphlet uses a question and answer format to provide people who have scleroderma with information on the nature and complications of localized scleroderma, as well as its treatment and prognosis. This condition, which has no known cause, is characterized by thickening of the skin from excessive collagen deposition. Localized scleroderma is limited to the skin and underlying muscle and tissue. Diagnosis is based on visual recognition and a skin biopsy, although several blood tests may be used to help determine how active the disease is and how extensive or prolonged it may become. There are four main types of localized scleroderma: morphea, generalized morphea, linear scleroderma, and en coup de sabre. The pamphlet describes their features and discusses the prognosis for patients who have each type. Several drugs may be used to help halt the spread of the disease, and various other treatments may be used to help the condition.

Healthfinder™

Healthfinder™ is sponsored by the U.S. Department of Health and Human Services and offers links to hundreds of other sites that contain healthcare information. This Web site is located at **http://www.healthfinder.gov**. Again, keyword searches can be used to find guidelines. The following was recently found in this database:

- **Handout on Health: Scleroderma**

  Summary: This booklet is for people who have scleroderma, as well as for their family members, friends, and others who want to find out more about the disease.

  Source: National Institute of Arthritis and Musculoskeletal and Skin Diseases, National Institutes of Health

  http://www.healthfinder.gov/scripts/recordpass.asp?RecordType=0&RecordID=6695

- **Scleroderma Fact Sheet**

  Summary: This consumer information mini-fact sheet provides basic information about this auto-immune disease of the connective tissue, generally classified as one of the rheumatic diseases.

  Source: Scleroderma Foundation

  http://www.healthfinder.gov/scripts/recordpass.asp?RecordType=0&RecordID=2433

- **Scleroderma Physician Referral List**

  Summary: Search by city, state, name, and specialty for a physician familiar with scleroderma.

  Source: Scleroderma Research Foundation

  http://www.healthfinder.gov/scripts/recordpass.asp?RecordType=0&RecordID=6825

- **Scleroderma Support Groups**

  Summary: Select a state to find a scleroderma support group in your area. A toll-free phone number is listed for further information if there is no support group in your area.

  Source: Scleroderma Foundation

  http://www.healthfinder.gov/scripts/recordpass.asp?RecordType=0&RecordID=2659

The NIH Search Utility

The NIH search utility allows you to search for documents on over 100 selected Web sites that comprise the NIH-WEB-SPACE. Each of these servers is "crawled" and indexed on an ongoing basis. Your search will produce a list of various documents, all of which will relate in some way to scleroderma. The drawbacks of this approach are that the information is not organized by theme and that the references are often a mix of information for professionals and patients. Nevertheless, a large number of the listed Web sites provide useful background information. We can only recommend this route, therefore, for relatively rare or specific disorders, or when using highly targeted searches. To use the NIH search utility, visit the following Web page: **http://search.nih.gov/index.html**.

NORD (The National Organization of Rare Disorders, Inc.)

NORD provides an invaluable service to the public by publishing short yet comprehensive guidelines on over 1,000 diseases. NORD primarily focuses on rare diseases that might not be covered by the previously listed sources. NORD's Web address is **http://www.rarediseases.org/**. A complete guide on scleroderma can be purchased from NORD for a nominal fee.

Additional Web Sources

A number of Web sites are available to the public that often link to government sites. These can also point you in the direction of essential information. The following is a representative sample:

- AOL: **http://search.aol.com/cat.adp?id=168&layer=&from=subcats**
- Family Village: **http://www.familyvillage.wisc.edu/specific.htm**
- Google: **http://directory.google.com/Top/Health/Conditions_and_Diseases/**
- Med Help International: **http://www.medhelp.org/HealthTopics/A.html**
- Open Directory Project: **http://dmoz.org/Health/Conditions_and_Diseases/**
- Yahoo.com: **http://dir.yahoo.com/Health/Diseases_and_Conditions/**
- WebMD®Health: **http://my.webmd.com/health_topics**

Associations and Scleroderma

The following is a list of associations that provide information on and resources relating to scleroderma:

- **Juvenile Scleroderma Network, Inc**

  Telephone: (310) 519-9511 Toll-free: (800) 297-4756

  Fax: (310) 519-9511

  Email: jsdinfo@jsdn.org

  Web Site: http://www.jsdn.org

  Background: The Juvenile **Scleroderma** Network, a voluntary organization, invites families nationwide to become involved and help provide support and friendship to children who have juvenile **scleroderma**. It also serves families in Canada, South America, Europe, the United Kingdom, and Australia. **Scleroderma** is a connective tissue disease involving skin, blood vessels, and the immune system. Children who have juvenile **scleroderma** may experience confusion about their illness, anger about changes in their appearance, and fear of the unknown. For parents to be able to help their children deal with such feelings, it is important for them to have a support network to exchange information and find emotional reassurance. The Network's services include advocacy, support groups, networking, publications, and research. Spanish language materials are available. The access code for the 24-hour 800 phone number is 74.

  Relevant area(s) of interest: Morphea

- **Scleroderma Foundation, Inc**

  Telephone: (978) 463-5843 Toll-free: (800) 722-4673

  Fax: (978) 463-5809

  Email: sfinfo@sceroderma.org

  Web Site: http://www.scleroderma.org

  Background: The **Scleroderma** Foundation, Inc. (SF) is a not-for-profit organization dedicated to providing educational and emotional support for people with **scleroderma** and their families; increasing awareness of **scleroderma;** and supporting research to determine the disorder's cause, treatment, and cure. The **Scleroderma** Foundation testifies before Congress concerning the needs of people with **scleroderma** and works to increase public awareness through all forms of media. The organization raises research funding; institutes research grants; and conducts an annual conference. The Foundation also networks with other national health agencies on common concerns; assists people with **scleroderma** in securing Social Security and Disability benefits; and works with the medical community to promote better care and treatment.

  Relevant area(s) of interest: Morphea, Scleroderma

- **Scleroderma Research Foundation**

  Telephone: (805) 563-9133 Toll-free: (800) 441-2873

  Fax: (805) 563-2402

  Email: srfcure@srfcure.org

  Web Site: www.sclerodermausa.org

  Background: The **Scleroderma** Research Foundation is a voluntary research non-profit organization dedicated to finding a cure for **scleroderma** by funding and facilitating ongoing medical research. The Foundation also seeks to increase public awareness and understanding of this disorder. Established in 1987, the **Scleroderma** Research Foundation created a team of scientific and biomedical advisors to identify and address key issues that may lead to a cure. The efforts of the Foundation and its advisory team have led to the opening of the Bay Area **Scleroderma** Research Center in San Francisco and the East Coast **Scleroderma** Research Center in Baltimore, both cross-institutional, multi-disciplinary research facilities. With participation of the National Institutes of Health (NIH) and several institutes and universities, the Foundation has also assisted in the creation of clinical laboratory tests that provide for the early diagnosis of several forms of **scleroderma.** The provides a variety of educational materials to affected individuals, family members, health care and research professionals, and the general public.

Relevant area(s) of interest: Morphea, Scleroderma

Finding Associations

There are several Internet directories that provide lists of medical associations with information on or resources relating to scleroderma. By consulting all of associations listed in this chapter, you will have nearly exhausted all sources for patient associations concerned with scleroderma.

The National Health Information Center (NHIC)

The National Health Information Center (NHIC) offers a free referral service to help people find organizations that provide information about scleroderma. For more information, see the NHIC's Web site at **http://www.health.gov/NHIC/** or contact an information specialist by calling 1-800-336-4797.

Directory of Health Organizations

The Directory of Health Organizations, provided by the National Library of Medicine Specialized Information Services, is a comprehensive source of information on associations. The Directory of Health Organizations database can be accessed via the Internet at **http://www.sis.nlm.nih.gov/Dir/DirMain.html**. It is composed of two parts: DIRLINE and Health Hotlines.

The DIRLINE database comprises some 10,000 records of organizations, research centers, and government institutes and associations that primarily focus on health and biomedicine. To access DIRLINE directly, go to the following Web site: **http://dirline.nlm.nih.gov/**. Simply type in "scleroderma" (or a synonym), and you will receive information on all relevant organizations listed in the database.

Health Hotlines directs you to toll-free numbers to over 300 organizations. You can access this database directly at **http://www.sis.nlm.nih.gov/hotlines/**. On this page, you are given the option to search by keyword or by browsing the subject list. When you have received your search results, click on the name of the organization for its description and contact information.

The Combined Health Information Database

Another comprehensive source of information on healthcare associations is the Combined Health Information Database. Using the "Detailed Search" option, you will need to limit your search to "Organizations" and "scleroderma". Type the following hyperlink into your Web browser: **http://chid.nih.gov/detail/detail.html**. To find associations, use the drop boxes at the bottom of the search page where "You may refine your search by." For publication date, select "All Years." Then, select your preferred language and the format option "Organization Resource Sheet." Type "scleroderma" (or synonyms) into the "For these words:" box. You should check back periodically with this database since it is updated every three months.

The National Organization for Rare Disorders, Inc.

The National Organization for Rare Disorders, Inc. has prepared a Web site that provides, at no charge, lists of associations organized by health topic. You can access this database at the following Web site: **http://www.rarediseases.org/search/orgsearch.html**. Type "scleroderma" (or a synonym) into the search box, and click "Submit Query."

APPENDIX C. FINDING MEDICAL LIBRARIES

Overview

In this Appendix, we show you how to quickly find a medical library in your area.

Preparation

Your local public library and medical libraries have interlibrary loan programs with the National Library of Medicine (NLM), one of the largest medical collections in the world. According to the NLM, most of the literature in the general and historical collections of the National Library of Medicine is available on interlibrary loan to any library. If you would like to access NLM medical literature, then visit a library in your area that can request the publications for you.[25]

Finding a Local Medical Library

The quickest method to locate medical libraries is to use the Internet-based directory published by the National Network of Libraries of Medicine (NN/LM). This network includes 4626 members and affiliates that provide many services to librarians, health professionals, and the public. To find a library in your area, simply visit http://nnlm.gov/members/adv.html or call 1-800-338-7657.

Medical Libraries in the U.S. and Canada

In addition to the NN/LM, the National Library of Medicine (NLM) lists a number of libraries with reference facilities that are open to the public. The following is the NLM's list and includes hyperlinks to each library's Web site. These Web pages can provide information on hours of operation and other restrictions. The list below is a small sample of

---

[25] Adapted from the NLM: http://www.nlm.nih.gov/psd/cas/interlibrary.html.

libraries recommended by the National Library of Medicine (sorted alphabetically by name of the U.S. state or Canadian province where the library is located)[26]:

- **Alabama:** Health InfoNet of Jefferson County (Jefferson County Library Cooperative, Lister Hill Library of the Health Sciences), **http://www.uab.edu/infonet/**

- **Alabama:** Richard M. Scrushy Library (American Sports Medicine Institute)

- **Arizona:** Samaritan Regional Medical Center: The Learning Center (Samaritan Health System, Phoenix, Arizona), **http://www.samaritan.edu/library/bannerlibs.htm**

- **California:** Kris Kelly Health Information Center (St. Joseph Health System, Humboldt), **http://www.humboldt1.com/~kkhic/index.html**

- **California:** Community Health Library of Los Gatos, **http://www.healthlib.org/orgresources.html**

- **California:** Consumer Health Program and Services (CHIPS) (County of Los Angeles Public Library, Los Angeles County Harbor-UCLA Medical Center Library) - Carson, CA, **http://www.colapublib.org/services/chips.html**

- **California:** Gateway Health Library (Sutter Gould Medical Foundation)

- **California:** Health Library (Stanford University Medical Center), **http://www-med.stanford.edu/healthlibrary/**

- **California:** Patient Education Resource Center - Health Information and Resources (University of California, San Francisco), **http://sfghdean.ucsf.edu/barnett/PERC/default.asp**

- **California:** Redwood Health Library (Petaluma Health Care District), **http://www.phcd.org/rdwdlib.html**

- **California:** Los Gatos PlaneTree Health Library, **http://planetreesanjose.org/**

- **California:** Sutter Resource Library (Sutter Hospitals Foundation, Sacramento), **http://suttermedicalcenter.org/library/**

- **California:** Health Sciences Libraries (University of California, Davis), **http://www.lib.ucdavis.edu/healthsci/**

- **California:** ValleyCare Health Library & Ryan Comer Cancer Resource Center (ValleyCare Health System, Pleasanton), **http://gaelnet.stmarys-ca.edu/other.libs/gbal/east/vchl.html**

- **California:** Washington Community Health Resource Library (Fremont), **http://www.healthlibrary.org/**

- **Colorado:** William V. Gervasini Memorial Library (Exempla Healthcare), **http://www.saintjosephdenver.org/yourhealth/libraries/**

- **Connecticut:** Hartford Hospital Health Science Libraries (Hartford Hospital), **http://www.harthosp.org/library/**

- **Connecticut:** Healthnet: Connecticut Consumer Health Information Center (University of Connecticut Health Center, Lyman Maynard Stowe Library), **http://library.uchc.edu/departm/hnet/**

---

[26] Abstracted from **http://www.nlm.nih.gov/medlineplus/libraries.html**.

- **Connecticut:** Waterbury Hospital Health Center Library (Waterbury Hospital, Waterbury), http://www.waterburyhospital.com/library/consumer.shtml

- **Delaware:** Consumer Health Library (Christiana Care Health System, Eugene du Pont Preventive Medicine & Rehabilitation Institute, Wilmington), http://www.christianacare.org/health_guide/health_guide_pmri_health_info.cfm

- **Delaware:** Lewis B. Flinn Library (Delaware Academy of Medicine, Wilmington), http://www.delamed.org/chls.html

- **Georgia:** Family Resource Library (Medical College of Georgia, Augusta), http://cmc.mcg.edu/kids_families/fam_resources/fam_res_lib/frl.htm

- **Georgia:** Health Resource Center (Medical Center of Central Georgia, Macon), http://www.mccg.org/hrc/hrchome.asp

- **Hawaii:** Hawaii Medical Library: Consumer Health Information Service (Hawaii Medical Library, Honolulu), http://hml.org/CHIS/

- **Idaho:** DeArmond Consumer Health Library (Kootenai Medical Center, Coeur d'Alene), http://www.nicon.org/DeArmond/index.htm

- **Illinois:** Health Learning Center of Northwestern Memorial Hospital (Chicago), http://www.nmh.org/health_info/hlc.html

- **Illinois:** Medical Library (OSF Saint Francis Medical Center, Peoria), http://www.osfsaintfrancis.org/general/library/

- **Kentucky:** Medical Library - Services for Patients, Families, Students & the Public (Central Baptist Hospital, Lexington), http://www.centralbap.com/education/community/library.cfm

- **Kentucky:** University of Kentucky - Health Information Library (Chandler Medical Center, Lexington), http://www.mc.uky.edu/PatientEd/

- **Louisiana:** Alton Ochsner Medical Foundation Library (Alton Ochsner Medical Foundation, New Orleans), http://www.ochsner.org/library/

- **Louisiana:** Louisiana State University Health Sciences Center Medical Library-Shreveport, http://lib-sh.lsuhsc.edu/

- **Maine:** Franklin Memorial Hospital Medical Library (Franklin Memorial Hospital, Farmington), http://www.fchn.org/fmh/lib.htm

- **Maine:** Gerrish-True Health Sciences Library (Central Maine Medical Center, Lewiston), http://www.cmmc.org/library/library.html

- **Maine:** Hadley Parrot Health Science Library (Eastern Maine Healthcare, Bangor), http://www.emh.org/hll/hpl/guide.htm

- **Maine:** Maine Medical Center Library (Maine Medical Center, Portland), http://www.mmc.org/library/

- **Maine:** Parkview Hospital (Brunswick), http://www.parkviewhospital.org/

- **Maine:** Southern Maine Medical Center Health Sciences Library (Southern Maine Medical Center, Biddeford), http://www.smmc.org/services/service.php3?choice=10

- **Maine:** Stephens Memorial Hospital's Health Information Library (Western Maine Health, Norway), http://www.wmhcc.org/Library/

- **Manitoba, Canada:** Consumer & Patient Health Information Service (University of Manitoba Libraries), http://www.umanitoba.ca/libraries/units/health/reference/chis.html

- **Manitoba, Canada:** J.W. Crane Memorial Library (Deer Lodge Centre, Winnipeg), http://www.deerlodge.mb.ca/crane_library/about.asp

- **Maryland:** Health Information Center at the Wheaton Regional Library (Montgomery County, Dept. of Public Libraries, Wheaton Regional Library), http://www.mont.lib.md.us/healthinfo/hic.asp

- **Massachusetts:** Baystate Medical Center Library (Baystate Health System), http://www.baystatehealth.com/1024/

- **Massachusetts:** Boston University Medical Center Alumni Medical Library (Boston University Medical Center), http://med-libwww.bu.edu/library/lib.html

- **Massachusetts:** Lowell General Hospital Health Sciences Library (Lowell General Hospital, Lowell), http://www.lowellgeneral.org/library/HomePageLinks/WWW.htm

- **Massachusetts:** Paul E. Woodard Health Sciences Library (New England Baptist Hospital, Boston), http://www.nebh.org/health_lib.asp

- **Massachusetts:** St. Luke's Hospital Health Sciences Library (St. Luke's Hospital, Southcoast Health System, New Bedford), http://www.southcoast.org/library/

- **Massachusetts:** Treadwell Library Consumer Health Reference Center (Massachusetts General Hospital), http://www.mgh.harvard.edu/library/chrcindex.html

- **Massachusetts:** UMass HealthNet (University of Massachusetts Medical School, Worchester), http://healthnet.umassmed.edu/

- **Michigan:** Botsford General Hospital Library - Consumer Health (Botsford General Hospital, Library & Internet Services), http://www.botsfordlibrary.org/consumer.htm

- **Michigan:** Helen DeRoy Medical Library (Providence Hospital and Medical Centers), http://www.providence-hospital.org/library/

- **Michigan:** Marquette General Hospital - Consumer Health Library (Marquette General Hospital, Health Information Center), http://www.mgh.org/center.html

- **Michigan:** Patient Education Resouce Center - University of Michigan Cancer Center (University of Michigan Comprehensive Cancer Center, Ann Arbor), http://www.cancer.med.umich.edu/learn/leares.htm

- **Michigan:** Sladen Library & Center for Health Information Resources - Consumer Health Information (Detroit), http://www.henryford.com/body.cfm?id=39330

- **Montana:** Center for Health Information (St. Patrick Hospital and Health Sciences Center, Missoula)

- **National:** Consumer Health Library Directory (Medical Library Association, Consumer and Patient Health Information Section), http://caphis.mlanet.org/directory/index.html

- **National:** National Network of Libraries of Medicine (National Library of Medicine) - provides library services for health professionals in the United States who do not have access to a medical library, http://nnlm.gov/

- **National:** NN/LM List of Libraries Serving the Public (National Network of Libraries of Medicine), http://nnlm.gov/members/

- **Nevada:** Health Science Library, West Charleston Library (Las Vegas-Clark County Library District, Las Vegas), **http://www.lvccld.org/special_collections/medical/index.htm**

- **New Hampshire:** Dartmouth Biomedical Libraries (Dartmouth College Library, Hanover), **http://www.dartmouth.edu/~biomed/resources.htmld/conshealth.htmld/**

- **New Jersey:** Consumer Health Library (Rahway Hospital, Rahway), **http://www.rahwayhospital.com/library.htm**

- **New Jersey:** Dr. Walter Phillips Health Sciences Library (Englewood Hospital and Medical Center, Englewood), **http://www.englewoodhospital.com/links/index.htm**

- **New Jersey:** Meland Foundation (Englewood Hospital and Medical Center, Englewood), **http://www.geocities.com/ResearchTriangle/9360/**

- **New York:** Choices in Health Information (New York Public Library) - NLM Consumer Pilot Project participant, **http://www.nypl.org/branch/health/links.html**

- **New York:** Health Information Center (Upstate Medical University, State University of New York, Syracuse), **http://www.upstate.edu/library/hic/**

- **New York:** Health Sciences Library (Long Island Jewish Medical Center, New Hyde Park), **http://www.lij.edu/library/library.html**

- **New York:** ViaHealth Medical Library (Rochester General Hospital), **http://www.nyam.org/library/**

- **Ohio:** Consumer Health Library (Akron General Medical Center, Medical & Consumer Health Library), **http://www.akrongeneral.org/hwlibrary.htm**

- **Oklahoma:** The Health Information Center at Saint Francis Hospital (Saint Francis Health System, Tulsa), **http://www.sfh-tulsa.com/services/healthinfo.asp**

- **Oregon:** Planetree Health Resource Center (Mid-Columbia Medical Center, The Dalles), **http://www.mcmc.net/phrc/**

- **Pennsylvania:** Community Health Information Library (Milton S. Hershey Medical Center, Hershey), **http://www.hmc.psu.edu/commhealth/**

- **Pennsylvania:** Community Health Resource Library (Geisinger Medical Center, Danville), **http://www.geisinger.edu/education/commlib.shtml**

- **Pennsylvania:** HealthInfo Library (Moses Taylor Hospital, Scranton), **http://www.mth.org/healthwellness.html**

- **Pennsylvania:** Hopwood Library (University of Pittsburgh, Health Sciences Library System, Pittsburgh), **http://www.hsls.pitt.edu/guides/chi/hopwood/index_html**

- **Pennsylvania:** Koop Community Health Information Center (College of Physicians of Philadelphia), **http://www.collphyphil.org/kooppg1.shtml**

- **Pennsylvania:** Learning Resources Center - Medical Library (Susquehanna Health System, Williamsport), **http://www.shscares.org/services/lrc/index.asp**

- **Pennsylvania:** Medical Library (UPMC Health System, Pittsburgh), **http://www.upmc.edu/passavant/library.htm**

- **Quebec, Canada:** Medical Library (Montreal General Hospital), **http://www.mghlib.mcgill.ca/**

- **South Dakota:** Rapid City Regional Hospital Medical Library (Rapid City Regional Hospital), **http://www.rcrh.org/Services/Library/Default.asp**

- **Texas:** Houston HealthWays (Houston Academy of Medicine-Texas Medical Center Library), **http://hhw.library.tmc.edu/**

- **Washington:** Community Health Library (Kittitas Valley Community Hospital), **http://www.kvch.com/**

- **Washington:** Southwest Washington Medical Center Library (Southwest Washington Medical Center, Vancouver), **http://www.swmedicalcenter.com/body.cfm?id=72**

ONLINE GLOSSARIES

The Internet provides access to a number of free-to-use medical dictionaries. The National Library of Medicine has compiled the following list of online dictionaries:

- ADAM Medical Encyclopedia (A.D.A.M., Inc.), comprehensive medical reference: **http://www.nlm.nih.gov/medlineplus/encyclopedia.html**

- MedicineNet.com Medical Dictionary (MedicineNet, Inc.): **http://www.medterms.com/Script/Main/hp.asp**

- Merriam-Webster Medical Dictionary (Inteli-Health, Inc.): **http://www.intelihealth.com/IH/**

- Multilingual Glossary of Technical and Popular Medical Terms in Eight European Languages (European Commission) - Danish, Dutch, English, French, German, Italian, Portuguese, and Spanish: **http://allserv.rug.ac.be/~rvdstich/eugloss/welcome.html**

- On-line Medical Dictionary (CancerWEB): **http://cancerweb.ncl.ac.uk/omd/**

- Rare Diseases Terms (Office of Rare Diseases): **http://ord.aspensys.com/asp/diseases/diseases.asp**

- Technology Glossary (National Library of Medicine) - Health Care Technology: **http://www.nlm.nih.gov/nichsr/ta101/ta10108.htm**

Beyond these, MEDLINEplus contains a very patient-friendly encyclopedia covering every aspect of medicine (licensed from A.D.A.M., Inc.). The ADAM Medical Encyclopedia can be accessed at **http://www.nlm.nih.gov/medlineplus/encyclopedia.html**. ADAM is also available on commercial Web sites such as drkoop.com (**http://www.drkoop.com/**) and Web MD (**http://my.webmd.com/adam/asset/adam_disease_articles/a_to_z/a**). The NIH suggests the following Web sites in the ADAM Medical Encyclopedia when searching for information on scleroderma:

- **Basic Guidelines for Scleroderma**

  Scleroderma - resources
  Web site: http://www.nlm.nih.gov/medlineplus/ency/article/002195.htm

  Systemic sclerosis (scleroderma)
  Web site: http://www.nlm.nih.gov/medlineplus/ency/article/000429.htm

- **Signs & Symptoms for Scleroderma**

  Blanching
  Web site: http://www.nlm.nih.gov/medlineplus/ency/article/003249.htm

  Bloating
  Web site: http://www.nlm.nih.gov/medlineplus/ency/article/003123.htm

  Constipation
  Web site: http://www.nlm.nih.gov/medlineplus/ency/article/003125.htm

Diarrhea
Web site: http://www.nlm.nih.gov/medlineplus/ency/article/003126.htm

Difficulty swallowing
Web site: http://www.nlm.nih.gov/medlineplus/ency/article/003115.htm

Dysphagia
Web site: http://www.nlm.nih.gov/medlineplus/ency/article/003115.htm

Dyspnea
Web site: http://www.nlm.nih.gov/medlineplus/ency/article/003075.htm

Eye burning, itching and discharge
Web site: http://www.nlm.nih.gov/medlineplus/ency/article/003034.htm

Hair loss
Web site: http://www.nlm.nih.gov/medlineplus/ency/article/003246.htm

Heartburn
Web site: http://www.nlm.nih.gov/medlineplus/ency/article/003114.htm

Hypopigmentation
Web site: http://www.nlm.nih.gov/medlineplus/ency/article/003224.htm

Joint pain
Web site: http://www.nlm.nih.gov/medlineplus/ency/article/003261.htm

Lung disease
Web site: http://www.nlm.nih.gov/medlineplus/ency/article/000066.htm

Muscle weakness
Web site: http://www.nlm.nih.gov/medlineplus/ency/article/003174.htm

Nausea and vomiting
Web site: http://www.nlm.nih.gov/medlineplus/ency/article/003117.htm

Pruritus
Web site: http://www.nlm.nih.gov/medlineplus/ency/article/003217.htm

Shortness of breath
Web site: http://www.nlm.nih.gov/medlineplus/ency/article/003075.htm

Skin, abnormally dark or light
Web site: http://www.nlm.nih.gov/medlineplus/ency/article/003242.htm

Stress
Web site: http://www.nlm.nih.gov/medlineplus/ency/article/003211.htm

Swelling
Web site: http://www.nlm.nih.gov/medlineplus/ency/article/003103.htm

Telangiectasia
Web site: http://www.nlm.nih.gov/medlineplus/ency/article/003284.htm

Vomiting
Web site: http://www.nlm.nih.gov/medlineplus/ency/article/003117.htm

Weakness
Web site: http://www.nlm.nih.gov/medlineplus/ency/article/003174.htm

Weight loss
Web site: http://www.nlm.nih.gov/medlineplus/ency/article/003107.htm

Wheezing
Web site: http://www.nlm.nih.gov/medlineplus/ency/article/003070.htm

Wrist pain
Web site: http://www.nlm.nih.gov/medlineplus/ency/article/003175.htm

- **Diagnostics and Tests for Scleroderma**

ACE levels
Web site: http://www.nlm.nih.gov/medlineplus/ency/article/003567.htm

ANA
Web site: http://www.nlm.nih.gov/medlineplus/ency/article/003535.htm

Antinuclear antibody
Web site: http://www.nlm.nih.gov/medlineplus/ency/article/003535.htm

Biopsy
Web site: http://www.nlm.nih.gov/medlineplus/ency/article/003416.htm

Chest X-ray
Web site: http://www.nlm.nih.gov/medlineplus/ency/article/003804.htm

CT
Web site: http://www.nlm.nih.gov/medlineplus/ency/article/003330.htm

Esophageal manometry
Web site: http://www.nlm.nih.gov/medlineplus/ency/article/003884.htm

ESR
Web site: http://www.nlm.nih.gov/medlineplus/ency/article/003638.htm

Febrile/cold agglutinins
Web site: http://www.nlm.nih.gov/medlineplus/ency/article/003549.htm

LE cell test
Web site: http://www.nlm.nih.gov/medlineplus/ency/article/003635.htm

Lung scan
Web site: http://www.nlm.nih.gov/medlineplus/ency/article/003824.htm

Pulmonary function
Web site: http://www.nlm.nih.gov/medlineplus/ency/article/003443.htm

Rheumatoid factor
Web site: http://www.nlm.nih.gov/medlineplus/ency/article/003548.htm

Skin biopsy
Web site: http://www.nlm.nih.gov/medlineplus/ency/article/003840.htm

Urinalysis
Web site: http://www.nlm.nih.gov/medlineplus/ency/article/003579.htm

X-ray
Web site: http://www.nlm.nih.gov/medlineplus/ency/article/003337.htm

- **Background Topics for Scleroderma**

  Cardiovascular
  Web site: http://www.nlm.nih.gov/medlineplus/ency/article/002310.htm

  Incidence
  Web site: http://www.nlm.nih.gov/medlineplus/ency/article/002387.htm

  Support group
  Web site: http://www.nlm.nih.gov/medlineplus/ency/article/002150.htm

  Systemic
  Web site: http://www.nlm.nih.gov/medlineplus/ency/article/002294.htm

Online Dictionary Directories

The following are additional online directories compiled by the National Library of Medicine, including a number of specialized medical dictionaries:

- Medical Dictionaries: Medical & Biological (World Health Organization):
  http://www.who.int/hlt/virtuallibrary/English/diction.htm#Medical

- MEL-Michigan Electronic Library List of Online Health and Medical Dictionaries
  (Michigan Electronic Library): **http://mel.lib.mi.us/health/health-dictionaries.html**

- Patient Education: Glossaries (DMOZ Open Directory Project):
  http://dmoz.org/Health/Education/Patient_Education/Glossaries/

- Web of Online Dictionaries (Bucknell University):
  http://www.yourdictionary.com/diction5.html#medicine

SCLERODERMA DICTIONARY

The definitions below are derived from official public sources, including the National Institutes of Health [NIH] and the European Union [EU].

1-phosphate: A drug that halts cell suicide in human white blood cells. [NIH]

Abdomen: That portion of the body that lies between the thorax and the pelvis. [NIH]

Abdominal: Having to do with the abdomen, which is the part of the body between the chest and the hips that contains the pancreas, stomach, intestines, liver, gallbladder, and other organs. [NIH]

Abdominal Pain: Sensation of discomfort, distress, or agony in the abdominal region. [NIH]

Aberrant: Wandering or deviating from the usual or normal course. [EU]

Acantholysis: Separation of the prickle cells of the stratum spinosum of the epidermis, resulting in atrophy of the prickle cell layer. It is seen in diseases such as pemphigus vulgaris (see pemphigus) and keratosis follicularis. [NIH]

Acceptor: A substance which, while normally not oxidized by oxygen or reduced by hydrogen, can be oxidized or reduced in presence of a substance which is itself undergoing oxidation or reduction. [NIH]

Acetylcholine: A neurotransmitter. Acetylcholine in vertebrates is the major transmitter at neuromuscular junctions, autonomic ganglia, parasympathetic effector junctions, a subset of sympathetic effector junctions, and at many sites in the central nervous system. It is generally not used as an administered drug because it is broken down very rapidly by cholinesterases, but it is useful in some ophthalmological applications. [NIH]

Acitretin: An oral retinoid effective in the treatment of psoriasis. It is the major metabolite of etretinate with the advantage of a much shorter half-life when compared with etretinate. [NIH]

Acne: A disorder of the skin marked by inflammation of oil glands and hair glands. [NIH]

Acne Vulgaris: A chronic disorder of the pilosebaceous apparatus associated with an increase in sebum secretion. It is characterized by open comedones (blackheads), closed comedones (whiteheads), and pustular nodules. The cause is unknown, but heredity and age are predisposing factors. [NIH]

Action Potentials: The electric response of a nerve or muscle to its stimulation. [NIH]

Acute renal: A condition in which the kidneys suddenly stop working. In most cases, kidneys can recover from almost complete loss of function. [NIH]

Adaptability: Ability to develop some form of tolerance to conditions extremely different from those under which a living organism evolved. [NIH]

Adaptation: 1. The adjustment of an organism to its environment, or the process by which it enhances such fitness. 2. The normal ability of the eye to adjust itself to variations in the intensity of light; the adjustment to such variations. 3. The decline in the frequency of firing of a neuron, particularly of a receptor, under conditions of constant stimulation. 4. In dentistry, (a) the proper fitting of a denture, (b) the degree of proximity and interlocking of restorative material to a tooth preparation, (c) the exact adjustment of bands to teeth. 5. In microbiology, the adjustment of bacterial physiology to a new environment. [EU]

Adenine: A purine base and a fundamental unit of adenine nucleotides. [NIH]

Adenosine: A nucleoside that is composed of adenine and d-ribose. Adenosine or adenosine derivatives play many important biological roles in addition to being components of DNA and RNA. Adenosine itself is a neurotransmitter. [NIH]

Adhesions: Pathological processes consisting of the union of the opposing surfaces of a wound. [NIH]

Adipose Tissue: Connective tissue composed of fat cells lodged in the meshes of areolar tissue. [NIH]

Adjustment: The dynamic process wherein the thoughts, feelings, behavior, and biophysiological mechanisms of the individual continually change to adjust to the environment. [NIH]

Adjuvant: A substance which aids another, such as an auxiliary remedy; in immunology, nonspecific stimulator (e.g., BCG vaccine) of the immune response. [EU]

Adolescence: The period of life beginning with the appearance of secondary sex characteristics and terminating with the cessation of somatic growth. The years usually referred to as adolescence lie between 13 and 18 years of age. [NIH]

Adoptive Transfer: Form of passive immunization where previously sensitized immunologic agents (cells or serum) are transferred to non-immune recipients. When transfer of cells is used as a therapy for the treatment of neoplasms, it is called adoptive immunotherapy (immunotherapy, adoptive). [NIH]

Adrenal Cortex: The outer layer of the adrenal gland. It secretes mineralocorticoids, androgens, and glucocorticoids. [NIH]

Adrenal Glands: Paired glands situated in the retroperitoneal tissues at the superior pole of each kidney. [NIH]

Adrenal Medulla: The inner part of the adrenal gland; it synthesizes, stores and releases catecholamines. [NIH]

Adrenergic: Activated by, characteristic of, or secreting epinephrine or substances with similar activity; the term is applied to those nerve fibres that liberate norepinephrine at a synapse when a nerve impulse passes, i.e., the sympathetic fibres. [EU]

Adverse Effect: An unwanted side effect of treatment. [NIH]

Affinity: 1. Inherent likeness or relationship. 2. A special attraction for a specific element, organ, or structure. 3. Chemical affinity; the force that binds atoms in molecules; the tendency of substances to combine by chemical reaction. 4. The strength of noncovalent chemical binding between two substances as measured by the dissociation constant of the complex. 5. In immunology, a thermodynamic expression of the strength of interaction between a single antigen-binding site and a single antigenic determinant (and thus of the stereochemical compatibility between them), most accurately applied to interactions among simple, uniform antigenic determinants such as haptens. Expressed as the association constant (K litres mole -1), which, owing to the heterogeneity of affinities in a population of antibody molecules of a given specificity, actually represents an average value (mean intrinsic association constant). 6. The reciprocal of the dissociation constant. [EU]

Agar: A complex sulfated polymer of galactose units, extracted from Gelidium cartilagineum, Gracilaria confervoides, and related red algae. It is used as a gel in the preparation of solid culture media for microorganisms, as a bulk laxative, in making emulsions, and as a supporting medium for immunodiffusion and immunoelectrophoresis. [NIH]

Age Groups: Persons classified by age from birth (infant, newborn) to octogenarians and older (aged, 80 and over). [NIH]

Aged, 80 and Over: A person 80 years of age and older. [NIH]

Agglutinins: Substances, usually of biological origin, that cause cells or other organic particles to aggregate and stick to each other. They also include those antibodies which cause aggregation or agglutination of a particulate or insoluble antigen. [NIH]

Agonist: In anatomy, a prime mover. In pharmacology, a drug that has affinity for and stimulates physiologic activity at cell receptors normally stimulated by naturally occurring substances. [EU]

Airway: A device for securing unobstructed passage of air into and out of the lungs during general anesthesia. [NIH]

Albumin: 1. Any protein that is soluble in water and moderately concentrated salt solutions and is coagulable by heat. 2. Serum albumin; the major plasma protein (approximately 60 per cent of the total), which is responsible for much of the plasma colloidal osmotic pressure and serves as a transport protein carrying large organic anions, such as fatty acids, bilirubin, and many drugs, and also carrying certain hormones, such as cortisol and thyroxine, when their specific binding globulins are saturated. Albumin is synthesized in the liver. Low serum levels occur in protein malnutrition, active inflammation and serious hepatic and renal disease. [EU]

Aldehydes: Organic compounds containing a carbonyl group in the form -CHO. [NIH]

Aldosterone: (11 beta)-11,21-Dihydroxy-3,20-dioxopregn-4-en-18-al. A hormone secreted by the adrenal cortex that functions in the regulation of electrolyte and water balance by increasing the renal retention of sodium and the excretion of potassium. [NIH]

Algorithms: A procedure consisting of a sequence of algebraic formulas and/or logical steps to calculate or determine a given task. [NIH]

Alimentary: Pertaining to food or nutritive material, or to the organs of digestion. [EU]

Alkaline: Having the reactions of an alkali. [EU]

Alkaloid: A member of a large group of chemicals that are made by plants and have nitrogen in them. Some alkaloids have been shown to work against cancer. [NIH]

Alkylating Agents: Highly reactive chemicals that introduce alkyl radicals into biologically active molecules and thereby prevent their proper functioning. Many are used as antineoplastic agents, but most are very toxic, with carcinogenic, mutagenic, teratogenic, and immunosuppressant actions. They have also been used as components in poison gases. [NIH]

Alleles: Mutually exclusive forms of the same gene, occupying the same locus on homologous chromosomes, and governing the same biochemical and developmental process. [NIH]

Allergic Rhinitis: Inflammation of the nasal mucous membrane associated with hay fever; fits may be provoked by substances in the working environment. [NIH]

Allogeneic: Taken from different individuals of the same species. [NIH]

Allografts: A graft of tissue obtained from the body of another animal of the same species but with genotype differing from that of the recipient; tissue graft from a donor of one genotype to a host of another genotype with host and donor being members of the same species. [NIH]

Alopecia: Absence of hair from areas where it is normally present. [NIH]

Alpha Particles: Positively charged particles composed of two protons and two neutrons, i.e., helium nuclei, emitted during disintegration of very heavy isotopes; a beam of alpha particles or an alpha ray has very strong ionizing power, but weak penetrability. [NIH]

Alternative medicine: Practices not generally recognized by the medical community as standard or conventional medical approaches and used instead of standard treatments. Alternative medicine includes the taking of dietary supplements, megadose vitamins, and herbal preparations; the drinking of special teas; and practices such as massage therapy, magnet therapy, spiritual healing, and meditation. [NIH]

Alveolar Process: The thickest and spongiest part of the maxilla and mandible hollowed out into deep cavities for the teeth. [NIH]

Alveolitis: Inflammation of an alveolus. Called also odontobothritis. [EU]

Ameliorating: A changeable condition which prevents the consequence of a failure or accident from becoming as bad as it otherwise would. [NIH]

Amine: An organic compound containing nitrogen; any member of a group of chemical compounds formed from ammonia by replacement of one or more of the hydrogen atoms by organic (hydrocarbon) radicals. The amines are distinguished as primary, secondary, and tertiary, according to whether one, two, or three hydrogen atoms are replaced. The amines include allylamine, amylamine, ethylamine, methylamine, phenylamine, propylamine, and many other compounds. [EU]

Amino Acid Sequence: The order of amino acids as they occur in a polypeptide chain. This is referred to as the primary structure of proteins. It is of fundamental importance in determining protein conformation. [NIH]

Amino Acids: Organic compounds that generally contain an amino (-NH2) and a carboxyl (-COOH) group. Twenty alpha-amino acids are the subunits which are polymerized to form proteins. [NIH]

Amino Acids: Organic compounds that generally contain an amino (-NH2) and a carboxyl (-COOH) group. Twenty alpha-amino acids are the subunits which are polymerized to form proteins. [NIH]

Amino-terminal: The end of a protein or polypeptide chain that contains a free amino group (-NH2). [NIH]

Amlodipine: 2-((2-Aminoethoxy)methyl)-4-(2-chlorophenyl)-1,4-dihydro-6-methyl-3,5-pyridinedicarboxylic acid 3-ethyl 5-methyl ester. A long-acting dihydropyridine calcium channel blocker. It is effective in the treatment of angina pectoris and hypertension. [NIH]

Ammonia: A colorless alkaline gas. It is formed in the body during decomposition of organic materials during a large number of metabolically important reactions. [NIH]

Amputation: Surgery to remove part or all of a limb or appendage. [NIH]

Amyloidosis: A group of diseases in which protein is deposited in specific organs (localized amyloidosis) or throughout the body (systemic amyloidosis). Amyloidosis may be either primary (with no known cause) or secondary (caused by another disease, including some types of cancer). Generally, primary amyloidosis affects the nerves, skin, tongue, joints, heart, and liver; secondary amyloidosis often affects the spleen, kidneys, liver, and adrenal glands. [NIH]

Anaemia: A reduction below normal in the number of erythrocytes per cu. mm., in the quantity of haemoglobin, or in the volume of packed red cells per 100 ml. of blood which occurs when the equilibrium between blood loss (through bleeding or destruction) and blood production is disturbed. [EU]

Anaesthesia: Loss of feeling or sensation. Although the term is used for loss of tactile sensibility, or of any of the other senses, it is applied especially to loss of the sensation of pain, as it is induced to permit performance of surgery or other painful procedures. [EU]

Anal: Having to do with the anus, which is the posterior opening of the large bowel. [NIH]

Analog: In chemistry, a substance that is similar, but not identical, to another. [NIH]

Analogous: Resembling or similar in some respects, as in function or appearance, but not in origin or development;. [EU]

Analytes: A component of a test sample the presence of which has to be demonstrated. The term "analyte" includes where appropriate formed from the analyte during the analyses. [NIH]

Anaphylatoxins: The family of peptides C3a, C4a, C5a, and C5a des-arginine produced in the serum during complement activation. They produce smooth muscle contraction, mast cell histamine release, affect platelet aggregation, and act as mediators of the local inflammatory process. The order of anaphylatoxin activity from strongest to weakest is C5a, C3a, C4a, and C5a des-arginine. The latter is the so-called "classical" anaphylatoxin but shows no spasmogenic activity though it contains some chemotactic ability. [NIH]

Anatomical: Pertaining to anatomy, or to the structure of the organism. [EU]

Androgens: A class of sex hormones associated with the development and maintenance of the secondary male sex characteristics, sperm induction, and sexual differentiation. In addition to increasing virility and libido, they also increase nitrogen and water retention and stimulate skeletal growth. [NIH]

Anemia: A reduction in the number of circulating erythrocytes or in the quantity of hemoglobin. [NIH]

Anergic: 1. Characterized by abnormal inactivity; inactive. 2. Marked by asthenia or lack of energy. 3. Pertaining to anergy. [EU]

Anergy: Absence of immune response to particular substances. [NIH]

Anesthesia: A state characterized by loss of feeling or sensation. This depression of nerve function is usually the result of pharmacologic action and is induced to allow performance of surgery or other painful procedures. [NIH]

Anesthetics: Agents that are capable of inducing a total or partial loss of sensation, especially tactile sensation and pain. They may act to induce general anesthesia, in which an unconscious state is achieved, or may act locally to induce numbness or lack of sensation at a targeted site. [NIH]

Aneurysm: A sac formed by the dilatation of the wall of an artery, a vein, or the heart. [NIH]

Angina: Chest pain that originates in the heart. [NIH]

Angina Pectoris: The symptom of paroxysmal pain consequent to myocardial ischemia usually of distinctive character, location and radiation, and provoked by a transient stressful situation during which the oxygen requirements of the myocardium exceed the capacity of the coronary circulation to supply it. [NIH]

Anginal: Pertaining to or characteristic of angina. [EU]

Angiogenesis: Blood vessel formation. Tumor angiogenesis is the growth of blood vessels from surrounding tissue to a solid tumor. This is caused by the release of chemicals by the tumor. [NIH]

Angiogenesis inhibitor: A substance that may prevent the formation of blood vessels. In anticancer therapy, an angiogenesis inhibitor prevents the growth of blood vessels from surrounding tissue to a solid tumor. [NIH]

Angiography: Radiography of blood vessels after injection of a contrast medium. [NIH]

Angioplasty: Endovascular reconstruction of an artery, which may include the removal of atheromatous plaque and/or the endothelial lining as well as simple dilatation. These are procedures performed by catheterization. When reconstruction of an artery is performed surgically, it is called endarterectomy. [NIH]

Angiotensin converting enzyme inhibitor: A drug used to decrease pressure inside blood vessels. [NIH]

Angiotensinogen: An alpha-globulin of which a fragment of 14 amino acids is converted by renin to angiotensin I, the inactive precursor of angiotensin II. It is a member of the serpin superfamily. [NIH]

Animal model: An animal with a disease either the same as or like a disease in humans. Animal models are used to study the development and progression of diseases and to test new treatments before they are given to humans. Animals with transplanted human cancers or other tissues are called xenograft models. [NIH]

Anions: Negatively charged atoms, radicals or groups of atoms which travel to the anode or positive pole during electrolysis. [NIH]

Anomalies: Birth defects; abnormalities. [NIH]

Anorexia: Lack or loss of appetite for food. Appetite is psychologic, dependent on memory and associations. Anorexia can be brought about by unattractive food, surroundings, or company. [NIH]

Antagonism: Interference with, or inhibition of, the growth of a living organism by another living organism, due either to creation of unfavorable conditions (e. g. exhaustion of food supplies) or to production of a specific antibiotic substance (e. g. penicillin). [NIH]

Antiallergic: Counteracting allergy or allergic conditions. [EU]

Antianginal: Counteracting angina or anginal conditions. [EU]

Antiarrhythmic: An agent that prevents or alleviates cardiac arrhythmia. [EU]

Antibacterial: A substance that destroys bacteria or suppresses their growth or reproduction. [EU]

Antibiotic: A drug used to treat infections caused by bacteria and other microorganisms. [NIH]

Antibodies: Immunoglobulin molecules having a specific amino acid sequence by virtue of which they interact only with the antigen that induced their synthesis in cells of the lymphoid series (especially plasma cells), or with an antigen closely related to it. [NIH]

Antibody: A type of protein made by certain white blood cells in response to a foreign substance (antigen). Each antibody can bind to only a specific antigen. The purpose of this binding is to help destroy the antigen. Antibodies can work in several ways, depending on the nature of the antigen. Some antibodies destroy antigens directly. Others make it easier for white blood cells to destroy the antigen. [NIH]

Antibody Affinity: A measure of the binding strength between antibody and a simple hapten or antigen determinant. It depends on the closeness of stereochemical fit between antibody combining sites and antigen determinants, on the size of the area of contact between them, and on the distribution of charged and hydrophobic groups. It includes the concept of "avidity," which refers to the strength of the antigen-antibody bond after formation of reversible complexes. [NIH]

Anticoagulant: A drug that helps prevent blood clots from forming. Also called a blood thinner. [NIH]

Antiemetic: An agent that prevents or alleviates nausea and vomiting. Also antinauseant. [EU]

Antigen: Any substance which is capable, under appropriate conditions, of inducing a specific immune response and of reacting with the products of that response, that is, with specific antibody or specifically sensitized T-lymphocytes, or both. Antigens may be soluble substances, such as toxins and foreign proteins, or particulate, such as bacteria and tissue cells; however, only the portion of the protein or polysaccharide molecule known as the antigenic determinant (q.v.) combines with antibody or a specific receptor on a lymphocyte. Abbreviated Ag. [EU]

Antigen-Antibody Complex: The complex formed by the binding of antigen and antibody molecules. The deposition of large antigen-antibody complexes leading to tissue damage causes immune complex diseases. [NIH]

Antigen-presenting cell: APC. A cell that shows antigen on its surface to other cells of the immune system. This is an important part of an immune response. [NIH]

Antihypertensive: An agent that reduces high blood pressure. [EU]

Anti-infective: An agent that so acts. [EU]

Anti-inflammatory: Having to do with reducing inflammation. [NIH]

Anti-Inflammatory Agents: Substances that reduce or suppress inflammation. [NIH]

Antimicrobial: Killing microorganisms, or suppressing their multiplication or growth. [EU]

Antineoplastic: Inhibiting or preventing the development of neoplasms, checking the maturation and proliferation of malignant cells. [EU]

Antineoplastic Agents: Substances that inhibit or prevent the proliferation of neoplasms. [NIH]

Antioxidant: A substance that prevents damage caused by free radicals. Free radicals are highly reactive chemicals that often contain oxygen. They are produced when molecules are split to give products that have unpaired electrons. This process is called oxidation. [NIH]

Antipruritic: Relieving or preventing itching. [EU]

Antipsychotic: Effective in the treatment of psychosis. Antipsychotic drugs (called also neuroleptic drugs and major tranquilizers) are a chemically diverse (including phenothiazines, thioxanthenes, butyrophenones, dibenzoxazepines, dibenzodiazepines, and diphenylbutylpiperidines) but pharmacologically similar class of drugs used to treat schizophrenic, paranoid, schizoaffective, and other psychotic disorders; acute delirium and dementia, and manic episodes (during induction of lithium therapy); to control the movement disorders associated with Huntington's chorea, Gilles de la Tourette's syndrome, and ballismus; and to treat intractable hiccups and severe nausea and vomiting. Antipsychotic agents bind to dopamine, histamine, muscarinic cholinergic, a-adrenergic, and serotonin receptors. Blockade of dopaminergic transmission in various areas is thought to be responsible for their major effects : antipsychotic action by blockade in the mesolimbic and mesocortical areas; extrapyramidal side effects (dystonia, akathisia, parkinsonism, and tardive dyskinesia) by blockade in the basal ganglia; and antiemetic effects by blockade in the chemoreceptor trigger zone of the medulla. Sedation and autonomic side effects (orthostatic hypotension, blurred vision, dry mouth, nasal congestion and constipation) are caused by blockade of histamine, cholinergic, and adrenergic receptors. [EU]

Antiviral: Destroying viruses or suppressing their replication. [EU]

Antiviral Agents: Agents used in the prophylaxis or therapy of virus diseases. Some of the ways they may act include preventing viral replication by inhibiting viral DNA polymerase; binding to specific cell-surface receptors and inhibiting viral penetration or uncoating; inhibiting viral protein synthesis; or blocking late stages of virus assembly. [NIH]

Anuria: Inability to form or excrete urine. [NIH]

Anus: The opening of the rectum to the outside of the body. [NIH]

Anxiety: Persistent feeling of dread, apprehension, and impending disaster. [NIH]

Aorta: The main trunk of the systemic arteries. [NIH]

Aortic Aneurysm: Aneurysm of the aorta. [NIH]

Aphakia: Absence of crystalline lens totally or partially from field of vision, from any cause except after cataract extraction. Aphakia is mainly congenital or as result of lens dislocation and subluxation. [NIH]

Aplastic anemia: A condition in which the bone marrow is unable to produce blood cells. [NIH]

Apoptosis: One of the two mechanisms by which cell death occurs (the other being the pathological process of necrosis). Apoptosis is the mechanism responsible for the physiological deletion of cells and appears to be intrinsically programmed. It is characterized by distinctive morphologic changes in the nucleus and cytoplasm, chromatin cleavage at regularly spaced sites, and the endonucleolytic cleavage of genomic DNA (DNA fragmentation) at internucleosomal sites. This mode of cell death serves as a balance to mitosis in regulating the size of animal tissues and in mediating pathologic processes associated with tumor growth. [NIH]

Aqueous: Having to do with water. [NIH]

Arachidonic Acid: An unsaturated, essential fatty acid. It is found in animal and human fat as well as in the liver, brain, and glandular organs, and is a constituent of animal phosphatides. It is formed by the synthesis from dietary linoleic acid and is a precursor in the biosynthesis of prostaglandins, thromboxanes, and leukotrienes. [NIH]

Arginine: An essential amino acid that is physiologically active in the L-form. [NIH]

Aromatic: Having a spicy odour. [EU]

Arrhythmia: Any variation from the normal rhythm or rate of the heart beat. [NIH]

Arterial: Pertaining to an artery or to the arteries. [EU]

Arteries: The vessels carrying blood away from the heart. [NIH]

Arteriolar: Pertaining to or resembling arterioles. [EU]

Arterioles: The smallest divisions of the arteries located between the muscular arteries and the capillaries. [NIH]

Arteriovenous: Both arterial and venous; pertaining to or affecting an artery and a vein. [EU]

Arthritis, Reactive: An abacterial form of arthritis developing after infection at a site distant from the affected joint or joints. The causative bacteria cannot be cultured from synovial specimens but bacterial antigens have been demonstrated in cells from the synovial fluid and membrane. It often follows Yersinia infection. [NIH]

Arthritis, Rheumatoid: A chronic systemic disease, primarily of the joints, marked by inflammatory changes in the synovial membranes and articular structures, widespread fibrinoid degeneration of the collagen fibers in mesenchymal tissues, and by atrophy and rarefaction of bony structures. Etiology is unknown, but autoimmune mechanisms have been implicated. [NIH]

Arthrosis: A disease of a joint. [EU]

Articular: Of or pertaining to a joint. [EU]

Ascites: Accumulation or retention of free fluid within the peritoneal cavity. [NIH]

Ascorbic Acid: A six carbon compound related to glucose. It is found naturally in citrus fruits and many vegetables. Ascorbic acid is an essential nutrient in human diets, and necessary to maintain connective tissue and bone. Its biologically active form, vitamin C, functions as a reducing agent and coenzyme in several metabolic pathways. Vitamin C is considered an antioxidant. [NIH]

Aspiration: The act of inhaling. [NIH]

Aspirin: A drug that reduces pain, fever, inflammation, and blood clotting. Aspirin belongs to the family of drugs called nonsteroidal anti-inflammatory agents. It is also being studied in cancer prevention. [NIH]

Assay: Determination of the amount of a particular constituent of a mixture, or of the biological or pharmacological potency of a drug. [EU]

Asthenia: Clinical sign or symptom manifested as debility, or lack or loss of strength and energy. [NIH]

Astringents: Agents, usually topical, that cause the contraction of tissues for the control of bleeding or secretions. [NIH]

Asymptomatic: Having no signs or symptoms of disease. [NIH]

Ataxia: Impairment of the ability to perform smoothly coordinated voluntary movements. This condition may affect the limbs, trunk, eyes, pharnyx, larnyx, and other structures. Ataxia may result from impaired sensory or motor function. Sensory ataxia may result from posterior column injury or peripheral nerve diseases. Motor ataxia may be associated with cerebellar diseases; cerebral cortex diseases; thalamic diseases; basal ganglia diseases; injury to the red nucleus; and other conditions. [NIH]

Atherectomy: Endovascular procedure in which atheromatous plaque is excised by a cutting or rotating catheter. It differs from balloon and laser angioplasty procedures which enlarge vessels by dilation but frequently do not remove much plaque. If the plaque is removed by surgical excision under general anesthesia rather than by an endovascular procedure through a catheter, it is called endarterectomy. [NIH]

Atmospheric Pressure: The pressure at any point in an atmosphere due solely to the weight of the atmospheric gases above the point concerned. [NIH]

Atopic: Pertaining to an atopen or to atopy; allergic. [EU]

Atrial: Pertaining to an atrium. [EU]

Atrial Fibrillation: Disorder of cardiac rhythm characterized by rapid, irregular atrial impulses and ineffective atrial contractions. [NIH]

Atrial Flutter: Rapid, irregular atrial contractions due to an abnormality of atrial excitation. [NIH]

Atrioventricular: Pertaining to an atrium of the heart and to a ventricle. [EU]

Atrioventricular Node: A small nodular mass of specialized muscle fibers located in the interatrial septum near the opening of the coronary sinus. It gives rise to the atrioventricular bundle of the conduction system of the heart. [NIH]

Atrium: A chamber; used in anatomical nomenclature to designate a chamber affording entrance to another structure or organ. Usually used alone to designate an atrium of the heart. [EU]

Atrophy: Decrease in the size of a cell, tissue, organ, or multiple organs, associated with a variety of pathological conditions such as abnormal cellular changes, ischemia, malnutrition, or hormonal changes. [NIH]

Attenuated: Strain with weakened or reduced virulence. [NIH]

Autoantibodies: Antibodies that react with self-antigens (autoantigens) of the organism that produced them. [NIH]

Autoantigens: Endogenous tissue constituents that have the ability to interact with autoantibodies and cause an immune response. [NIH]

Autoimmune disease: A condition in which the body recognizes its own tissues as foreign and directs an immune response against them. [NIH]

Autoimmunity: Process whereby the immune system reacts against the body's own tissues. Autoimmunity may produce or be caused by autoimmune diseases. [NIH]

Autologous: Taken from an individual's own tissues, cells, or DNA. [NIH]

Autonomic: Self-controlling; functionally independent. [EU]

Autonomic Nervous System: The enteric, parasympathetic, and sympathetic nervous systems taken together. Generally speaking, the autonomic nervous system regulates the internal environment during both peaceful activity and physical or emotional stress. Autonomic activity is controlled and integrated by the central nervous system, especially the hypothalamus and the solitary nucleus, which receive information relayed from visceral afferents; these and related central and sensory structures are sometimes (but not here) considered to be part of the autonomic nervous system itself. [NIH]

Autopsy: Postmortem examination of the body. [NIH]

Autoradiography: A process in which radioactive material within an object produces an image when it is in close proximity to a radiation sensitive emulsion. [NIH]

Avian: A plasmodial infection in birds. [NIH]

Avidity: The strength of the interaction of an antiserum with a multivalent antigen. [NIH]

Azotemia: An excess of urea or other nitrogenous compounds in the blood. [EU]

Bacillus: A genus of Bacillaceae that are spore-forming, rod-shaped cells. Most species are saprophytic soil forms with only a few species being pathogenic. [NIH]

Backcross: A cross between a hybrid and either one of its parents. [NIH]

Bacteria: Unicellular prokaryotic microorganisms which generally possess rigid cell walls, multiply by cell division, and exhibit three principal forms: round or coccal, rodlike or bacillary, and spiral or spirochetal. [NIH]

Bacterial Infections: Infections by bacteria, general or unspecified. [NIH]

Bacteriophage: A virus whose host is a bacterial cell; A virus that exclusively infects bacteria. It generally has a protein coat surrounding the genome (DNA or RNA). One of the coliphages most extensively studied is the lambda phage, which is also one of the most important. [NIH]

Bacterium: Microscopic organism which may have a spherical, rod-like, or spiral unicellular or non-cellular body. Bacteria usually reproduce through asexual processes. [NIH]

Bacteriuria: The presence of bacteria in the urine with or without consequent urinary tract infection. Since bacteriuria is a clinical entity, the term does not preclude the use of urine/microbiology for technical discussions on the isolation and segregation of bacteria in the urine. [NIH]

Barbiturate: A drug with sedative and hypnotic effects. Barbiturates have been used as sedatives and anesthetics, and they have been used to treat the convulsions associated with epilepsy. [NIH]

Basal Ganglia: Large subcortical nuclear masses derived from the telencephalon and located in the basal regions of the cerebral hemispheres. [NIH]

Basal Ganglia Diseases: Diseases of the basal ganglia including the putamen; globus pallidus; claustrum; amygdala; and caudate nucleus. Dyskinesias (most notably involuntary movements and alterations of the rate of movement) represent the primary clinical manifestations of these disorders. Common etiologies include cerebrovascular disease; neurodegenerative diseases; and craniocerebral trauma. [NIH]

Base: In chemistry, the nonacid part of a salt; a substance that combines with acids to form salts; a substance that dissociates to give hydroxide ions in aqueous solutions; a substance whose molecule or ion can combine with a proton (hydrogen ion); a substance capable of donating a pair of electrons (to an acid) for the formation of a coordinate covalent bond. [EU]

Basement Membrane: Ubiquitous supportive tissue adjacent to epithelium and around smooth and striated muscle cells. This tissue contains intrinsic macromolecular components such as collagen, laminin, and sulfated proteoglycans. As seen by light microscopy one of its subdivisions is the basal (basement) lamina. [NIH]

Basophil: A type of white blood cell. Basophils are granulocytes. [NIH]

Benign: Not cancerous; does not invade nearby tissue or spread to other parts of the body. [NIH]

Benzene: Toxic, volatile, flammable liquid hydrocarbon biproduct of coal distillation. It is used as an industrial solvent in paints, varnishes, lacquer thinners, gasoline, etc. Benzene causes central nervous system damage acutely and bone marrow damage chronically and is carcinogenic. It was formerly used as parasiticide. [NIH]

Bewilderment: Impairment or loss of will power. [NIH]

Bile: An emulsifying agent produced in the liver and secreted into the duodenum. Its composition includes bile acids and salts, cholesterol, and electrolytes. It aids digestion of fats in the duodenum. [NIH]

Bile Acids: Acids made by the liver that work with bile to break down fats. [NIH]

Bile Acids and Salts: Steroid acids and salts. The primary bile acids are derived from cholesterol in the liver and usually conjugated with glycine or taurine. The secondary bile acids are further modified by bacteria in the intestine. They play an important role in the digestion and absorption of fat. They have also been used pharmacologically, especially in the treatment of gallstones. [NIH]

Bile Ducts: Tubes that carry bile from the liver to the gallbladder for storage and to the small intestine for use in digestion. [NIH]

Biliary: Having to do with the liver, bile ducts, and/or gallbladder. [NIH]

Bilirubin: A bile pigment that is a degradation product of heme. [NIH]

Binding Sites: The reactive parts of a macromolecule that directly participate in its specific combination with another molecule. [NIH]

Biochemical: Relating to biochemistry; characterized by, produced by, or involving chemical reactions in living organisms. [EU]

Biogenesis: The origin of life. It includes studies of the potential basis for life in organic compounds but excludes studies of the development of altered forms of life through mutation and natural selection, which is evolution. [NIH]

Biological response modifier: BRM. A substance that stimulates the body's response to infection and disease. [NIH]

Biological therapy: Treatment to stimulate or restore the ability of the immune system to fight infection and disease. Also used to lessen side effects that may be caused by some cancer treatments. Also known as immunotherapy, biotherapy, or biological response modifier (BRM) therapy. [NIH]

Biomarkers: Substances sometimes found in an increased amount in the blood, other body fluids, or tissues and that may suggest the presence of some types of cancer. Biomarkers include CA 125 (ovarian cancer), CA 15-3 (breast cancer), CEA (ovarian, lung, breast, pancreas, and GI tract cancers), and PSA (prostate cancer). Also called tumor markers. [NIH]

Biopsy: Removal and pathologic examination of specimens in the form of small pieces of tissue from the living body. [NIH]

Biopsy specimen: Tissue removed from the body and examined under a microscope to determine whether disease is present. [NIH]

Biosynthesis: The building up of a chemical compound in the physiologic processes of a living organism. [EU]

Biotechnology: Body of knowledge related to the use of organisms, cells or cell-derived constituents for the purpose of developing products which are technically, scientifically and clinically useful. Alteration of biologic function at the molecular level (i.e., genetic engineering) is a central focus; laboratory methods used include transfection and cloning technologies, sequence and structure analysis algorithms, computer databases, and gene and protein structure function analysis and prediction. [NIH]

Biotransformation: The chemical alteration of an exogenous substance by or in a biological system. The alteration may inactivate the compound or it may result in the production of an active metabolite of an inactive parent compound. The alteration may be either non-synthetic (oxidation-reduction, hydrolysis) or synthetic (glucuronide formation, sulfate conjugation, acetylation, methylation). This also includes metabolic detoxication and clearance. [NIH]

Bladder: The organ that stores urine. [NIH]

Blebs: Cysts on or near the surface of the lungs. [NIH]

Bleomycin: A complex of related glycopeptide antibiotics from Streptomyces verticillus consisting of bleomycin A2 and B2. It inhibits DNA metabolism and is used as an antineoplastic, especially for solid tumors. [NIH]

Blister: Visible accumulations of fluid within or beneath the epidermis. [NIH]

Bloating: Fullness or swelling in the abdomen that often occurs after meals. [NIH]

Blood Coagulation: The process of the interaction of blood coagulation factors that results in an insoluble fibrin clot. [NIH]

Blood Glucose: Glucose in blood. [NIH]

Blood Platelets: Non-nucleated disk-shaped cells formed in the megakaryocyte and found in the blood of all mammals. They are mainly involved in blood coagulation. [NIH]

Blood pressure: The pressure of blood against the walls of a blood vessel or heart chamber. Unless there is reference to another location, such as the pulmonary artery or one of the heart chambers, it refers to the pressure in the systemic arteries, as measured, for example, in the forearm. [NIH]

Blood vessel: A tube in the body through which blood circulates. Blood vessels include a network of arteries, arterioles, capillaries, venules, and veins. [NIH]

Blood-Brain Barrier: Specialized non-fenestrated tightly-joined endothelial cells (tight junctions) that form a transport barrier for certain substances between the cerebral capillaries and the brain tissue. [NIH]

Blot: To transfer DNA, RNA, or proteins to an immobilizing matrix such as nitrocellulose. [NIH]

Blotting, Western: Identification of proteins or peptides that have been electrophoretically separated by blotting and transferred to strips of nitrocellulose paper. The blots are then detected by radiolabeled antibody probes. [NIH]

Body Fluids: Liquid components of living organisms. [NIH]

Bone Density: The amount of mineral per square centimeter of bone. This is the definition used in clinical practice. Actual bone density would be expressed in grams per milliliter. It is most frequently measured by photon absorptiometry or x-ray computed tomography. [NIH]

Bone Marrow: The soft tissue filling the cavities of bones. Bone marrow exists in two types, yellow and red. Yellow marrow is found in the large cavities of large bones and consists mostly of fat cells and a few primitive blood cells. Red marrow is a hematopoietic tissue and is the site of production of erythrocytes and granular leukocytes. Bone marrow is made up of a framework of connective tissue containing branching fibers with the frame being filled with marrow cells. [NIH]

Bone Marrow Transplantation: The transference of bone marrow from one human or animal to another. [NIH]

Bone Resorption: Bone loss due to osteoclastic activity. [NIH]

Bone scan: A technique to create images of bones on a computer screen or on film. A small amount of radioactive material is injected into a blood vessel and travels through the bloodstream; it collects in the bones and is detected by a scanner. [NIH]

Boron: A trace element with the atomic symbol B, atomic number 5, and atomic weight 10.81. Boron-10, an isotope of boron, is used as a neutron absorber in boron neutron capture therapy. [NIH]

Bowel: The long tube-shaped organ in the abdomen that completes the process of digestion. There is both a small and a large bowel. Also called the intestine. [NIH]

Bowel Movement: Body wastes passed through the rectum and anus. [NIH]

Brachytherapy: A collective term for interstitial, intracavity, and surface radiotherapy. It uses small sealed or partly-sealed sources that may be placed on or near the body surface or within a natural body cavity or implanted directly into the tissues. [NIH]

Bradykinin: A nonapeptide messenger that is enzymatically produced from kallidin in the blood where it is a potent but short-lived agent of arteriolar dilation and increased capillary permeability. Bradykinin is also released from mast cells during asthma attacks, from gut walls as a gastrointestinal vasodilator, from damaged tissues as a pain signal, and may be a neurotransmitter. [NIH]

Branch: Most commonly used for branches of nerves, but applied also to other structures. [NIH]

Breakdown: A physical, metal, or nervous collapse. [NIH]

Broadband: A wide frequency range. Sound whose energy is distributed over a broad range of frequency (generally, more than one octave). [NIH]

Bronchi: The larger air passages of the lungs arising from the terminal bifurcation of the trachea. [NIH]

Bronchial: Pertaining to one or more bronchi. [EU]

Bronchitis: Inflammation (swelling and reddening) of the bronchi. [NIH]

Bronchoalveolar Lavage: Washing out of the lungs with saline or mucolytic agents for diagnostic or therapeutic purposes. It is very useful in the diagnosis of diffuse pulmonary infiltrates in immunosuppressed patients. [NIH]

Bronchoalveolar Lavage Fluid: Fluid obtained by washout of the alveolar compartment of the lung. It is used to assess biochemical and inflammatory changes in and effects of therapy on the interstitial lung tissue. [NIH]

Bronchoconstriction: Diminution of the caliber of a bronchus physiologically or as a result of pharmacological intervention. [NIH]

Bronchoscopy: Endoscopic examination, therapy or surgery of the bronchi. [NIH]

Bronchus: A large air passage that leads from the trachea (windpipe) to the lung. [NIH]

Buccal: Pertaining to or directed toward the cheek. In dental anatomy, used to refer to the buccal surface of a tooth. [EU]

Bullous: Pertaining to or characterized by bullae. [EU]

Burns: Injuries to tissues caused by contact with heat, steam, chemicals (burns, chemical), electricity (burns, electric), or the like. [NIH]

Burns, Electric: Burns produced by contact with electric current or from a sudden discharge of electricity. [NIH]

Bypass: A surgical procedure in which the doctor creates a new pathway for the flow of body fluids. [NIH]

Calcifediol: The major circulating metabolite of vitamin D3 produced in the liver and the best indicator of the body's vitamin D stores. It is effective in the treatment of rickets and osteomalacia, both in azotemic and non-azotemic patients. Calcifediol also has mineralizing properties. [NIH]

Calcification: Deposits of calcium in the tissues of the breast. Calcification in the breast can be seen on a mammogram, but cannot be detected by touch. There are two types of breast calcification, macrocalcification and microcalcification. Macrocalcifications are large deposits and are usually not related to cancer. Microcalcifications are specks of calcium that may be found in an area of rapidly dividing cells. Many microcalcifications clustered together may be a sign of cancer. [NIH]

Calcinosis: Pathologic deposition of calcium salts in tissues. [NIH]

Calcitriol: The physiologically active form of vitamin D. It is formed primarily in the kidney by enzymatic hydroxylation of 25-hydroxycholecalciferol (calcifediol). Its production is stimulated by low blood calcium levels and parathyroid hormone. Calcitriol increases intestinal absorption of calcium and phosphorus, and in concert with parathyroid hormone increases bone resorption. [NIH]

Calcium: A basic element found in nearly all organized tissues. It is a member of the alkaline earth family of metals with the atomic symbol Ca, atomic number 20, and atomic weight 40. Calcium is the most abundant mineral in the body and combines with phosphorus to form calcium phosphate in the bones and teeth. It is essential for the normal functioning of nerves and muscles and plays a role in blood coagulation (as factor IV) and in many enzymatic processes. [NIH]

Calcium channel blocker: A drug used to relax the blood vessel and heart muscle, causing pressure inside blood vessels to drop. It also can regulate heart rhythm. [NIH]

Calcium Channel Blockers: A class of drugs that act by selective inhibition of calcium influx through cell membranes or on the release and binding of calcium in intracellular pools. Since they are inducers of vascular and other smooth muscle relaxation, they are used in the drug therapy of hypertension and cerebrovascular spasms, as myocardial protective agents, and in the relaxation of uterine spasms. [NIH]

Calcium Channels: Voltage-dependent cell membrane glycoproteins selectively permeable to calcium ions. They are categorized as L-, T-, N-, P-, Q-, and R-types based on the activation and inactivation kinetics, ion specificity, and sensitivity to drugs and toxins. The L- and T-types are present throughout the cardiovascular and central nervous systems and the N-, P-, Q-, & R-types are located in neuronal tissue. [NIH]

Calmodulin: A heat-stable, low-molecular-weight activator protein found mainly in the brain and heart. The binding of calcium ions to this protein allows this protein to bind to cyclic nucleotide phosphodiesterases and to adenyl cyclase with subsequent activation. Thereby this protein modulates cyclic AMP and cyclic GMP levels. [NIH]

Camptothecin: An alkaloid isolated from the stem wood of the Chinese tree, Camptotheca acuminata. This compound selectively inhibits the nuclear enzyme DNA topoisomerase. Several semisynthetic analogs of camptothecin have demonstrated antitumor activity. [NIH]

Candidiasis: Infection with a fungus of the genus Candida. It is usually a superficial infection of the moist cutaneous areas of the body, and is generally caused by C. albicans; it most commonly involves the skin (dermatocandidiasis), oral mucous membranes (thrush, def. 1), respiratory tract (bronchocandidiasis), and vagina (vaginitis). Rarely there is a systemic infection or endocarditis. Called also moniliasis, candidosis, oidiomycosis, and formerly blastodendriosis. [EU]

Candidosis: An infection caused by an opportunistic yeasts that tends to proliferate and become pathologic when the environment is favorable and the host resistance is weakened. [NIH]

Capillary: Any one of the minute vessels that connect the arterioles and venules, forming a network in nearly all parts of the body. Their walls act as semipermeable membranes for the interchange of various substances, including fluids, between the blood and tissue fluid; called also vas capillare. [EU]

Capillary Permeability: Property of blood capillary walls that allows for the selective exchange of substances. Small lipid-soluble molecules such as carbon dioxide and oxygen move freely by diffusion. Water and water-soluble molecules cannot pass through the endothelial walls and are dependent on microscopic pores. These pores show narrow areas (tight junctions) which may limit large molecule movement. [NIH]

Capsules: Hard or soft soluble containers used for the oral administration of medicine. [NIH]

Captopril: A potent and specific inhibitor of peptidyl-dipeptidase A. It blocks the conversion of angiotensin I to angiotensin II, a vasoconstrictor and important regulator of arterial blood pressure. Captopril acts to suppress the renin-angiotensin system and inhibits pressure responses to exogenous angiotensin. [NIH]

Carbidopa: A peripheral inhibitor of dopa decarboxylase. It is given in parkinsonism along with levodopa to inhibit the conversion of levodopa to dopamine in the periphery, thereby reducing the peripheral adverse effects, increasing the amount of levodopa that reaches the central nervous system, and reducing the dose needed. It has no antiparkinson actions when given alone. [NIH]

Carbohydrate: An aldehyde or ketone derivative of a polyhydric alcohol, particularly of the pentahydric and hexahydric alcohols. They are so named because the hydrogen and oxygen are usually in the proportion to form water, $(CH2O)n$. The most important carbohydrates are the starches, sugars, celluloses, and gums. They are classified into mono-, di-, tri-, poly- and heterosaccharides. [EU]

Carbon Dioxide: A colorless, odorless gas that can be formed by the body and is necessary for the respiration cycle of plants and animals. [NIH]

Carboplatin: An organoplatinum compound that possesses antineoplastic activity. [NIH]

Carboxy: Cannabinoid. [NIH]

Carcinogenic: Producing carcinoma. [EU]

Carcinogens: Substances that increase the risk of neoplasms in humans or animals. Both genotoxic chemicals, which affect DNA directly, and nongenotoxic chemicals, which induce neoplasms by other mechanism, are included. [NIH]

Carcinoma: Cancer that begins in the skin or in tissues that line or cover internal organs. [NIH]

Cardiac: Having to do with the heart. [NIH]

Cardiac Output: The volume of blood passing through the heart per unit of time. It is usually expressed as liters (volume) per minute so as not to be confused with stroke volume (volume per beat). [NIH]

Cardiomyopathy: A general diagnostic term designating primary myocardial disease, often of obscure or unknown etiology. [EU]

Cardiovascular: Having to do with the heart and blood vessels. [NIH]

Cardiovascular System: The heart and the blood vessels by which blood is pumped and circulated through the body. [NIH]

Carotene: The general name for a group of pigments found in green, yellow, and leafy vegetables, and yellow fruits. The pigments are fat-soluble, unsaturated aliphatic hydrocarbons functioning as provitamins and are converted to vitamin A through enzymatic processes in the intestinal wall. [NIH]

Case report: A detailed report of the diagnosis, treatment, and follow-up of an individual patient. Case reports also contain some demographic information about the patient (for example, age, gender, ethnic origin). [NIH]

Catalyse: To speed up a chemical reaction. [EU]

Cataract: An opacity, partial or complete, of one or both eyes, on or in the lens or capsule, especially an opacity impairing vision or causing blindness. The many kinds of cataract are classified by their morphology (size, shape, location) or etiology (cause and time of occurrence). [EU]

Catecholamine: A group of chemical substances manufactured by the adrenal medulla and secreted during physiological stress. [NIH]

Catheterization: Use or insertion of a tubular device into a duct, blood vessel, hollow organ, or body cavity for injecting or withdrawing fluids for diagnostic or therapeutic purposes. It differs from intubation in that the tube here is used to restore or maintain patency in obstructions. [NIH]

Catheters: A small, flexible tube that may be inserted into various parts of the body to inject or remove liquids. [NIH]

Cations: Postively charged atoms, radicals or groups of atoms which travel to the cathode or negative pole during electrolysis. [NIH]

Cause of Death: Factors which produce cessation of all vital bodily functions. They can be analyzed from an epidemiologic viewpoint. [NIH]

Caustic: An escharotic or corrosive agent. Called also cauterant. [EU]

Cecum: The beginning of the large intestine. The cecum is connected to the lower part of the small intestine, called the ileum. [NIH]

Cell: The individual unit that makes up all of the tissues of the body. All living things are made up of one or more cells. [NIH]

Cell Adhesion: Adherence of cells to surfaces or to other cells. [NIH]

Cell Cycle: The complex series of phenomena, occurring between the end of one cell division and the end of the next, by which cellular material is divided between daughter cells. [NIH]

Cell Death: The termination of the cell's ability to carry out vital functions such as metabolism, growth, reproduction, responsiveness, and adaptability. [NIH]

Cell Differentiation: Progressive restriction of the developmental potential and increasing specialization of function which takes place during the development of the embryo and leads to the formation of specialized cells, tissues, and organs. [NIH]

Cell Division: The fission of a cell. [NIH]

Cell membrane: Cell membrane = plasma membrane. The structure enveloping a cell, enclosing the cytoplasm, and forming a selective permeability barrier; it consists of lipids, proteins, and some carbohydrates, the lipids thought to form a bilayer in which integral proteins are embedded to varying degrees. [EU]

Cell Nucleolus: A small dense body (sub organelle) within the nucleus of eukaryotic cells, visible by phase contrast and interference microscopy in live cells throughout interphase. Contains RNA and protein and is the site of synthesis of ribosomal RNA. [NIH]

Cell proliferation: An increase in the number of cells as a result of cell growth and cell division. [NIH]

Cell Size: The physical dimensions of a cell. It refers mainly to changes in dimensions correlated with physiological or pathological changes in cells. [NIH]

Cell Survival: The span of viability of a cell characterized by the capacity to perform certain functions such as metabolism, growth, reproduction, some form of responsiveness, and adaptability. [NIH]

Cell Transplantation: Transference of cells within an individual, between individuals of the same species, or between individuals of different species. [NIH]

Cellular metabolism: The sum of all chemical changes that take place in a cell through which energy and basic components are provided for essential processes, including the synthesis of new molecules and the breakdown and removal of others. [NIH]

Cellular Structures: Components of a cell. [NIH]

Cellulose: A polysaccharide with glucose units linked as in cellobiose. It is the chief constituent of plant fibers, cotton being the purest natural form of the substance. As a raw material, it forms the basis for many derivatives used in chromatography, ion exchange materials, explosives manufacturing, and pharmaceutical preparations. [NIH]

Central Nervous System: The main information-processing organs of the nervous system, consisting of the brain, spinal cord, and meninges. [NIH]

Central Nervous System Infections: Pathogenic infections of the brain, spinal cord, and meninges. DNA virus infections; RNA virus infections; bacterial infections; mycoplasma infections; Spirochaetales infections; fungal infections; protozoan infections; helminthiasis; and prion diseases may involve the central nervous system as a primary or secondary process. [NIH]

Centromere: The clear constricted portion of the chromosome at which the chromatids are joined and by which the chromosome is attached to the spindle during cell division. [NIH]

Ceramide: A type of fat produced in the body. It may cause some types of cells to die, and is being studied in cancer treatment. [NIH]

Cerebellar: Pertaining to the cerebellum. [EU]

Cerebral: Of or pertaining of the cerebrum or the brain. [EU]

Cerebrovascular: Pertaining to the blood vessels of the cerebrum, or brain. [EU]

Cerebrum: The largest part of the brain. It is divided into two hemispheres, or halves, called the cerebral hemispheres. The cerebrum controls muscle functions of the body and also controls speech, emotions, reading, writing, and learning. [NIH]

Cervical: Relating to the neck, or to the neck of any organ or structure. Cervical lymph nodes are located in the neck; cervical cancer refers to cancer of the uterine cervix, which is the lower, narrow end (the "neck") of the uterus. [NIH]

Cervix: The lower, narrow end of the uterus that forms a canal between the uterus and vagina. [NIH]

Character: In current usage, approximately equivalent to personality. The sum of the relatively fixed personality traits and habitual modes of response of an individual. [NIH]

Chelation: Combination with a metal in complexes in which the metal is part of a ring. [EU]

Chemokines: Class of pro-inflammatory cytokines that have the ability to attract and activate leukocytes. They can be divided into at least three structural branches: C (chemokines, C), CC (chemokines, CC), and CXC (chemokines, CXC), according to variations in a shared cysteine motif. [NIH]

Chemotactic Factors: Chemical substances that attract or repel cells or organisms. The concept denotes especially those factors released as a result of tissue injury, invasion, or immunologic activity, that attract leukocytes, macrophages, or other cells to the site of infection or insult. [NIH]

Chemotaxis: The movement of cells or organisms toward or away from a substance in response to its concentration gradient. [NIH]

Chemotherapy: Treatment with anticancer drugs. [NIH]

Chenodeoxycholic Acid: A bile acid, usually conjugated with either glycine or taurine. It acts as a detergent to solubilize fats for intestinal absorption and is reabsorbed by the small intestine. It is used as cholagogue, a choleretic laxative, and to prevent or dissolve gallstones. [NIH]

Chest Pain: Pressure, burning, or numbness in the chest. [NIH]

Chlamydia: A genus of the family Chlamydiaceae whose species cause a variety of diseases in vertebrates including humans, mice, and swine. Chlamydia species are gram-negative and produce glycogen. The type species is Chlamydia trachomatis. [NIH]

Chlorophyll: Porphyrin derivatives containing magnesium that act to convert light energy in photosynthetic organisms. [NIH]

Cholangitis: Inflammation of a bile duct. [NIH]

Choleretic: A choleretic agent. [EU]

Cholesterol: The principal sterol of all higher animals, distributed in body tissues, especially the brain and spinal cord, and in animal fats and oils. [NIH]

Chondroitin sulfate: The major glycosaminoglycan (a type of sugar molecule) in cartilage. [NIH]

Chromatin: The material of chromosomes. It is a complex of DNA, histones, and nonhistone proteins (chromosomal proteins, non-histone) found within the nucleus of a cell. [NIH]

Chromosomal: Pertaining to chromosomes. [EU]

Chromosome: Part of a cell that contains genetic information. Except for sperm and eggs, all human cells contain 46 chromosomes. [NIH]

Chronic: A disease or condition that persists or progresses over a long period of time. [NIH]

Chronic Disease: Disease or ailment of long duration. [NIH]

Chronic Obstructive Pulmonary Disease: Collective term for chronic bronchitis and emphysema. [NIH]

Chronic renal: Slow and progressive loss of kidney function over several years, often resulting in end-stage renal disease. People with end-stage renal disease need dialysis or transplantation to replace the work of the kidneys. [NIH]

Cicatrix: The formation of new tissue in the process of wound healing. [NIH]

Circulatory system: The system that contains the heart and the blood vessels and moves blood throughout the body. This system helps tissues get enough oxygen and nutrients, and it helps them get rid of waste products. The lymph system, which connects with the blood system, is often considered part of the circulatory system. [NIH]

CIS: Cancer Information Service. The CIS is the National Cancer Institute's link to the public, interpreting and explaining research findings in a clear and understandable manner, and providing personalized responses to specific questions about cancer. Access the CIS by calling 1-800-4-CANCER, or by using the Web site at http://cis.nci.nih.gov. [NIH]

Citrus: Any tree or shrub of the Rue family or the fruit of these plants. [NIH]

Clinical Medicine: The study and practice of medicine by direct examination of the patient. [NIH]

Clinical trial: A research study that tests how well new medical treatments or other interventions work in people. Each study is designed to test new methods of screening, prevention, diagnosis, or treatment of a disease. [NIH]

Clonal Deletion: Removal, via cell death, of immature lymphocytes that interact with antigens during maturation. For T-lymphocytes this occurs in the thymus and ensures that mature T-lymphocytes are self tolerant. B-lymphocytes may also undergo clonal deletion. [NIH]

Clone: The term "clone" has acquired a new meaning. It is applied specifically to the bits of inserted foreign DNA in the hybrid molecules of the population. Each inserted segment originally resided in the DNA of a complex genome amid millions of other DNA segment. [NIH]

Cloning: The production of a number of genetically identical individuals; in genetic engineering, a process for the efficient replication of a great number of identical DNA molecules. [NIH]

Cluster Analysis: A set of statistical methods used to group variables or observations into strongly inter-related subgroups. In epidemiology, it may be used to analyze a closely grouped series of events or cases of disease or other health-related phenomenon with well-defined distribution patterns in relation to time or place or both. [NIH]

Coagulation: 1. The process of clot formation. 2. In colloid chemistry, the solidification of a sol into a gelatinous mass; an alteration of a disperse phase or of a dissolved solid which causes the separation of the system into a liquid phase and an insoluble mass called the clot or curd. Coagulation is usually irreversible. 3. In surgery, the disruption of tissue by physical means to form an amorphous residuum, as in electrocoagulation and photocoagulation. [EU]

Coculture: The culturing of normal cells or tissues with infected or latently infected cells or tissues of the same kind (From Dorland, 28th ed, entry for cocultivation). It also includes culturing of normal cells or tissues with other normal cells or tissues. [NIH]

Coenzyme: An organic nonprotein molecule, frequently a phosphorylated derivative of a water-soluble vitamin, that binds with the protein molecule (apoenzyme) to form the active enzyme (holoenzyme). [EU]

Cofactor: A substance, microorganism or environmental factor that activates or enhances the action of another entity such as a disease-causing agent. [NIH]

Cognitive restructuring: A method of identifying and replacing fear-promoting, irrational beliefs with more realistic and functional ones. [NIH]

Colitis: Inflammation of the colon. [NIH]

Collagen: A polypeptide substance comprising about one third of the total protein in mammalian organisms. It is the main constituent of skin, connective tissue, and the organic substance of bones and teeth. Different forms of collagen are produced in the body but all consist of three alpha-polypeptide chains arranged in a triple helix. Collagen is differentiated from other fibrous proteins, such as elastin, by the content of proline, hydroxyproline, and hydroxylysine; by the absence of tryptophan; and particularly by the high content of polar groups which are responsible for its swelling properties. [NIH]

Collagen disease: A term previously used to describe chronic diseases of the connective tissue (e.g., rheumatoid arthritis, systemic lupus erythematosus, and systemic sclerosis), but now is thought to be more appropriate for diseases associated with defects in collagen, which is a component of the connective tissue. [NIH]

Colloidal: Of the nature of a colloid. [EU]

Combination Therapy: Association of 3 drugs to treat AIDS (AZT + DDC or DDI + protease inhibitor). [NIH]

Combinatorial: A cut-and-paste process that churns out thousands of potentially valuable compounds at once. [NIH]

Comedo: A plug of keratin and sebum within the dilated orifice of a hair follicle, frequently containing the bacteria Propionibacterium acnes, Staphylococcus albus, and Pityrosporon ovale; called also blackhead. [EU]

Complement: A term originally used to refer to the heat-labile factor in serum that causes immune cytolysis, the lysis of antibody-coated cells, and now referring to the entire functionally related system comprising at least 20 distinct serum proteins that is the effector not only of immune cytolysis but also of other biologic functions. Complement activation occurs by two different sequences, the classic and alternative pathways. The proteins of the classic pathway are termed 'components of complement' and are designated by the symbols C1 through C9. C1 is a calcium-dependent complex of three distinct proteins C1q, C1r and C1s. The proteins of the alternative pathway (collectively referred to as the properdin system) and complement regulatory proteins are known by semisystematic or trivial names. Fragments resulting from proteolytic cleavage of complement proteins are designated with lower-case letter suffixes, e.g., C3a. Inactivated fragments may be designated with the suffix 'i', e.g. C3bi. Activated components or complexes with biological activity are designated by a bar over the symbol e.g. C1 or C4b,2a. The classic pathway is activated by the binding of C1 to classic pathway activators, primarily antigen-antibody complexes containing IgM, IgG1, IgG3; C1q binds to a single IgM molecule or two adjacent IgG molecules. The alternative pathway can be activated by IgA immune complexes and also by nonimmunologic materials including bacterial endotoxins, microbial polysaccharides, and cell walls. Activation of the classic pathway triggers an enzymatic cascade involving C1, C4, C2 and C3; activation of the alternative pathway triggers a cascade involving C3 and factors B, D and P. Both result in the cleavage of C5 and the formation of the membrane attack complex. Complement activation also results in the formation of many biologically active complement fragments that act as anaphylatoxins, opsonins, or chemotactic factors. [EU]

Complementary and alternative medicine: CAM. Forms of treatment that are used in addition to (complementary) or instead of (alternative) standard treatments. These practices are not considered standard medical approaches. CAM includes dietary supplements, megadose vitamins, herbal preparations, special teas, massage therapy, magnet therapy, spiritual healing, and meditation. [NIH]

Complementary medicine: Practices not generally recognized by the medical community as standard or conventional medical approaches and used to enhance or complement the standard treatments. Complementary medicine includes the taking of dietary supplements, megadose vitamins, and herbal preparations; the drinking of special teas; and practices such as massage therapy, magnet therapy, spiritual healing, and meditation. [NIH]

Computational Biology: A field of biology concerned with the development of techniques for the collection and manipulation of biological data, and the use of such data to make biological discoveries or predictions. This field encompasses all computational methods and theories applicable to molecular biology and areas of computer-based techniques for solving biological problems including manipulation of models and datasets. [NIH]

Computed tomography: CT scan. A series of detailed pictures of areas inside the body, taken from different angles; the pictures are created by a computer linked to an x-ray machine. Also called computerized tomography and computerized axial tomography (CAT) scan. [NIH]

Computerized axial tomography: A series of detailed pictures of areas inside the body, taken from different angles; the pictures are created by a computer linked to an x-ray machine. Also called CAT scan, computed tomography (CT scan), or computerized tomography. [NIH]

Computerized tomography: A series of detailed pictures of areas inside the body, taken from different angles; the pictures are created by a computer linked to an x-ray machine. Also called computerized axial tomography (CAT) scan and computed tomography (CT scan). [NIH]

Concentric: Having a common center of curvature or symmetry. [NIH]

Conception: The onset of pregnancy, marked by implantation of the blastocyst; the formation of a viable zygote. [EU]

Concomitant: Accompanying; accessory; joined with another. [EU]

Condoms: A sheath that is worn over the penis during sexual behavior in order to prevent pregnancy or spread of sexually transmitted disease. [NIH]

Cones: One type of specialized light-sensitive cells (photoreceptors) in the retina that provide sharp central vision and color vision. [NIH]

Confusion: A mental state characterized by bewilderment, emotional disturbance, lack of clear thinking, and perceptual disorientation. [NIH]

Congestive heart failure: Weakness of the heart muscle that leads to a buildup of fluid in body tissues. [NIH]

Conjugated: Acting or operating as if joined; simultaneous. [EU]

Conjunctiva: The mucous membrane that lines the inner surface of the eyelids and the anterior part of the sclera. [NIH]

Connective Tissue: Tissue that supports and binds other tissues. It consists of connective tissue cells embedded in a large amount of extracellular matrix. [NIH]

Connective Tissue: Tissue that supports and binds other tissues. It consists of connective tissue cells embedded in a large amount of extracellular matrix. [NIH]

Connective Tissue Cells: A group of cells that includes fibroblasts, cartilage cells, adipocytes, smooth muscle cells, and bone cells. [NIH]

Connective Tissue Diseases: A heterogeneous group of disorders, some hereditary, others acquired, characterized by abnormal structure or function of one or more of the elements of connective tissue, i.e., collagen, elastin, or the mucopolysaccharides. [NIH]

Consciousness: Sense of awareness of self and of the environment. [NIH]

Constipation: Infrequent or difficult evacuation of feces. [NIH]

Constitutional: 1. Affecting the whole constitution of the body; not local. 2. Pertaining to the constitution. [EU]

Constrict: Tighten; narrow. [NIH]

Constriction: The act of constricting. [NIH]

Constriction, Pathologic: The condition of an anatomical structure's being constricted beyond normal dimensions. [NIH]

Consumption: Pulmonary tuberculosis. [NIH]

Contamination: The soiling or pollution by inferior material, as by the introduction of organisms into a wound, or sewage into a stream. [EU]

Contraception: Use of agents, devices, methods, or procedures which diminish the likelihood of or prevent conception. [NIH]

Contractility: Capacity for becoming short in response to a suitable stimulus. [EU]

Contracture: A condition of fixed high resistance to passive stretch of a muscle, resulting from fibrosis of the tissues supporting the muscles or the joints, or from disorders of the muscle fibres. [EU]

Contraindications: Any factor or sign that it is unwise to pursue a certain kind of action or treatment, e. g. giving a general anesthetic to a person with pneumonia. [NIH]

Control group: In a clinical trial, the group that does not receive the new treatment being studied. This group is compared to the group that receives the new treatment, to see if the new treatment works. [NIH]

Controlled study: An experiment or clinical trial that includes a comparison (control) group. [NIH]

Conventional therapy: A currently accepted and widely used treatment for a certain type of disease, based on the results of past research. Also called conventional treatment. [NIH]

Conventional treatment: A currently accepted and widely used treatment for a certain type of disease, based on the results of past research. Also called conventional therapy. [NIH]

Convulsions: A general term referring to sudden and often violent motor activity of cerebral or brainstem origin. Convulsions may also occur in the absence of an electrical cerebral discharge (e.g., in response to hypotension). [NIH]

Coordination: Muscular or motor regulation or the harmonious cooperation of muscles or groups of muscles, in a complex action or series of actions. [NIH]

Cornea: The transparent part of the eye that covers the iris and the pupil and allows light to enter the inside. [NIH]

Corneum: The superficial layer of the epidermis containing keratinized cells. [NIH]

Coronary: Encircling in the manner of a crown; a term applied to vessels; nerves, ligaments, etc. The term usually denotes the arteries that supply the heart muscle and, by extension, a pathologic involvement of them. [EU]

Coronary Circulation: The circulation of blood through the coronary vessels of the heart. [NIH]

Coronary Thrombosis: Presence of a thrombus in a coronary artery, often causing a myocardial infarction. [NIH]

Corpus: The body of the uterus. [NIH]

Corpus Luteum: The yellow glandular mass formed in the ovary by an ovarian follicle that has ruptured and discharged its ovum. [NIH]

Cortex: The outer layer of an organ or other body structure, as distinguished from the internal substance. [EU]

Corticosteroid: Any of the steroids elaborated by the adrenal cortex (excluding the sex hormones of adrenal origin) in response to the release of corticotrophin (adrenocorticotropic hormone) by the pituitary gland, to any of the synthetic equivalents of these steroids, or to angiotensin II. They are divided, according to their predominant biological activity, into three major groups: glucocorticoids, chiefly influencing carbohydrate, fat, and protein metabolism; mineralocorticoids, affecting the regulation of electrolyte and water balance; and C19 androgens. Some corticosteroids exhibit both types of activity in varying degrees, and others exert only one type of effect. The corticosteroids are used clinically for hormonal replacement therapy, for suppression of ACTH secretion by the anterior pituitary, as antineoplastic, antiallergic, and anti-inflammatory agents, and to suppress the immune response. Called also adrenocortical hormone and corticoid. [EU]

Cortisol: A steroid hormone secreted by the adrenal cortex as part of the body's response to stress. [NIH]

Cortisone: A natural steroid hormone produced in the adrenal gland. It can also be made in the laboratory. Cortisone reduces swelling and can suppress immune responses. [NIH]

Cost Savings: Reductions in all or any portion of the costs of providing goods or services. Savings may be incurred by the provider or the consumer. [NIH]

Coumarin: A fluorescent dye. [NIH]

Cranial: Pertaining to the cranium, or to the anterior (in animals) or superior (in humans) end of the body. [EU]

Craniocerebral Trauma: Traumatic injuries involving the cranium and intracranial structures (i.e., brain; cranial nerves; meninges; and other structures). Injuries may be classified by whether or not the skull is penetrated (i.e., penetrating vs. nonpenetrating) or whether there is an associated hemorrhage. [NIH]

Creatinine: A compound that is excreted from the body in urine. Creatinine levels are measured to monitor kidney function. [NIH]

Crossing-over: The exchange of corresponding segments between chromatids of homologous chromosomes during meiosia, forming a chiasma. [NIH]

Crystallins: A heterogeneous family of water-soluble structural proteins found in cells of the vertebrate lens. The presence of these proteins accounts for the transparency of the lens. The family is composed of four major groups, alpha, beta, gamma, and delta, and several minor groups, which are classed on the basis of size, charge, immunological properties, and vertebrate source. Alpha, beta, and delta crystallins occur in avian and reptilian lenses, while alpha, beta, and gamma crystallins occur in all other lenses. [NIH]

Cues: Signals for an action; that specific portion of a perceptual field or pattern of stimuli to which a subject has learned to respond. [NIH]

Curative: Tending to overcome disease and promote recovery. [EU]

Curcumin: A dye obtained from tumeric, the powdered root of Curcuma longa Linn. It is used in the preparation of curcuma paper and the detection of boron. Curcumin appears to possess a spectrum of pharmacological properties, due primarily to its inhibitory effects on metabolic enzymes. [NIH]

Cutaneous: Having to do with the skin. [NIH]

Cyanogen Bromide: Cyanogen bromide (CNBr). A compound used in molecular biology to digest some proteins and as a coupling reagent for phosphoroamidate or pyrophosphate internucleotide bonds in DNA duplexes. [NIH]

Cyanosis: A bluish or purplish discoloration of the skin and mucous membranes due to an increase in the amount of deoxygenated hemoglobin in the blood or a structural defect in the hemoglobin molecule. [NIH]

Cyclic: Pertaining to or occurring in a cycle or cycles; the term is applied to chemical compounds that contain a ring of atoms in the nucleus. [EU]

Cyclophosphamide: Precursor of an alkylating nitrogen mustard antineoplastic and immunosuppressive agent that must be activated in the liver to form the active aldophosphamide. It is used in the treatment of lymphomas, leukemias, etc. Its side effect, alopecia, has been made use of in defleecing sheep. Cyclophosphamide may also cause sterility, birth defects, mutations, and cancer. [NIH]

Cysteine: A thiol-containing non-essential amino acid that is oxidized to form cystine. [NIH]

Cystine: A covalently linked dimeric nonessential amino acid formed by the oxidation of cysteine. Two molecules of cysteine are joined together by a disulfide bridge to form cystine. [NIH]

Cystitis: Inflammation of the urinary bladder. [EU]

Cytogenetic Analysis: Examination of chromosomes to diagnose, classify, screen for, or manage genetic diseases and abnormalities. Following preparation of the sample, karyotyping is performed and/or the specific chromosomes are analyzed. [NIH]

Cytokine: Small but highly potent protein that modulates the activity of many cell types, including T and B cells. [NIH]

Cytomegalovirus: A genus of the family Herpesviridae, subfamily Betaherpesvirinae, infecting the salivary glands, liver, spleen, lungs, eyes, and other organs, in which they produce characteristically enlarged cells with intranuclear inclusions. Infection with Cytomegalovirus is also seen as an opportunistic infection in AIDS. [NIH]

Cytoplasm: The protoplasm of a cell exclusive of that of the nucleus; it consists of a continuous aqueous solution (cytosol) and the organelles and inclusions suspended in it (phaneroplasm), and is the site of most of the chemical activities of the cell. [EU]

Cytotoxic: Cell-killing. [NIH]

Data Collection: Systematic gathering of data for a particular purpose from various sources, including questionnaires, interviews, observation, existing records, and electronic devices. The process is usually preliminary to statistical analysis of the data. [NIH]

Databases, Bibliographic: Extensive collections, reputedly complete, of references and citations to books, articles, publications, etc., generally on a single subject or specialized subject area. Databases can operate through automated files, libraries, or computer disks. The concept should be differentiated from factual databases which is used for collections of data and facts apart from bibliographic references to them. [NIH]

De novo: In cancer, the first occurrence of cancer in the body. [NIH]

Deamination: The removal of an amino group (NH2) from a chemical compound. [NIH]

Decarboxylation: The removal of a carboxyl group, usually in the form of carbon dioxide, from a chemical compound. [NIH]

Degenerative: Undergoing degeneration : tending to degenerate; having the character of or involving degeneration; causing or tending to cause degeneration. [EU]

Dehydration: The condition that results from excessive loss of body water. [NIH]

Deletion: A genetic rearrangement through loss of segments of DNA (chromosomes), bringing sequences, which are normally separated, into close proximity. [NIH]

Delusions: A false belief regarding the self or persons or objects outside the self that persists despite the facts, and is not considered tenable by one's associates. [NIH]

Dementia: An acquired organic mental disorder with loss of intellectual abilities of sufficient severity to interfere with social or occupational functioning. The dysfunction is multifaceted and involves memory, behavior, personality, judgment, attention, spatial relations, language, abstract thought, and other executive functions. The intellectual decline is usually progressive, and initially spares the level of consciousness. [NIH]

Dendrites: Extensions of the nerve cell body. They are short and branched and receive stimuli from other neurons. [NIH]

Dendritic: 1. Branched like a tree. 2. Pertaining to or possessing dendrites. [EU]

Dendritic cell: A special type of antigen-presenting cell (APC) that activates T lymphocytes. [NIH]

Density: The logarithm to the base 10 of the opacity of an exposed and processed film. [NIH]

Dental Care: The total of dental diagnostic, preventive, and restorative services provided to meet the needs of a patient (from Illustrated Dictionary of Dentistry, 1982). [NIH]

Dental Caries: Localized destruction of the tooth surface initiated by decalcification of the enamel followed by enzymatic lysis of organic structures and leading to cavity formation. If left unchecked, the cavity may penetrate the enamel and dentin and reach the pulp. The three most prominent theories used to explain the etiology of the disase are that acids produced by bacteria lead to decalcification; that micro-organisms destroy the enamel protein; or that keratolytic micro-organisms produce chelates that lead to decalcification. [NIH]

Depigmentation: Removal or loss of pigment, especially melanin. [EU]

Depolarization: The process or act of neutralizing polarity. In neurophysiology, the reversal of the resting potential in excitable cell membranes when stimulated, i.e., the tendency of the cell membrane potential to become positive with respect to the potential outside the cell. [EU]

Dermal: Pertaining to or coming from the skin. [NIH]

Dermatitis: Any inflammation of the skin. [NIH]

Dermatitis Herpetiformis: Rare, chronic, papulo-vesicular disease characterized by an intensely pruritic eruption consisting of various combinations of symmetrical, erythematous, papular, vesicular, or bullous lesions. The disease is strongly associated with the presence of HLA-B8 and HLA-DR3 antigens. A variety of different autoantibodies has been detected in small numbers in patients with dermatitis herpetiformis. [NIH]

Dermatologist: A doctor who specializes in the diagnosis and treatment of skin problems. [NIH]

Dermatosis: Any skin disease, especially one not characterized by inflammation. [EU]

Detergents: Purifying or cleansing agents, usually salts of long-chain aliphatic bases or acids, that exert cleansing (oil-dissolving) and antimicrobial effects through a surface action that depends on possessing both hydrophilic and hydrophobic properties. [NIH]

Deuterium: Deuterium. The stable isotope of hydrogen. It has one neutron and one proton in the nucleus. [NIH]

Diabetes Mellitus: A heterogeneous group of disorders that share glucose intolerance in common. [NIH]

Diabetic Retinopathy: Retinopathy associated with diabetes mellitus, which may be of the background type, progressively characterized by microaneurysms, interretinal punctuate macular edema, or of the proliferative type, characterized by neovascularization of the retina and optic disk, which may project into the vitreous, proliferation of fibrous tissue, vitreous hemorrhage, and retinal detachment. [NIH]

Diagnostic procedure: A method used to identify a disease. [NIH]

Diarrhea: Passage of excessively liquid or excessively frequent stools. [NIH]

Diarrhoea: Abnormal frequency and liquidity of faecal discharges. [EU]

Diastolic: Of or pertaining to the diastole. [EU]

Diffusion: The tendency of a gas or solute to pass from a point of higher pressure or concentration to a point of lower pressure or concentration and to distribute itself throughout the available space; a major mechanism of biological transport. [NIH]

Digestion: The process of breakdown of food for metabolism and use by the body. [NIH]

Digestive system: The organs that take in food and turn it into products that the body can use to stay healthy. Waste products the body cannot use leave the body through bowel movements. The digestive system includes the salivary glands, mouth, esophagus, stomach, liver, pancreas, gallbladder, small and large intestines, and rectum. [NIH]

Digestive tract: The organs through which food passes when food is eaten. These organs are the mouth, esophagus, stomach, small and large intestines, and rectum. [NIH]

Dihydrotestosterone: Anabolic agent. [NIH]

Dihydroxy: AMPA/Kainate antagonist. [NIH]

Dilatation: The act of dilating. [NIH]

Dilatation, Pathologic: The condition of an anatomical structure's being dilated beyond normal dimensions. [NIH]

Dilation: A process by which the pupil is temporarily enlarged with special eye drops (mydriatic); allows the eye care specialist to better view the inside of the eye. [NIH]

Diltiazem: A benzothiazepine derivative with vasodilating action due to its antagonism of the actions of the calcium ion in membrane functions. It is also teratogenic. [NIH]

Dilution: A diluted or attenuated medicine; in homeopathy, the diffusion of a given quantity of a medicinal agent in ten or one hundred times the same quantity of water. [NIH]

Dimethyl: A volatile metabolite of the amino acid methionine. [NIH]

Dipyridamole: A drug that prevents blood cell clumping and enhances the effectiveness of fluorouracil and other chemotherapeutic agents. [NIH]

Direct: 1. Straight; in a straight line. 2. Performed immediately and without the intervention of subsidiary means. [EU]

Disease Progression: The worsening of a disease over time. This concept is most often used for chronic and incurable diseases where the stage of the disease is an important determinant of therapy and prognosis. [NIH]

Disease Susceptibility: A constitution or condition of the body which makes the tissues react in special ways to certain extrinsic stimuli and thus tends to make the individual more than usually susceptible to certain diseases. [NIH]

Dislocation: The displacement of any part, more especially of a bone. Called also luxation. [EU]

Disorientation: The loss of proper bearings, or a state of mental confusion as to time, place, or identity. [EU]

Dissection: Cutting up of an organism for study. [NIH]

Dissociation: 1. The act of separating or state of being separated. 2. The separation of a molecule into two or more fragments (atoms, molecules, ions, or free radicals) produced by the absorption of light or thermal energy or by solvation. 3. In psychology, a defense mechanism in which a group of mental processes are segregated from the rest of a person's mental activity in order to avoid emotional distress, as in the dissociative disorders (q.v.), or in which an idea or object is segregated from its emotional significance; in the first sense it is roughly equivalent to splitting, in the second, to isolation. 4. A defect of mental integration in which one or more groups of mental processes become separated off from normal consciousness and, thus separated, function as a unitary whole. [EU]

Distal: Remote; farther from any point of reference; opposed to proximal. In dentistry, used to designate a position on the dental arch farther from the median line of the jaw. [EU]

Diuresis: Increased excretion of urine. [EU]

Diuretic: A drug that increases the production of urine. [NIH]

Dizziness: An imprecise term which may refer to a sense of spatial disorientation, motion of the environment, or lightheadedness. [NIH]

Docetaxel: An anticancer drug that belongs to the family of drugs called mitotic inhibitors. [NIH]

Dopa: The racemic or DL form of DOPA, an amino acid found in various legumes. The dextro form has little physiologic activity but the levo form (levodopa) is a very important physiologic mediator and precursor and pharmacological agent. [NIH]

Dopa Decarboxylase: One of the aromatic-l-amino-acid decarboxylases, this enzyme is responsible for the conversion of dopa to dopamine. It is of clinical importance in the treatment of Parkinson's disease. EC 4.1.1.28. [NIH]

Dopamine: An endogenous catecholamine and prominent neurotransmitter in several systems of the brain. In the synthesis of catecholamines from tyrosine, it is the immediate precursor to norepinephrine and epinephrine. Dopamine is a major transmitter in the extrapyramidal system of the brain, and important in regulating movement. A family of dopaminergic receptor subtypes mediate its action. Dopamine is used pharmacologically for its direct (beta adrenergic agonist) and indirect (adrenergic releasing) sympathomimetic effects including its actions as an inotropic agent and as a renal vasodilator. [NIH]

Drive: A state of internal activity of an organism that is a necessary condition before a given stimulus will elicit a class of responses; e.g., a certain level of hunger (drive) must be present before food will elicit an eating response. [NIH]

Drug Design: The molecular designing of drugs for specific purposes (such as DNA-binding, enzyme inhibition, anti-cancer efficacy, etc.) based on knowledge of molecular properties such as activity of functional groups, molecular geometry, and electronic structure, and also on information cataloged on analogous molecules. Drug design is generally computer-assisted molecular modeling and does not include pharmacokinetics, dosage analysis, or drug administration analysis. [NIH]

Drug Interactions: The action of a drug that may affect the activity, metabolism, or toxicity of another drug. [NIH]

Drug Tolerance: Progressive diminution of the susceptibility of a human or animal to the effects of a drug, resulting from its continued administration. It should be differentiated from drug resistance wherein an organism, disease, or tissue fails to respond to the intended effectiveness of a chemical or drug. It should also be differentiated from maximum tolerated dose and no-observed-adverse-effect level. [NIH]

Dry Eye Syndrome: A common condition that occurs when the eyes do not produce enough tears to keep the eye moist and comfortable. Common symptoms of dry eye include pain, stinging, burning, scratchiness, and intermittent blurring of vision. [NIH]

Duct: A tube through which body fluids pass. [NIH]

Duodenum: The first part of the small intestine. [NIH]

Dysplasia: Cells that look abnormal under a microscope but are not cancer. [NIH]

Dyspnea: Difficult or labored breathing. [NIH]

Dystrophic: Pertaining to toxic habitats low in nutrients. [NIH]

Dystrophy: Any disorder arising from defective or faulty nutrition, especially the muscular dystrophies. [EU]

Ecteinascidin 743: An anticancer drug that inhibits the growth of cancer cells by disrupting the structure of tumor-cell DNA. [NIH]

Ectopia Lentis: Congenital displacement of the lens resulting from defective zonule formation. [NIH]

Ectopic: Pertaining to or characterized by ectopia. [EU]

Eczema: A pruritic papulovesicular dermatitis occurring as a reaction to many endogenous and exogenous agents (Dorland, 27th ed). [NIH]

Edema: Excessive amount of watery fluid accumulated in the intercellular spaces, most commonly present in subcutaneous tissue. [NIH]

Effector: It is often an enzyme that converts an inactive precursor molecule into an active second messenger. [NIH]

Effector cell: A cell that performs a specific function in response to a stimulus; usually used to describe cells in the immune system. [NIH]

Efficacy: The extent to which a specific intervention, procedure, regimen, or service produces a beneficial result under ideal conditions. Ideally, the determination of efficacy is based on the results of a randomized control trial. [NIH]

Effusion: The escape of fluid into a part or tissue, as an exudation or a transudation. [EU]

Ejection fraction: A measure of ventricular contractility, equal to normally 65 8 per cent; lower values indicate ventricular dysfunction. [EU]

Elasticity: Resistance and recovery from distortion of shape. [NIH]

Elastin: The protein that gives flexibility to tissues. [NIH]

Elective: Subject to the choice or decision of the patient or physician; applied to procedures that are advantageous to the patient but not urgent. [EU]

Electrolyte: A substance that dissociates into ions when fused or in solution, and thus becomes capable of conducting electricity; an ionic solute. [EU]

Electrons: Stable elementary particles having the smallest known negative charge, present in all elements; also called negatrons. Positively charged electrons are called positrons. The numbers, energies and arrangement of electrons around atomic nuclei determine the chemical identities of elements. Beams of electrons are called cathode rays or beta rays, the latter being a high-energy biproduct of nuclear decay. [NIH]

Emboli: Bit of foreign matter which enters the blood stream at one point and is carried until it is lodged or impacted in an artery and obstructs it. It may be a blood clot, an air bubble, fat or other tissue, or clumps of bacteria. [NIH]

Embolism: Blocking of a blood vessel by a blood clot or foreign matter that has been transported from a distant site by the blood stream. [NIH]

Embolization: The blocking of an artery by a clot or foreign material. Embolization can be done as treatment to block the flow of blood to a tumor. [NIH]

Embryo: The prenatal stage of mammalian development characterized by rapid morphological changes and the differentiation of basic structures. [NIH]

Emollient: Softening or soothing; called also malactic. [EU]

Emphysema: A pathological accumulation of air in tissues or organs. [NIH]

Emulsion: A preparation of one liquid distributed in small globules throughout the body of a second liquid. The dispersed liquid is the discontinuous phase, and the dispersion medium is the continuous phase. When oil is the dispersed liquid and an aqueous solution is the continuous phase, it is known as an oil-in-water emulsion, whereas when water or aqueous solution is the dispersed phase and oil or oleaginous substance is the continuous phase, it is known as a water-in-oil emulsion. Pharmaceutical emulsions for which official standards have been promulgated include cod liver oil emulsion, cod liver oil emulsion with malt, liquid petrolatum emulsion, and phenolphthalein in liquid petrolatum emulsion. [EU]

Enamel: A very hard whitish substance which covers the dentine of the anatomical crown of a tooth. [NIH]

Endarterectomy: Surgical excision, performed under general anesthesia, of the atheromatous tunica intima of an artery. When reconstruction of an artery is performed as an endovascular procedure through a catheter, it is called atherectomy. [NIH]

Endemic: Present or usually prevalent in a population or geographical area at all times; said of a disease or agent. Called also endemial. [EU]

Endocarditis: Exudative and proliferative inflammatory alterations of the endocardium, characterized by the presence of vegetations on the surface of the endocardium or in the endocardium itself, and most commonly involving a heart valve, but sometimes affecting the inner lining of the cardiac chambers or the endocardium elsewhere. It may occur as a primary disorder or as a complication of or in association with another disease. [EU]

Endometrial: Having to do with the endometrium (the layer of tissue that lines the uterus). [NIH]

Endometriosis: A condition in which tissue more or less perfectly resembling the uterine mucous membrane (the endometrium) and containing typical endometrial granular and stromal elements occurs aberrantly in various locations in the pelvic cavity. [NIH]

Endometrium: The layer of tissue that lines the uterus. [NIH]

Endostatin: A drug that is being studied for its ability to prevent the growth of new blood vessels into a solid tumor. Endostatin belongs to the family of drugs called angiogenesis inhibitors. [NIH]

Endothelial cell: The main type of cell found in the inside lining of blood vessels, lymph vessels, and the heart. [NIH]

Endothelium: A layer of epithelium that lines the heart, blood vessels (endothelium, vascular), lymph vessels (endothelium, lymphatic), and the serous cavities of the body. [NIH]

Endothelium, Lymphatic: Unbroken cellular lining (intima) of the lymph vessels (e.g., the high endothelial lymphatic venules). It is more permeable than vascular endothelium, lacking selective absorption and functioning mainly to remove plasma proteins that have filtered through the capillaries into the tissue spaces. [NIH]

Endothelium, Vascular: Single pavement layer of cells which line the luminal surface of the entire vascular system and regulate the transport of macromolecules and blood components from interstitium to lumen; this function has been most intensively studied in the blood capillaries. [NIH]

Endothelium-derived: Small molecule that diffuses to the adjacent muscle layer and relaxes it. [NIH]

Endotoxic: Of, relating to, or acting as an endotoxin (= a heat-stable toxin, associated with the outer membranes of certain gram-negative bacteria. Endotoxins are not secreted and are released only when the cells are disrupted). [EU]

Endotoxin: Toxin from cell walls of bacteria. [NIH]

End-stage renal: Total chronic kidney failure. When the kidneys fail, the body retains fluid and harmful wastes build up. A person with ESRD needs treatment to replace the work of the failed kidneys. [NIH]

Enhancer: Transcriptional element in the virus genome. [NIH]

Enteritis: Inflammation of the intestine, applied chiefly to inflammation of the small intestine; see also enterocolitis. [EU]

Enterocolitis: Inflammation of the intestinal mucosa of the small and large bowel. [NIH]

Environmental Exposure: The exposure to potentially harmful chemical, physical, or biological agents in the environment or to environmental factors that may include ionizing radiation, pathogenic organisms, or toxic chemicals. [NIH]

Environmental Health: The science of controlling or modifying those conditions, influences, or forces surrounding man which relate to promoting, establishing, and maintaining health. [NIH]

Enzymatic: Phase where enzyme cuts the precursor protein. [NIH]

Enzyme: A protein that speeds up chemical reactions in the body. [NIH]

Eosinophil: A polymorphonuclear leucocyte with large eosinophilic granules in its cytoplasm, which plays a role in hypersensitivity reactions. [NIH]

Eosinophilia: Abnormal increase in eosinophils in the blood, tissues or organs. [NIH]

Eosinophilic: A condition found primarily in grinding workers caused by a reaction of the pulmonary tissue, in particular the eosinophilic cells, to dust that has entered the lung. [NIH]

Epidemic: Occurring suddenly in numbers clearly in excess of normal expectancy; said especially of infectious diseases but applied also to any disease, injury, or other health-related event occurring in such outbreaks. [EU]

Epidemiological: Relating to, or involving epidemiology. [EU]

Epidermal: Pertaining to or resembling epidermis. Called also epidermic or epidermoid. [EU]

Epidermal Growth Factor: A 6 kD polypeptide growth factor initially discovered in mouse submaxillary glands. Human epidermal growth factor was originally isolated from urine based on its ability to inhibit gastric secretion and called urogastrone. epidermal growth factor exerts a wide variety of biological effects including the promotion of proliferation and differentiation of mesenchymal and epithelial cells. [NIH]

Epidermis: Nonvascular layer of the skin. It is made up, from within outward, of five layers: 1) basal layer (stratum basale epidermidis); 2) spinous layer (stratum spinosum epidermidis); 3) granular layer (stratum granulosum epidermidis); 4) clear layer (stratum lucidum epidermidis); and 5) horny layer (stratum corneum epidermidis). [NIH]

Epigastric: Having to do with the upper middle area of the abdomen. [NIH]

Epinephrine: The active sympathomimetic hormone from the adrenal medulla in most species. It stimulates both the alpha- and beta- adrenergic systems, causes systemic vasoconstriction and gastrointestinal relaxation, stimulates the heart, and dilates bronchi and cerebral vessels. It is used in asthma and cardiac failure and to delay absorption of local anesthetics. [NIH]

Episcleritis: Inflammation of the episclera and/or the outer layers of the sclera itself. [NIH]

Epithelial: Refers to the cells that line the internal and external surfaces of the body. [NIH]

Epithelial Cells: Cells that line the inner and outer surfaces of the body. [NIH]

Epithelium: One or more layers of epithelial cells, supported by the basal lamina, which covers the inner or outer surfaces of the body. [NIH]

Epitope: A molecule or portion of a molecule capable of binding to the combining site of an antibody. For every given antigenic determinant, the body can construct a variety of antibody-combining sites, some of which fit almost perfectly, and others which barely fit. [NIH]

Epoprostenol: A prostaglandin that is biosynthesized enzymatically from prostaglandin endoperoxides in human vascular tissue. It is a potent inhibitor of platelet aggregation. The sodium salt has been also used to treat primary pulmonary hypertension. [NIH]

Erythema: Redness of the skin produced by congestion of the capillaries. This condition may result from a variety of causes. [NIH]

Erythrocytes: Red blood cells. Mature erythrocytes are non-nucleated, biconcave disks containing hemoglobin whose function is to transport oxygen. [NIH]

Escalation: Progressive use of more harmful drugs. [NIH]

Esophageal: Having to do with the esophagus, the muscular tube through which food passes from the throat to the stomach. [NIH]

Esophagitis: Inflammation, acute or chronic, of the esophagus caused by bacteria, chemicals, or trauma. [NIH]

Esophagus: The muscular tube through which food passes from the throat to the stomach. [NIH]

Essential Tremor: A rhythmic, involuntary, purposeless, oscillating movement resulting from the alternate contraction and relaxation of opposing groups of muscles. [NIH]

Estrogen: One of the two female sex hormones. [NIH]

Ethnic Groups: A group of people with a common cultural heritage that sets them apart from others in a variety of social relationships. [NIH]

Ethylene Glycol: A colorless, odorless, viscous dihydroxy alcohol. It has a sweet taste, but is poisonous if ingested. Ethylene glycol is the most important glycol commercially available and is manufactured on a large scale in the United States. It is used as an antifreeze and coolant, in hydraulic fluids, and in the manufacture of low-freezing dynamites and resins. [NIH]

Etretinate: An oral retinoid used in the treatment of keratotic genodermatosis, lichen planus, and psoriasis. Beneficial effects have also been claimed in the prophylaxis of epithelial neoplasia. The compound may be teratogenic. [NIH]

Eukaryotic Cells: Cells of the higher organisms, containing a true nucleus bounded by a nuclear membrane. [NIH]

Evacuation: An emptying, as of the bowels. [EU]

Excitation: An act of irritation or stimulation or of responding to a stimulus; the addition of energy, as the excitation of a molecule by absorption of photons. [EU]

Excrete: To get rid of waste from the body. [NIH]

Exfoliation: A falling off in scales or layers. [EU]

Exocrine: Secreting outwardly, via a duct. [EU]

Exocytosis: Cellular release of material within membrane-limited vesicles by fusion of the vesicles with the cell membrane. [NIH]

Exogenous: Developed or originating outside the organism, as exogenous disease. [EU]

Exon: The part of the DNA that encodes the information for the actual amino acid sequence of the protein. In many eucaryotic genes, the coding sequences consist of a series of exons alternating with intron sequences. [NIH]

Exoribonucleases: A family of enzymes that catalyze the exonucleolytic cleavage of RNA. It includes EC 3.1.13.-, EC 3.1.14.-, EC 3.1.15.-, and EC 3.1.16.-. EC 3.1.- [NIH]

Expiration: The act of breathing out, or expelling air from the lungs. [EU]

Expressed Sequence Tags: Sequence tags derived from cDNAs. Expressed sequence tags (ESTs) are partial DNA sequences from clones. [NIH]

Extensor: A muscle whose contraction tends to straighten a limb; the antagonist of a flexor. [NIH]

External-beam radiation: Radiation therapy that uses a machine to aim high-energy rays at the cancer. Also called external radiation. [NIH]

Extracellular: Outside a cell or cells. [EU]

Extracellular Matrix: A meshwork-like substance found within the extracellular space and in association with the basement membrane of the cell surface. It promotes cellular proliferation and provides a supporting structure to which cells or cell lysates in culture dishes adhere. [NIH]

Extracellular Matrix Proteins: Macromolecular organic compounds that contain carbon, hydrogen, oxygen, nitrogen, and usually, sulfur. These macromolecules (proteins) form an intricate meshwork in which cells are embedded to construct tissues. Variations in the relative types of macromolecules and their organization determine the type of extracellular matrix, each adapted to the functional requirements of the tissue. The two main classes of macromolecules that form the extracellular matrix are: glycosaminoglycans, usually linked to proteins (proteoglycans), and fibrous proteins (e.g., collagen, elastin, fibronectins and laminin). [NIH]

Extracellular Space: Interstitial space between cells, occupied by fluid as well as amorphous and fibrous substances. [NIH]

Extracorporeal: Situated or occurring outside the body. [EU]

Extraction: The process or act of pulling or drawing out. [EU]

Extrapyramidal: Outside of the pyramidal tracts. [EU]

Extravascular: Situated or occurring outside a vessel or the vessels. [EU]

Facial: Of or pertaining to the face. [EU]

Facial Hemiatrophy: A syndrome characterized by slowly progressive unilateral atrophy of facial subcutaneous fat, muscle tissue, skin, cartilage, and bone. The condition typically progresses over a period of 2-10 years and then stabilizes. [NIH]

Family Planning: Programs or services designed to assist the family in controlling reproduction by either improving or diminishing fertility. [NIH]

Family Relations: Behavioral, psychological, and social relations among various members of the nuclear family and the extended family. [NIH]

Famotidine: A competitive histamine H2-receptor antagonist. Its main pharmacodynamic effect is the inhibition of gastric secretion. [NIH]

Fasciitis: Inflammation of the fascia. There are three major types: 1) Eosinophilic fasciitis, an inflammatory reaction with eosinophilia, producing hard thickened skin with an orange-peel configuration suggestive of scleroderma and considered by some a variant of scleroderma; 2) Necrotizing fasciitis, a serious fulminating infection (usually by a beta hemolytic Streptococcus) causing extensive necrosis of superficial fascia; 3) Nodular/Pseudosarcomatous/Proliferative fasciitis, characterized by a rapid growth of fibroblasts with mononuclear inflammatory cells and proliferating capillaries in soft tissue, often the forearm; it is not malignant but is sometimes mistaken for fibrosarcoma. [NIH]

Fascioliasis: Helminth infection of the liver caused by species of Fasciola. [NIH]

Fat: Total lipids including phospholipids. [NIH]

Fatigue: The state of weariness following a period of exertion, mental or physical, characterized by a decreased capacity for work and reduced efficiency to respond to stimuli. [NIH]

Fatty acids: A major component of fats that are used by the body for energy and tissue development. [NIH]

Feces: The excrement discharged from the intestines, consisting of bacteria, cells exfoliated from the intestines, secretions, chiefly of the liver, and a small amount of food residue. [EU]

Felodipine: A dihydropyridine calcium antagonist with positive inotropic effects. It lowers blood pressure by reducing peripheral vascular resistance through a highly selective action on smooth muscle in arteriolar resistance vessels. [NIH]

Femoral: Pertaining to the femur, or to the thigh. [EU]

Femur: The longest and largest bone of the skeleton, it is situated between the hip and the knee. [NIH]

Fendiline: Coronary vasodilator; inhibits calcium function in muscle cells in excitation-contraction coupling; proposed as antiarrhythmic and antianginal agents. [NIH]

Fenfluramine: A centrally active drug that apparently both blocks serotonin uptake and provokes transport-mediated serotonin release. [NIH]

Fetal Blood: Blood of the fetus. Exchange of nutrients and waste between the fetal and maternal blood occurs via the placenta. The cord blood is blood contained in the umbilical vessels at the time of delivery. [NIH]

Fetus: The developing offspring from 7 to 8 weeks after conception until birth. [NIH]

Fibrin: A protein derived from fibrinogen in the presence of thrombin, which forms part of the blood clot. [NIH]

Fibrinogen: Plasma glycoprotein clotted by thrombin, composed of a dimer of three non-identical pairs of polypeptide chains (alpha, beta, gamma) held together by disulfide bonds. Fibrinogen clotting is a sol-gel change involving complex molecular arrangements: whereas fibrinogen is cleaved by thrombin to form polypeptides A and B, the proteolytic action of other enzymes yields different fibrinogen degradation products. [NIH]

Fibroblasts: Connective tissue cells which secrete an extracellular matrix rich in collagen and other macromolecules. [NIH]

Fibronectin: An adhesive glycoprotein. One form circulates in plasma, acting as an opsonin; another is a cell-surface protein which mediates cellular adhesive interactions. [NIH]

Fibrosarcoma: A type of soft tissue sarcoma that begins in fibrous tissue, which holds bones, muscles, and other organs in place. [NIH]

Fibrosis: Any pathological condition where fibrous connective tissue invades any organ, usually as a consequence of inflammation or other injury. [NIH]

Fibrositis: Aching, soreness or stiffness of muscles; often caused by inexpedient work postures. [NIH]

Fibrotic tissue: Inflamed tissue that has become scarred. [NIH]

Fistula: Abnormal communication most commonly seen between two internal organs, or between an internal organ and the surface of the body. [NIH]

Fixation: 1. The act or operation of holding, suturing, or fastening in a fixed position. 2. The condition of being held in a fixed position. 3. In psychiatry, a term with two related but distinct meanings : (1) arrest of development at a particular stage, which like regression (return to an earlier stage), if temporary is a normal reaction to setbacks and difficulties but if protracted or frequent is a cause of developmental failures and emotional problems, and (2) a close and suffocating attachment to another person, especially a childhood figure, such as one's mother or father. Both meanings are derived from psychoanalytic theory and refer to 'fixation' of libidinal energy either in a specific erogenous zone, hence fixation at the oral, anal, or phallic stage, or in a specific object, hence mother or father fixation. 4. The use of a fixative (q.v.) to preserve histological or cytological specimens. 5. In chemistry, the process whereby a substance is removed from the gaseous or solution phase and localized, as in carbon dioxide fixation or nitrogen fixation. 6. In ophthalmology, direction of the gaze so that the visual image of the object falls on the fovea centralis. 7. In film processing, the chemical removal of all undeveloped salts of the film emulsion, leaving only the developed silver to form a permanent image. [EU]

Flatus: Gas passed through the rectum. [NIH]

Flexor: Muscles which flex a joint. [NIH]

Flow Cytometry: Technique using an instrument system for making, processing, and displaying one or more measurements on individual cells obtained from a cell suspension. Cells are usually stained with one or more fluorescent dyes specific to cell components of interest, e.g., DNA, and fluorescence of each cell is measured as it rapidly transverses the excitation beam (laser or mercury arc lamp). Fluorescence provides a quantitative measure of various biochemical and biophysical properties of the cell, as well as a basis for cell sorting. Other measurable optical parameters include light absorption and light scattering, the latter being applicable to the measurement of cell size, shape, density, granularity, and stain uptake. [NIH]

Flunarizine: Flunarizine is a selective calcium entry blocker with calmodulin binding properties and histamine H1 blocking activity. It is effective in the prophylaxis of migraine, occlusive peripheral vascular disease, vertigo of central and peripheral origin, and as an adjuvant in the therapy of epilepsy. [NIH]

Fluorescence: The property of emitting radiation while being irradiated. The radiation emitted is usually of longer wavelength than that incident or absorbed, e.g., a substance can be irradiated with invisible radiation and emit visible light. X-ray fluorescence is used in diagnosis. [NIH]

Fluorescent Dyes: Dyes that emit light when exposed to light. The wave length of the emitted light is usually longer than that of the incident light. Fluorochromes are substances that cause fluorescence in other substances, i.e., dyes used to mark or label other compounds with fluorescent tags. They are used as markers in biochemistry and immunology. [NIH]

Fluorouracil: A pyrimidine analog that acts as an antineoplastic antimetabolite and also has immunosuppressant. It interferes with DNA synthesis by blocking the thymidylate synthetase conversion of deoxyuridylic acid to thymidylic acid. [NIH]

Fold: A plication or doubling of various parts of the body. [NIH]

Follicles: Shafts through which hair grows. [NIH]

Forearm: The part between the elbow and the wrist. [NIH]

Fovea: The central part of the macula that provides the sharpest vision. [NIH]

Fractionation: Dividing the total dose of radiation therapy into several smaller, equal doses delivered over a period of several days. [NIH]

Friction: Surface resistance to the relative motion of one body against the rubbing, sliding, rolling, or flowing of another with which it is in contact. [NIH]

Fructose: A type of sugar found in many fruits and vegetables and in honey. Fructose is used to sweeten some diet foods. It is considered a nutritive sweetener because it has calories. [NIH]

Fungi: A kingdom of eukaryotic, heterotrophic organisms that live as saprobes or parasites, including mushrooms, yeasts, smuts, molds, etc. They reproduce either sexually or asexually, and have life cycles that range from simple to complex. Filamentous fungi refer to those that grow as multicelluar colonies (mushrooms and molds). [NIH]

Fungus: A general term used to denote a group of eukaryotic protists, including mushrooms, yeasts, rusts, moulds, smuts, etc., which are characterized by the absence of chlorophyll and by the presence of a rigid cell wall composed of chitin, mannans, and sometimes cellulose. They are usually of simple morphological form or show some reversible cellular specialization, such as the formation of pseudoparenchymatous tissue in the fruiting body of a mushroom. The dimorphic fungi grow, according to environmental conditions, as moulds or yeasts. [EU]

Gallbladder: The pear-shaped organ that sits below the liver. Bile is concentrated and stored in the gallbladder. [NIH]

Gallopamil: Coronary vasodilator that is an analog of iproveratril (verapamil) with one more methoxy group on the benzene ring. [NIH]

Gallstones: The solid masses or stones made of cholesterol or bilirubin that form in the gallbladder or bile ducts. [NIH]

Gamma Rays: Very powerful and penetrating, high-energy electromagnetic radiation of shorter wavelength than that of x-rays. They are emitted by a decaying nucleus, usually between 0.01 and 10 MeV. They are also called nuclear x-rays. [NIH]

Ganglia: Clusters of multipolar neurons surrounded by a capsule of loosely organized connective tissue located outside the central nervous system. [NIH]

Gap Junctions: Connections between cells which allow passage of small molecules and electric current. Gap junctions were first described anatomically as regions of close apposition between cells with a narrow (1-2 nm) gap between cell membranes. The variety in the properties of gap junctions is reflected in the number of connexins, the family of proteins which form the junctions. [NIH]

Gas: Air that comes from normal breakdown of food. The gases are passed out of the body through the rectum (flatus) or the mouth (burp). [NIH]

Gas exchange: Primary function of the lungs; transfer of oxygen from inhaled air into the blood and of carbon dioxide from the blood into the lungs. [NIH]

Gastric: Having to do with the stomach. [NIH]

Gastric Acid: Hydrochloric acid present in gastric juice. [NIH]

Gastrin: A hormone released after eating. Gastrin causes the stomach to produce more acid. [NIH]

Gastrointestinal: Refers to the stomach and intestines. [NIH]

Gastrointestinal tract: The stomach and intestines. [NIH]

Gene: The functional and physical unit of heredity passed from parent to offspring. Genes are pieces of DNA, and most genes contain the information for making a specific protein. [NIH]

Gene Expression: The phenotypic manifestation of a gene or genes by the processes of gene action. [NIH]

Gene Rearrangement: The ordered rearrangement of gene regions by DNA recombination such as that which occurs normally during development. [NIH]

Gene Silencing: Interruption or suppression of the expression of a gene at transcriptional or translational levels. [NIH]

Genetic Code: The specifications for how information, stored in nucleic acid sequence (base sequence), is translated into protein sequence (amino acid sequence). The start, stop, and order of amino acids of a protein is specified by consecutive triplets of nucleotides called codons (codon). [NIH]

Genetic Engineering: Directed modification of the gene complement of a living organism by such techniques as altering the DNA, substituting genetic material by means of a virus, transplanting whole nuclei, transplanting cell hybrids, etc. [NIH]

Genetic Markers: A phenotypically recognizable genetic trait which can be used to identify a genetic locus, a linkage group, or a recombination event. [NIH]

Genetic Techniques: Chromosomal, biochemical, intracellular, and other methods used in the study of genetics. [NIH]

Genetics: The biological science that deals with the phenomena and mechanisms of heredity. [NIH]

Genital: Pertaining to the genitalia. [EU]

Genotype: The genetic constitution of the individual; the characterization of the genes. [NIH]

Germ Cells: The reproductive cells in multicellular organisms. [NIH]

Giant Cells: Multinucleated masses produced by the fusion of many cells; often associated with viral infections. In AIDS, they are induced when the envelope glycoprotein of the HIV virus binds to the CD4 antigen of uninfected neighboring T4 cells. The resulting syncytium leads to cell death and thus may account for the cytopathic effect of the virus. [NIH]

Gingival Recession: The exposure of root surface by an apical shift in the position of the gingiva. [NIH]

Gland: An organ that produces and releases one or more substances for use in the body. Some glands produce fluids that affect tissues or organs. Others produce hormones or participate in blood production. [NIH]

Glomerular: Pertaining to or of the nature of a glomerulus, especially a renal glomerulus. [EU]

Glomerular Filtration Rate: The volume of water filtered out of plasma through glomerular capillary walls into Bowman's capsules per unit of time. It is considered to be equivalent to inulin clearance. [NIH]

Glomeruli: Plural of glomerulus. [NIH]

Glomerulonephritis: Glomerular disease characterized by an inflammatory reaction, with leukocyte infiltration and cellular proliferation of the glomeruli, or that appears to be the result of immune glomerular injury. [NIH]

Glomerulus: A tiny set of looping blood vessels in the nephron where blood is filtered in the kidney. [NIH]

Glucocorticoid: A compound that belongs to the family of compounds called corticosteroids (steroids). Glucocorticoids affect metabolism and have anti-inflammatory and immunosuppressive effects. They may be naturally produced (hormones) or synthetic (drugs). [NIH]

Glucose: D-Glucose. A primary source of energy for living organisms. It is naturally occurring and is found in fruits and other parts of plants in its free state. It is used therapeutically in fluid and nutrient replacement. [NIH]

Glucose Intolerance: A pathological state in which the fasting plasma glucose level is less than 140 mg per deciliter and the 30-, 60-, or 90-minute plasma glucose concentration following a glucose tolerance test exceeds 200 mg per deciliter. This condition is seen frequently in diabetes mellitus but also occurs with other diseases. [NIH]

Glucuronic Acid: Derivatives of uronic acid found throughout the plant and animal kingdoms. They detoxify drugs and toxins by conjugating with them to form glucuronides in the liver which are more water-soluble metabolites that can be easily eliminated from the body. [NIH]

Glycine: A non-essential amino acid. It is found primarily in gelatin and silk fibroin and used therapeutically as a nutrient. It is also a fast inhibitory neurotransmitter. [NIH]

Glycogen: A sugar stored in the liver and muscles. It releases glucose into the blood when cells need it for energy. Glycogen is the chief source of stored fuel in the body. [NIH]

Glycoprotein: A protein that has sugar molecules attached to it. [NIH]

Glycosaminoglycan: A type of long, unbranched polysaccharide molecule. Glycosaminoglycans are major structural components of cartilage and are also found in the cornea of the eye. [NIH]

Glycoside: Any compound that contains a carbohydrate molecule (sugar), particularly any such natural product in plants, convertible, by hydrolytic cleavage, into sugar and a nonsugar component (aglycone), and named specifically for the sugar contained, as glucoside (glucose), pentoside (pentose), fructoside (fructose) etc. [EU]

Glycosylation: The chemical or biochemical addition of carbohydrate or glycosyl groups to other chemicals, especially peptides or proteins. Glycosyl transferases are used in this biochemical reaction. [NIH]

Gonadal: Pertaining to a gonad. [EU]

Governing Board: The group in which legal authority is vested for the control of health-related institutions and organizations. [NIH]

Gp120: 120-kD HIV envelope glycoprotein which is involved in the binding of the virus to its membrane receptor, the CD4 molecule, found on the surface of certain cells in the body. [NIH]

Graft: Healthy skin, bone, or other tissue taken from one part of the body and used to replace diseased or injured tissue removed from another part of the body. [NIH]

Graft Rejection: An immune response with both cellular and humoral components, directed against an allogeneic transplant, whose tissue antigens are not compatible with those of the recipient. [NIH]

Grafting: The operation of transfer of tissue from one site to another. [NIH]

Graft-versus-host disease: GVHD. A reaction of donated bone marrow or peripheral stem cells against a person's tissue. [NIH]

Gram-negative: Losing the stain or decolorized by alcohol in Gram's method of staining, a primary characteristic of bacteria having a cell wall composed of a thin layer of peptidoglycan covered by an outer membrane of lipoprotein and lipopolysaccharide. [EU]

Granule: A small pill made from sucrose. [EU]

Granulocytes: Leukocytes with abundant granules in the cytoplasm. They are divided into three groups: neutrophils, eosinophils, and basophils. [NIH]

Gravis: Eruption of watery blisters on the skin among those handling animals and animal products. [NIH]

Growth: The progressive development of a living being or part of an organism from its earliest stage to maturity. [NIH]

Growth factors: Substances made by the body that function to regulate cell division and cell survival. Some growth factors are also produced in the laboratory and used in biological therapy. [NIH]

Guanylate Cyclase: An enzyme that catalyzes the conversion of GTP to 3',5'-cyclic GMP and pyrophosphate. It also acts on ITP and dGTP. (From Enzyme Nomenclature, 1992) EC 4.6.1.2. [NIH]

Hair follicles: Shafts or openings on the surface of the skin through which hair grows. [NIH]

Half-Life: The time it takes for a substance (drug, radioactive nuclide, or other) to lose half of its pharmacologic, physiologic, or radiologic activity. [NIH]

Hand Deformities: Alterations or deviations from normal shape or size which result in a disfigurement of the hand. [NIH]

Haploid: An organism with one basic chromosome set, symbolized by n; the normal condition of gametes in diploids. [NIH]

Haplotypes: The genetic constitution of individuals with respect to one member of a pair of allelic genes, or sets of genes that are closely linked and tend to be inherited together such as those of the major histocompatibility complex. [NIH]

Haptens: Small antigenic determinants capable of eliciting an immune response only when coupled to a carrier. Haptens bind to antibodies but by themselves cannot elicit an antibody response. [NIH]

Headache: Pain in the cranial region that may occur as an isolated and benign symptom or as a manifestation of a wide variety of conditions including subarachnoid hemorrhage; craniocerebral trauma; central nervous system infections; intracranial hypertension; and other disorders. In general, recurrent headaches that are not associated with a primary disease process are referred to as headache disorders (e.g., migraine). [NIH]

Headache Disorders: Common conditions characterized by persistent or recurrent headaches. Headache syndrome classification systems may be based on etiology (e.g., vascular headache, post-traumatic headaches, etc.), temporal pattern (e.g., cluster headache, paroxysmal hemicrania, etc.), and precipitating factors (e.g., cough headache). [NIH]

Health Education: Education that increases the awareness and favorably influences the attitudes and knowledge relating to the improvement of health on a personal or community basis. [NIH]

Health Services: Services for the diagnosis and treatment of disease and the maintenance of health. [NIH]

Heart Catheterization: Procedure which includes placement of catheter, recording of intracardiac and intravascular pressure, obtaining blood samples for chemical analysis, and cardiac output measurement, etc. Specific angiographic injection techniques are also involved. [NIH]

Heart failure: Loss of pumping ability by the heart, often accompanied by fatigue, breathlessness, and excess fluid accumulation in body tissues. [NIH]

Heartburn: Substernal pain or burning sensation, usually associated with regurgitation of gastric juice into the esophagus. [NIH]

Hematologic malignancies: Cancers of the blood or bone marrow, including leukemia and lymphoma. Also called hematologic cancers. [NIH]

Hemodialysis: The use of a machine to clean wastes from the blood after the kidneys have failed. The blood travels through tubes to a dialyzer, which removes wastes and extra fluid. The cleaned blood then flows through another set of tubes back into the body. [NIH]

Hemoglobin: One of the fractions of glycosylated hemoglobin A1c. Glycosylated hemoglobin is formed when linkages of glucose and related monosaccharides bind to hemoglobin A and its concentration represents the average blood glucose level over the previous several weeks. HbA1c levels are used as a measure of long-term control of plasma glucose (normal, 4 to 6 percent). In controlled diabetes mellitus, the concentration of glycosylated hemoglobin A is within the normal range, but in uncontrolled cases the level may be 3 to 4 times the normal conentration. Generally, complications are substantially lower among patients with Hb levels of 7 percent or less than in patients with HbA1c levels of 9 percent or more. [NIH]

Hemoglobin M: A group of abnormal hemoglobins in which amino acid substitutions take place in either the alpha or beta chains but near the heme iron. This results in facilitated oxidation of the hemoglobin to yield excess methemoglobin which leads to cyanosis. [NIH]

Hemoglobinuria: The presence of free hemoglobin in the urine. [NIH]

Hemolytic: A disease that affects the blood and blood vessels. It destroys red blood cells, cells that cause the blood to clot, and the lining of blood vessels. HUS is often caused by the Escherichia coli bacterium in contaminated food. People with HUS may develop acute renal failure. [NIH]

Hemorrhage: Bleeding or escape of blood from a vessel. [NIH]

Hemostasis: The process which spontaneously arrests the flow of blood from vessels carrying blood under pressure. It is accomplished by contraction of the vessels, adhesion and aggregation of formed blood elements, and the process of blood or plasma coagulation. [NIH]

Heparin: Heparinic acid. A highly acidic mucopolysaccharide formed of equal parts of sulfated D-glucosamine and D-glucuronic acid with sulfaminic bridges. The molecular weight ranges from six to twenty thousand. Heparin occurs in and is obtained from liver, lung, mast cells, etc., of vertebrates. Its function is unknown, but it is used to prevent blood clotting in vivo and vitro, in the form of many different salts. [NIH]

Hepatic: Refers to the liver. [NIH]

Hepatitis: Inflammation of the liver and liver disease involving degenerative or necrotic alterations of hepatocytes. [NIH]

Hepatocytes: The main structural component of the liver. They are specialized epithelial cells that are organized into interconnected plates called lobules. [NIH]

Hereditary: Of, relating to, or denoting factors that can be transmitted genetically from one generation to another. [NIH]

Heredity: 1. The genetic transmission of a particular quality or trait from parent to offspring. 2. The genetic constitution of an individual. [EU]

Herpes: Any inflammatory skin disease caused by a herpesvirus and characterized by the formation of clusters of small vesicles. When used alone, the term may refer to herpes simplex or to herpes zoster. [EU]

Herpes virus: A member of the herpes family of viruses. [NIH]

Herpes Zoster: Acute vesicular inflammation. [NIH]

Heterogeneity: The property of one or more samples or populations which implies that they are not identical in respect of some or all of their parameters, e. g. heterogeneity of variance. [NIH]

Hirsutism: Excess hair in females and children with an adult male pattern of distribution. The concept does not include hypertrichosis, which is localized or generalized excess hair. [NIH]

Histamine: 1H-Imidazole-4-ethanamine. A depressor amine derived by enzymatic decarboxylation of histidine. It is a powerful stimulant of gastric secretion, a constrictor of bronchial smooth muscle, a vasodilator, and also a centrally acting neurotransmitter. [NIH]

Histamine Release: The secretion of histamine from mast cell and basophil granules by exocytosis. This can be initiated by a number of factors, all of which involve binding of IgE, cross-linked by antigen, to the mast cell or basophil's Fc receptors. Once released, histamine binds to a number of different target cell receptors and exerts a wide variety of effects. [NIH]

Histidine: An essential amino acid important in a number of metabolic processes. It is required for the production of histamine. [NIH]

Histidine Decarboxylase: An enzyme that catalyzes the decarboxylation of histidine to histamine and carbon dioxide. It requires pyridoxal phosphate in animal tissues, but not in microorganisms. EC 4.1.1.22. [NIH]

Histocompatibility: The degree of antigenic similarity between the tissues of different individuals, which determines the acceptance or rejection of allografts. [NIH]

Histocompatibility Antigens: A group of antigens that includes both the major and minor histocompatibility antigens. The former are genetically determined by the major histocompatibility complex. They determine tissue type for transplantation and cause allograft rejections. The latter are systems of allelic alloantigens that can cause weak transplant rejection. [NIH]

Histology: The study of tissues and cells under a microscope. [NIH]

Homeostasis: The processes whereby the internal environment of an organism tends to remain balanced and stable. [NIH]

Homodimer: Protein-binding "activation domains" always combine with identical proteins. [NIH]

Homologous: Corresponding in structure, position, origin, etc., as (a) the feathers of a bird and the scales of a fish, (b) antigen and its specific antibody, (c) allelic chromosomes. [EU]

Hormonal: Pertaining to or of the nature of a hormone. [EU]

Hormone: A substance in the body that regulates certain organs. Hormones such as gastrin help in breaking down food. Some hormones come from cells in the stomach and small intestine. [NIH]

Horny layer: The superficial layer of the epidermis containing keratinized cells. [NIH]

Host: Any animal that receives a transplanted graft. [NIH]

Humoral: Of, relating to, proceeding from, or involving a bodily humour - now often used of endocrine factors as opposed to neural or somatic. [EU]

Humour: 1. A normal functioning fluid or semifluid of the body (as the blood, lymph or bile) especially of vertebrates. 2. A secretion that is itself an excitant of activity (as certain hormones). [EU]

Hybrid: Cross fertilization between two varieties or, more usually, two species of vines, see also crossing. [NIH]

Hybridization: The genetic process of crossbreeding to produce a hybrid. Hybrid nucleic acids can be formed by nucleic acid hybridization of DNA and RNA molecules. Protein hybridization allows for hybrid proteins to be formed from polypeptide chains. [NIH]

Hybridoma: A hybrid cell resulting from the fusion of a specific antibody-producing spleen cell with a myeloma cell. [NIH]

Hydrochloric Acid: A strong corrosive acid that is commonly used as a laboratory reagent. It is formed by dissolving hydrogen chloride in water. Gastric acid is the hydrochloric acid component of gastric juice. [NIH]

Hydrogen: The first chemical element in the periodic table. It has the atomic symbol H, atomic number 1, and atomic weight 1. It exists, under normal conditions, as a colorless, odorless, tasteless, diatomic gas. Hydrogen ions are protons. Besides the common H1 isotope, hydrogen exists as the stable isotope deuterium and the unstable, radioactive isotope tritium. [NIH]

Hydrogen Peroxide: A strong oxidizing agent used in aqueous solution as a ripening agent, bleach, and topical anti-infective. It is relatively unstable and solutions deteriorate over time unless stabilized by the addition of acetanilide or similar organic materials. [NIH]

Hydrolysis: The process of cleaving a chemical compound by the addition of a molecule of water. [NIH]

Hydrophilic: Readily absorbing moisture; hygroscopic; having strongly polar groups that readily interact with water. [EU]

Hydrophobic: Not readily absorbing water, or being adversely affected by water, as a hydrophobic colloid. [EU]

Hydroxylation: Hydroxylate, to introduce hydroxyl into (a compound or radical) usually by replacement of hydrogen. [EU]

Hydroxylysine: A hydroxylated derivative of the amino acid lysine that is present in certain collagens. [NIH]

Hydroxyproline: A hydroxylated form of the imino acid proline. A deficiency in ascorbic acid can result in impaired hydroxyproline formation. [NIH]

Hyperaldosteronism: Aldosteronism. [EU]

Hyperbaric: Characterized by greater than normal pressure or weight; applied to gases under greater than atmospheric pressure, as hyperbaric oxygen, or to a solution of greater specific gravity than another taken as a standard of reference. [EU]

Hyperbaric oxygen: Oxygen that is at an atmospheric pressure higher than the pressure at sea level. Breathing hyperbaric oxygen to enhance the effectiveness of radiation therapy is being studied. [NIH]

Hyperkeratosis: 1. Hypertrophy of the corneous layer of the skin. 2a. Any of various conditions marked by hyperkeratosis. 2b. A disease of cattle marked by thickening and wringling of the hide and formation of papillary outgrowths on the buccal mucous membranes, often accompanied by watery discharge from eyes and nose, diarrhoea, loss of condition, and abortion of pregnant animals, and now believed to result from ingestion of the chlorinated naphthalene of various lubricating oils. [EU]

Hyperplasia: An increase in the number of cells in a tissue or organ, not due to tumor formation. It differs from hypertrophy, which is an increase in bulk without an increase in the number of cells. [NIH]

Hypersecretion: Excessive secretion. [EU]

Hypersensitivity: Altered reactivity to an antigen, which can result in pathologic reactions upon subsequent exposure to that particular antigen. [NIH]

Hypertension: Persistently high arterial blood pressure. Currently accepted threshold levels are 140 mm Hg systolic and 90 mm Hg diastolic pressure. [NIH]

Hypertension, Pulmonary: Increased pressure within the pulmonary circulation, usually secondary to cardiac or pulmonary disease. [NIH]

Hypertrichosis: Localized or generalized excess hair. The concept does not include hirsutism, which is excess hair in females and children with an adult male pattern of distribution. [NIH]

Hypertrophic cardiomyopathy: Heart muscle disease that leads to thickening of the heart walls, interfering with the heart's ability to fill with and pump blood. [NIH]

Hypertrophy: General increase in bulk of a part or organ, not due to tumor formation, nor to an increase in the number of cells. [NIH]

Hypnotic: A drug that acts to induce sleep. [EU]

Hypoplasia: Incomplete development or underdevelopment of an organ or tissue. [EU]

Hypotension: Abnormally low blood pressure. [NIH]

Hypothalamus: Ventral part of the diencephalon extending from the region of the optic chiasm to the caudal border of the mammillary bodies and forming the inferior and lateral walls of the third ventricle. [NIH]

Id: The part of the personality structure which harbors the unconscious instinctive desires and strivings of the individual. [NIH]

Idiopathic: Describes a disease of unknown cause. [NIH]

Ileitis: Inflammation of the ileum. [EU]

Ileum: The lower end of the small intestine. [NIH]

Iloprost: An eicosanoid, derived from the cyclooxygenase pathway of arachidonic acid metabolism. It is a stable and synthetic analog of epoprostenol, but with a longer half-life than the parent compound. Its actions are similar to prostacyclin. Iloprost produces vasodilation and inhibits platelet aggregation. [NIH]

Imidazole: C3H4N2. The ring is present in polybenzimidazoles. [NIH]

Immune Complex Diseases: Group of diseases mediated by the deposition of large soluble complexes of antigen and antibody with resultant damage to tissue. Besides serum sickness and the arthus reaction, evidence supports a pathogenic role for immune complexes in many other systemic immunologic diseases including glomerulonephritis, systemic lupus erythematosus and polyarteritis nodosa. [NIH]

Immune function: Production and action of cells that fight disease or infection. [NIH]

Immune response: The activity of the immune system against foreign substances (antigens). [NIH]

Immune Sera: Serum that contains antibodies. It is obtained from an animal that has been immunized either by antigen injection or infection with microorganisms containing the antigen. [NIH]

Immune system: The organs, cells, and molecules responsible for the recognition and disposal of foreign ("non-self") material which enters the body. [NIH]

Immune Tolerance: The specific failure of a normally responsive individual to make an immune response to a known antigen. It results from previous contact with the antigen by an immunologically immature individual (fetus or neonate) or by an adult exposed to extreme high-dose or low-dose antigen, or by exposure to radiation, antimetabolites, antilymphocytic serum, etc. [NIH]

Immunity: Nonsusceptibility to the invasive or pathogenic effects of foreign microorganisms or to the toxic effect of antigenic substances. [NIH]

Immunization: Deliberate stimulation of the host's immune response. Active immunization involves administration of antigens or immunologic adjuvants. Passive immunization involves administration of immune sera or lymphocytes or their extracts (e.g., transfer factor, immune RNA) or transplantation of immunocompetent cell producing tissue (thymus or bone marrow). [NIH]

Immunoassay: Immunochemical assay or detection of a substance by serologic or immunologic methods. Usually the substance being studied serves as antigen both in antibody production and in measurement of antibody by the test substance. [NIH]

Immunoblotting: Immunologic methods for isolating and quantitatively measuring immunoreactive substances. When used with immune reagents such as monoclonal antibodies, the process is known generically as western blot analysis (blotting, western). [NIH]

Immunochemistry: Field of chemistry that pertains to immunological phenomena and the study of chemical reactions related to antigen stimulation of tissues. It includes physicochemical interactions between antigens and antibodies. [NIH]

Immunodeficiency: The decreased ability of the body to fight infection and disease. [NIH]

Immunofluorescence: A technique for identifying molecules present on the surfaces of cells or in tissues using a highly fluorescent substance coupled to a specific antibody. [NIH]

Immunogenic: Producing immunity; evoking an immune response. [EU]

Immunoglobulin: A protein that acts as an antibody. [NIH]

Immunohistochemistry: Histochemical localization of immunoreactive substances using labeled antibodies as reagents. [NIH]

Immunologic: The ability of the antibody-forming system to recall a previous experience with an antigen and to respond to a second exposure with the prompt production of large amounts of antibody. [NIH]

Immunology: The study of the body's immune system. [NIH]

Immunophenotyping: Process of classifying cells of the immune system based on structural and functional differences. The process is commonly used to analyze and sort T-lymphocytes into subsets based on CD antigens by the technique of flow cytometry. [NIH]

Immunosuppressive: Describes the ability to lower immune system responses. [NIH]

Immunosuppressive Agents: Agents that suppress immune function by one of several mechanisms of action. Classical cytotoxic immunosuppressants act by inhibiting DNA synthesis. Others may act through activation of suppressor T-cell populations or by inhibiting the activation of helper cells. While immunosuppression has been brought about in the past primarily to prevent rejection of transplanted organs, new applications involving mediation of the effects of interleukins and other cytokines are emerging. [NIH]

Immunotherapy: Manipulation of the host's immune system in treatment of disease. It includes both active and passive immunization as well as immunosuppressive therapy to prevent graft rejection. [NIH]

Impairment: In the context of health experience, an impairment is any loss or abnormality of psychological, physiological, or anatomical structure or function. [NIH]

Implant radiation: A procedure in which radioactive material sealed in needles, seeds, wires, or catheters is placed directly into or near the tumor. Also called [NIH]

Implantation: The insertion or grafting into the body of biological, living, inert, or radioactive material. [EU]

In vitro: In the laboratory (outside the body). The opposite of in vivo (in the body). [NIH]

In vivo: In the body. The opposite of in vitro (outside the body or in the laboratory). [NIH]

Incision: A cut made in the body during surgery. [NIH]

Incisor: Anything adapted for cutting; any one of the four front teeth in each jaw. [NIH]

Incontinence: Inability to control the flow of urine from the bladder (urinary incontinence) or the escape of stool from the rectum (fecal incontinence). [NIH]

Incubated: Grown in the laboratory under controlled conditions. (For instance, white blood cells can be grown in special conditions so that they attack specific cancer cells when returned to the body.) [NIH]

Incubation: The development of an infectious disease from the entrance of the pathogen to the appearance of clinical symptoms. [EU]

Incubation period: The period of time likely to elapse between exposure to the agent of the disease and the onset of clinical symptoms. [NIH]

Indicative: That indicates; that points out more or less exactly; that reveals fairly clearly. [EU]

Induction: The act or process of inducing or causing to occur, especially the production of a specific morphogenetic effect in the developing embryo through the influence of evocators or organizers, or the production of anaesthesia or unconsciousness by use of appropriate agents. [EU]

Induration: 1. The quality of being hard; the process of hardening. 2. An abnormally hard spot or place. [EU]

Infant, Newborn: An infant during the first month after birth. [NIH]

Infarction: A pathological process consisting of a sudden insufficient blood supply to an area, which results in necrosis of that area. It is usually caused by a thrombus, an embolus, or a vascular torsion. [NIH]

Infection: 1. Invasion and multiplication of microorganisms in body tissues, which may be clinically unapparent or result in local cellular injury due to competitive metabolism, toxins, intracellular replication, or antigen-antibody response. The infection may remain localized, subclinical, and temporary if the body's defensive mechanisms are effective. A local infection may persist and spread by extension to become an acute, subacute, or chronic clinical infection or disease state. A local infection may also become systemic when the microorganisms gain access to the lymphatic or vascular system. 2. An infectious disease. [EU]

Infiltration: The diffusion or accumulation in a tissue or cells of substances not normal to it or in amounts of the normal. Also, the material so accumulated. [EU]

Inflammation: A pathological process characterized by injury or destruction of tissues caused by a variety of cytologic and chemical reactions. It is usually manifested by typical signs of pain, heat, redness, swelling, and loss of function. [NIH]

Inflammatory bowel disease: A general term that refers to the inflammation of the colon and rectum. Inflammatory bowel disease includes ulcerative colitis and Crohn's disease. [NIH]

Informed Consent: Voluntary authorization, given to the physician by the patient, with full comprehension of the risks involved, for diagnostic or investigative procedures and medical and surgical treatment. [NIH]

Infusion: A method of putting fluids, including drugs, into the bloodstream. Also called intravenous infusion. [NIH]

Ingestion: Taking into the body by mouth [NIH]

Inhalation: The drawing of air or other substances into the lungs. [EU]

Initiation: Mutation induced by a chemical reactive substance causing cell changes; being a step in a carcinogenic process. [NIH]

Inorganic: Pertaining to substances not of organic origin. [EU]

Inotropic: Affecting the force or energy of muscular contractions. [EU]

Insight: The capacity to understand one's own motives, to be aware of one's own psychodynamics, to appreciate the meaning of symbolic behavior. [NIH]

Insulator: Material covering the metal conductor of the lead. It is usually polyurethane or silicone. [NIH]

Insulin: A protein hormone secreted by beta cells of the pancreas. Insulin plays a major role in the regulation of glucose metabolism, generally promoting the cellular utilization of glucose. It is also an important regulator of protein and lipid metabolism. Insulin is used as a drug to control insulin-dependent diabetes mellitus. [NIH]

Insulin-dependent diabetes mellitus: A disease characterized by high levels of blood glucose resulting from defects in insulin secretion, insulin action, or both. Autoimmune, genetic, and environmental factors are involved in the development of type I diabetes. [NIH]

Insulin-like: Muscular growth factor. [NIH]

Interferon: A biological response modifier (a substance that can improve the body's natural response to disease). Interferons interfere with the division of cancer cells and can slow tumor growth. There are several types of interferons, including interferon-alpha, -beta, and -gamma. These substances are normally produced by the body. They are also made in the laboratory for use in treating cancer and other diseases. [NIH]

Interferon-alpha: One of the type I interferons produced by peripheral blood leukocytes or lymphoblastoid cells when exposed to live or inactivated virus, double-stranded RNA, or bacterial products. It is the major interferon produced by virus-induced leukocyte cultures and, in addition to its pronounced antiviral activity, it causes activation of NK cells. [NIH]

Interleukin-1: A soluble factor produced by monocytes, macrophages, and other cells which activates T-lymphocytes and potentiates their response to mitogens or antigens. IL-1 consists of two distinct forms, IL-1 alpha and IL-1 beta which perform the same functions but are distinct proteins. The biological effects of IL-1 include the ability to replace macrophage requirements for T-cell activation. The factor is distinct from interleukin-2. [NIH]

Interleukin-13: T-lymphocyte-derived cytokine that produces proliferation, immunoglobulin isotype switching, and immunoglobulin production by immature B-lymphocytes. It appears to play a role in regulating inflammatory and immune responses. [NIH]

Interleukin-2: Chemical mediator produced by activated T lymphocytes and which regulates the proliferation of T cells, as well as playing a role in the regulation of NK cell activity. [NIH]

Interleukin-4: Soluble factor produced by activated T-lymphocytes that causes proliferation and differentiation of B-cells. Interleukin-4 induces the expression of class II major histocompatibility complex and Fc receptors on B-cells. It also acts on T-lymphocytes, mast cell lines, and several other hematopoietic lineage cells including granulocyte, megakaryocyte, and erythroid precursors, as well as macrophages. [NIH]

Interleukin-6: Factor that stimulates the growth and differentiation of human B-cells and is also a growth factor for hybridomas and plasmacytomas. It is produced by many different cells including T-cells, monocytes, and fibroblasts. [NIH]

Intermittent: Occurring at separated intervals; having periods of cessation of activity. [EU]

Internal Medicine: A medical specialty concerned with the diagnosis and treatment of diseases of the internal organ systems of adults. [NIH]

Internal radiation: A procedure in which radioactive material sealed in needles, seeds, wires, or catheters is placed directly into or near the tumor. Also called brachytherapy, implant radiation, or interstitial radiation therapy. [NIH]

Interphase: The interval between two successive cell divisions during which the chromosomes are not individually distinguishable and DNA replication occurs. [NIH]

Interstitial: Pertaining to or situated between parts or in the interspaces of a tissue. [EU]

Interstitial Collagenase: A member of the metalloproteinase family of enzymes that is principally responsible for cleaving fibrillar collagen. It can degrade interstitial collagens, types I, II and III. EC 3.4.24.7. [NIH]

Intestinal: Having to do with the intestines. [NIH]

Intestine: A long, tube-shaped organ in the abdomen that completes the process of digestion. There is both a large intestine and a small intestine. Also called the bowel. [NIH]

Intoxication: Poisoning, the state of being poisoned. [EU]

Intracellular: Inside a cell. [NIH]

Intramuscular: IM. Within or into muscle. [NIH]

Intrathecal: Describes the fluid-filled space between the thin layers of tissue that cover the brain and spinal cord. Drugs can be injected into the fluid or a sample of the fluid can be removed for testing. [NIH]

Intravascular: Within a vessel or vessels. [EU]

Intravenous: IV. Into a vein. [NIH]

Intrinsic: Situated entirely within or pertaining exclusively to a part. [EU]

Inulin: A starch found in the tubers and roots of many plants. Since it is hydrolyzable to fructose, it is classified as a fructosan. It has been used in physiologic investigation for determination of the rate of glomerular function. [NIH]

Invasive: 1. Having the quality of invasiveness. 2. Involving puncture or incision of the skin or insertion of an instrument or foreign material into the body; said of diagnostic techniques. [EU]

Invertebrates: Animals that have no spinal column. [NIH]

Involuntary: Reaction occurring without intention or volition. [NIH]

Ion Channels: Gated, ion-selective glycoproteins that traverse membranes. The stimulus for channel gating can be a membrane potential, drug, transmitter, cytoplasmic messenger, or a mechanical deformation. Ion channels which are integral parts of ionotropic neurotransmitter receptors are not included. [NIH]

Ionizing: Radiation comprising charged particles, e. g. electrons, protons, alpha-particles, etc., having sufficient kinetic energy to produce ionization by collision. [NIH]

Ions: An atom or group of atoms that have a positive or negative electric charge due to a gain (negative charge) or loss (positive charge) of one or more electrons. Atoms with a positive charge are known as cations; those with a negative charge are anions. [NIH]

Irradiation: The use of high-energy radiation from x-rays, neutrons, and other sources to kill cancer cells and shrink tumors. Radiation may come from a machine outside the body (external-beam radiation therapy) or from materials called radioisotopes. Radioisotopes produce radiation and can be placed in or near the tumor or in the area near cancer cells. This type of radiation treatment is called internal radiation therapy, implant radiation, interstitial radiation, or brachytherapy. Systemic radiation therapy uses a radioactive substance, such as a radiolabeled monoclonal antibody, that circulates throughout the body. Irradiation is also called radiation therapy, radiotherapy, and x-ray therapy. [NIH]

Ischemia: Deficiency of blood in a part, due to functional constriction or actual obstruction of a blood vessel. [EU]

Islet: Cell producing insulin in pancreas. [NIH]

Isoelectric: Separation of amphoteric substances, dissolved in water, based on their isoelectric behavior. The amphoteric substances are a mixture of proteins to be separated and of auxiliary "carrier ampholytes". [NIH]

Isoelectric Point: The pH in solutions of proteins and related compounds at which the dipolar ions are at a maximum. [NIH]

Isradipine: 4-(4-Benzofurazanyl)-1,4-dihydro-2,6-dimethyl-3,5-pyridinedicarboxylic acid methyl 1-methyl ethyl ester. A potent calcium channel antagonist that is highly selective for vascular smooth muscle. It is effective in the treatment of chronic stable angina pectoris, hypertension, and congestive cardiac failure. [NIH]

Joint: The point of contact between elements of an animal skeleton with the parts that surround and support it. [NIH]

Kallidin: A decapeptide bradykinin homolog produced by the action of tissue and glandular kallikreins on low-molecular-weight kininogen. It is a smooth-muscle stimulant and hypotensive agent that functions through vasodilatation. [NIH]

Kb: A measure of the length of DNA fragments, 1 Kb = 1000 base pairs. The largest DNA fragments are up to 50 kilobases long. [NIH]

Keloid: A sharply elevated, irregularly shaped, progressively enlarging scar resulting from formation of excessive amounts of collagen in the dermis during connective tissue repair. It is differentiated from a hypertrophic scar (cicatrix, hypertrophic) in that the former does not spread to surrounding tissues. [NIH]

Keratin: A class of fibrous proteins or scleroproteins important both as structural proteins and as keys to the study of protein conformation. The family represents the principal constituent of epidermis, hair, nails, horny tissues, and the organic matrix of tooth enamel. Two major conformational groups have been characterized, alpha-keratin, whose peptide backbone forms an alpha-helix, and beta-keratin, whose backbone forms a zigzag or pleated sheet structure. [NIH]

Keratinocytes: Epidermal cells which synthesize keratin and undergo characteristic changes as they move upward from the basal layers of the epidermis to the cornified (horny) layer of the skin. Successive stages of differentiation of the keratinocytes forming the epidermal layers are basal cell, spinous or prickle cell, and the granular cell. [NIH]

Keratoconjunctivitis: Simultaneous inflammation of the cornea and conjunctiva. [NIH]

Keratoconjunctivitis Sicca: Drying and inflammation of the conjunctiva as a result of insufficient lacrimal secretion. When found in association with xerostomia and polyarthritis, it is called Sjogren's syndrome. [NIH]

Keratolytic: An agent that promotes keratolysis. [EU]

Kidney Disease: Any one of several chronic conditions that are caused by damage to the cells of the kidney. People who have had diabetes for a long time may have kidney damage. Also called nephropathy. [NIH]

Kidney Failure: The inability of a kidney to excrete metabolites at normal plasma levels under conditions of normal loading, or the inability to retain electrolytes under conditions of normal intake. In the acute form (kidney failure, acute), it is marked by uremia and usually by oliguria or anuria, with hyperkalemia and pulmonary edema. The chronic form (kidney failure, chronic) is irreversible and requires hemodialysis. [NIH]

Kidney Failure, Acute: A clinical syndrome characterized by a sudden decrease in glomerular filtration rate, often to values of less than 1 to 2 ml per minute. It is usually associated with oliguria (urine volumes of less than 400 ml per day) and is always associated with biochemical consequences of the reduction in glomerular filtration rate such as a rise in blood urea nitrogen (BUN) and serum creatinine concentrations. [NIH]

Kidney Failure, Chronic: An irreversible and usually progressive reduction in renal function in which both kidneys have been damaged by a variety of diseases to the extent that they are unable to adequately remove the metabolic products from the blood and regulate the body's electrolyte composition and acid-base balance. Chronic kidney failure requires hemodialysis or surgery, usually kidney transplantation. [NIH]

Kinetic: Pertaining to or producing motion. [EU]

Labetalol: Blocker of both alpha- and beta-adrenergic receptors that is used as an antihypertensive. [NIH]

Labile: 1. Gliding; moving from point to point over the surface; unstable; fluctuating. 2. Chemically unstable. [EU]

Lacrimal: Pertaining to the tears. [EU]

Laminin: Large, noncollagenous glycoprotein with antigenic properties. It is localized in the basement membrane lamina lucida and functions to bind epithelial cells to the basement membrane. Evidence suggests that the protein plays a role in tumor invasion. [NIH]

Large Intestine: The part of the intestine that goes from the cecum to the rectum. The large intestine absorbs water from stool and changes it from a liquid to a solid form. The large intestine is 5 feet long and includes the appendix, cecum, colon, and rectum. Also called colon. [NIH]

Larynx: An irregularly shaped, musculocartilaginous tubular structure, lined with mucous membrane, located at the top of the trachea and below the root of the tongue and the hyoid bone. It is the essential sphincter guarding the entrance into the trachea and functioning secondarily as the organ of voice. [NIH]

Latency: The period of apparent inactivity between the time when a stimulus is presented and the moment a response occurs. [NIH]

Latent: Phoria which occurs at one distance or another and which usually has no troublesome effect. [NIH]

Lavage: A cleaning of the stomach and colon. Uses a special drink and enemas. [NIH]

Lens: The transparent, double convex (outward curve on both sides) structure suspended between the aqueous and vitreous; helps to focus light on the retina. [NIH]

Lentivirus: A genus of the family Retroviridae consisting of non-oncogenic retroviruses that produce multi-organ diseases characterized by long incubation periods and persistent infection. Lentiviruses are unique in that they contain open reading frames (ORFs) between the pol and env genes and in the 3' env region. Five serogroups are recognized, reflecting the mammalian hosts with which they are associated. HIV-1 is the type species. [NIH]

Lesion: An area of abnormal tissue change. [NIH]

Lethal: Deadly, fatal. [EU]

Leucine: An essential branched-chain amino acid important for hemoglobin formation. [NIH]

Leucocyte: All the white cells of the blood and their precursors (myeloid cell series, lymphoid cell series) but commonly used to indicate granulocytes exclusive of lymphocytes. [NIH]

Leukemia: Cancer of blood-forming tissue. [NIH]

Leukocytes: White blood cells. These include granular leukocytes (basophils, eosinophils, and neutrophils) as well as non-granular leukocytes (lymphocytes and monocytes). [NIH]

Leukotrienes: A family of biologically active compounds derived from arachidonic acid by oxidative metabolism through the 5-lipoxygenase pathway. They participate in host defense reactions and pathophysiological conditions such as immediate hypersensitivity and inflammation. They have potent actions on many essential organs and systems, including the cardiovascular, pulmonary, and central nervous system as well as the gastrointestinal tract and the immune system. [NIH]

Levodopa: The naturally occurring form of dopa and the immediate precursor of dopamine. Unlike dopamine itself, it can be taken orally and crosses the blood-brain barrier. It is rapidly taken up by dopaminergic neurons and converted to dopamine. It is used for the treatment of parkinsonism and is usually given with agents that inhibit its conversion to dopamine outside of the central nervous system. [NIH]

Library Services: Services offered to the library user. They include reference and circulation. [NIH]

Life Expectancy: A figure representing the number of years, based on known statistics, to which any person of a given age may reasonably expect to live. [NIH]

Ligament: A band of fibrous tissue that connects bones or cartilages, serving to support and strengthen joints. [EU]

Ligands: A RNA simulation method developed by the MIT. [NIH]

Ligation: Application of a ligature to tie a vessel or strangulate a part. [NIH]

Linkage: The tendency of two or more genes in the same chromosome to remain together from one generation to the next more frequently than expected according to the law of independent assortment. [NIH]

Lip: Either of the two fleshy, full-blooded margins of the mouth. [NIH]

Lipid: Fat. [NIH]

Lipid A: Lipid A is the biologically active component of lipopolysaccharides. It shows strong endotoxic activity and exhibits immunogenic properties. [NIH]

Lipid Peroxidation: Peroxidase catalyzed oxidation of lipids using hydrogen peroxide as an electron acceptor. [NIH]

Lipopolysaccharides: Substance consisting of polysaccharide and lipid. [NIH]

Lipoprotein: Any of the lipid-protein complexes in which lipids are transported in the blood; lipoprotein particles consist of a spherical hydrophobic core of triglycerides or cholesterol esters surrounded by an amphipathic monolayer of phospholipids, cholesterol, and apolipoproteins; the four principal classes are high-density, low-density, and very-low-density lipoproteins and chylomicrons. [EU]

Lipoxygenase: An enzyme of the oxidoreductase class that catalyzes reactions between linoleate and other fatty acids and oxygen to form hydroperoxy-fatty acid derivatives. Related enzymes in this class include the arachidonate lipoxygenases, arachidonate 5-

lipoxygenase, arachidonate 12-lipoxygenase, and arachidonate 15-lipoxygenase. EC 1.13.11.12. [NIH]

Liver: A large, glandular organ located in the upper abdomen. The liver cleanses the blood and aids in digestion by secreting bile. [NIH]

Liver Cirrhosis: Liver disease in which the normal microcirculation, the gross vascular anatomy, and the hepatic architecture have been variably destroyed and altered with fibrous septa surrounding regenerated or regenerating parenchymal nodules. [NIH]

Liver scan: An image of the liver created on a computer screen or on film. A radioactive substance is injected into a blood vessel and travels through the bloodstream. It collects in the liver, especially in abnormal areas, and can be detected by the scanner. [NIH]

Liver Transplantation: The transference of a part of or an entire liver from one human or animal to another. [NIH]

Localization: The process of determining or marking the location or site of a lesion or disease. May also refer to the process of keeping a lesion or disease in a specific location or site. [NIH]

Localized: Cancer which has not metastasized yet. [NIH]

Longitudinal Studies: Studies in which variables relating to an individual or group of individuals are assessed over a period of time. [NIH]

Loop: A wire usually of platinum bent at one end into a small loop (usually 4 mm inside diameter) and used in transferring microorganisms. [NIH]

Low-density lipoprotein: Lipoprotein that contains most of the cholesterol in the blood. LDL carries cholesterol to the tissues of the body, including the arteries. A high level of LDL increases the risk of heart disease. LDL typically contains 60 to 70 percent of the total serum cholesterol and both are directly correlated with CHD risk. [NIH]

Lower Esophageal Sphincter: The muscle between the esophagus and stomach. When a person swallows, this muscle relaxes to let food pass from the esophagus to the stomach. It stays closed at other times to keep stomach contents from flowing back into the esophagus. [NIH]

Lubricants: Oily or slippery substances. [NIH]

Lubrication: The application of a substance to diminish friction between two surfaces. It may refer to oils, greases, and similar substances for the lubrication of medical equipment but it can be used for the application of substances to tissue to reduce friction, such as lotions for skin and vaginal lubricants. [NIH]

Lucida: An instrument, invented by Wollaton, consisting essentially of a prism or a mirror through which an object can be viewed so as to appear on a plane surface seen in direct view and on which the outline of the object may be traced. [NIH]

Lupus: A form of cutaneous tuberculosis. It is seen predominantly in women and typically involves the nasal, buccal, and conjunctival mucosa. [NIH]

Lupus Nephritis: Glomerulonephritis associated with systemic lupus erythematosus. It is classified into four histologic types: mesangial, focal, diffuse, and membranous. [NIH]

Luxation: The displacement of the particular surface of a bone from its normal joint, without fracture. [NIH]

Lymph: The almost colorless fluid that travels through the lymphatic system and carries cells that help fight infection and disease. [NIH]

Lymph node: A rounded mass of lymphatic tissue that is surrounded by a capsule of connective tissue. Also known as a lymph gland. Lymph nodes are spread out along lymphatic vessels and contain many lymphocytes, which filter the lymphatic fluid (lymph). [NIH]

Lymphatic: The tissues and organs, including the bone marrow, spleen, thymus, and lymph nodes, that produce and store cells that fight infection and disease. [NIH]

Lymphatic system: The tissues and organs that produce, store, and carry white blood cells that fight infection and other diseases. This system includes the bone marrow, spleen, thymus, lymph nodes and a network of thin tubes that carry lymph and white blood cells. These tubes branch, like blood vessels, into all the tissues of the body. [NIH]

Lymphocyte: A white blood cell. Lymphocytes have a number of roles in the immune system, including the production of antibodies and other substances that fight infection and diseases. [NIH]

Lymphocytic: Referring to lymphocytes, a type of white blood cell. [NIH]

Lymphoid: Referring to lymphocytes, a type of white blood cell. Also refers to tissue in which lymphocytes develop. [NIH]

Lymphoma: A general term for various neoplastic diseases of the lymphoid tissue. [NIH]

Lysine: An essential amino acid. It is often added to animal feed. [NIH]

Lytic: 1. Pertaining to lysis or to a lysin. 2. Producing lysis. [EU]

Macrophage: A type of white blood cell that surrounds and kills microorganisms, removes dead cells, and stimulates the action of other immune system cells. [NIH]

Magnetic Resonance Imaging: Non-invasive method of demonstrating internal anatomy based on the principle that atomic nuclei in a strong magnetic field absorb pulses of radiofrequency energy and emit them as radiowaves which can be reconstructed into computerized images. The concept includes proton spin tomographic techniques. [NIH]

Maintenance therapy: Treatment that is given to help a primary (original) treatment keep working. Maintenance therapy is often given to help keep cancer in remission. [NIH]

Major Histocompatibility Complex: The genetic region which contains the loci of genes which determine the structure of the serologically defined (SD) and lymphocyte-defined (LD) transplantation antigens, genes which control the structure of the immune response-associated (Ia) antigens, the immune response (Ir) genes which control the ability of an animal to respond immunologically to antigenic stimuli, and genes which determine the structure and/or level of the first four components of complement. [NIH]

Malabsorption: Impaired intestinal absorption of nutrients. [EU]

Malignant: Cancerous; a growth with a tendency to invade and destroy nearby tissue and spread to other parts of the body. [NIH]

Malignant tumor: A tumor capable of metastasizing. [NIH]

Malnutrition: A condition caused by not eating enough food or not eating a balanced diet. [NIH]

Mammary: Pertaining to the mamma, or breast. [EU]

Mammogram: An x-ray of the breast. [NIH]

Mandible: The largest and strongest bone of the face constituting the lower jaw. It supports the lower teeth. [NIH]

Manic: Affected with mania. [EU]

Manic-depressive psychosis: One of a group of psychotic reactions, fundamentally marked by severe mood swings and a tendency to remission and recurrence. [NIH]

Manifest: Being the part or aspect of a phenomenon that is directly observable : concretely expressed in behaviour. [EU]

Mannans: Polysaccharides consisting of mannose units. [NIH]

Manometry: Tests that measure muscle pressure and movements in the GI tract. [NIH]

Maternal-Fetal Exchange: Exchange of substances between the maternal blood and the fetal blood through the placental barrier. It excludes microbial or viral transmission. [NIH]

Matrix metalloproteinase: A member of a group of enzymes that can break down proteins, such as collagen, that are normally found in the spaces between cells in tissues (i.e., extracellular matrix proteins). Because these enzymes need zinc or calcium atoms to work properly, they are called metalloproteinases. Matrix metalloproteinases are involved in wound healing, angiogenesis, and tumor cell metastasis. [NIH]

Maxillary: Pertaining to the maxilla : the irregularly shaped bone that with its fellow forms the upper jaw. [EU]

McMaster: Index used to measure painful syndromes linked to arthrosis. [NIH]

Mediate: Indirect; accomplished by the aid of an intervening medium. [EU]

Mediator: An object or substance by which something is mediated, such as (1) a structure of the nervous system that transmits impulses eliciting a specific response; (2) a chemical substance (transmitter substance) that induces activity in an excitable tissue, such as nerve or muscle; or (3) a substance released from cells as the result of the interaction of antigen with antibody or by the action of antigen with a sensitized lymphocyte. [EU]

Medical Records: Recording of pertinent information concerning patient's illness or illnesses. [NIH]

MEDLINE: An online database of MEDLARS, the computerized bibliographic Medical Literature Analysis and Retrieval System of the National Library of Medicine. [NIH]

Meiosis: A special method of cell division, occurring in maturation of the germ cells, by means of which each daughter nucleus receives half the number of chromosomes characteristic of the somatic cells of the species. [NIH]

Melanin: The substance that gives the skin its color. [NIH]

Melanocytes: Epidermal dendritic pigment cells which control long-term morphological color changes by alteration in their number or in the amount of pigment they produce and store in the pigment containing organelles called melanosomes. Melanophores are larger cells which do not exist in mammals. [NIH]

Melanoma: A form of skin cancer that arises in melanocytes, the cells that produce pigment. Melanoma usually begins in a mole. [NIH]

Melanosomes: Melanin-containing organelles found in melanocytes and melanophores. [NIH]

Membrane: A very thin layer of tissue that covers a surface. [NIH]

Memory: Complex mental function having four distinct phases: (1) memorizing or learning, (2) retention, (3) recall, and (4) recognition. Clinically, it is usually subdivided into immediate, recent, and remote memory. [NIH]

Meninges: The three membranes that cover and protect the brain and spinal cord. [NIH]

Menopause: Permanent cessation of menstruation. [NIH]

Mental Disorders: Psychiatric illness or diseases manifested by breakdowns in the adaptational process expressed primarily as abnormalities of thought, feeling, and behavior producing either distress or impairment of function. [NIH]

Mercury: A silver metallic element that exists as a liquid at room temperature. It has the atomic symbol Hg (from hydrargyrum, liquid silver), atomic number 80, and atomic weight 200.59. Mercury is used in many industrial applications and its salts have been employed therapeutically as purgatives, antisyphilitics, disinfectants, and astringents. It can be absorbed through the skin and mucous membranes which leads to mercury poisoning. Because of its toxicity, the clinical use of mercury and mercurials is diminishing. [NIH]

Mesenchymal: Refers to cells that develop into connective tissue, blood vessels, and lymphatic tissue. [NIH]

Metabolite: Any substance produced by metabolism or by a metabolic process. [EU]

Metastasis: The spread of cancer from one part of the body to another. Tumors formed from cells that have spread are called "secondary tumors" and contain cells that are like those in the original (primary) tumor. The plural is metastases. [NIH]

Methanol: A colorless, flammable liquid used in the manufacture of formaldehyde and acetic acid, in chemical synthesis, antifreeze, and as a solvent. Ingestion of methanol is toxic and may cause blindness. [NIH]

Methoxsalen: A naturally occurring furocoumarin compound found in several species of plants, including Psoralea corylifolia. It is a photoactive substance that forms DNA adducts in the presence of ultraviolet A irradiation. [NIH]

Metoclopramide: A dopamine D2 antagonist that is used as an antiemetic. [NIH]

MI: Myocardial infarction. Gross necrosis of the myocardium as a result of interruption of the blood supply to the area; it is almost always caused by atherosclerosis of the coronary arteries, upon which coronary thrombosis is usually superimposed. [NIH]

Mibefradil: A benzimidazoyl-substituted tetraline that binds selectively to and inhibits calcium channels, T-type. [NIH]

Microbe: An organism which cannot be observed with the naked eye; e. g. unicellular animals, lower algae, lower fungi, bacteria. [NIH]

Microcalcifications: Tiny deposits of calcium in the breast that cannot be felt but can be detected on a mammogram. A cluster of these very small specks of calcium may indicate that cancer is present. [NIH]

Microcirculation: The vascular network lying between the arterioles and venules; includes capillaries, metarterioles and arteriovenous anastomoses. Also, the flow of blood through this network. [NIH]

Microfibrils: Components of the extracellular matrix consisting primarily of fibrillin. They are essential for the integrity of elastic fibers. [NIH]

Microorganism: An organism that can be seen only through a microscope. Microorganisms include bacteria, protozoa, algae, and fungi. Although viruses are not considered living organisms, they are sometimes classified as microorganisms. [NIH]

Micro-organism: An organism which cannot be observed with the naked eye; e. g. unicellular animals, lower algae, lower fungi, bacteria. [NIH]

Microscopy: The application of microscope magnification to the study of materials that cannot be properly seen by the unaided eye. [NIH]

Microtubules: Slender, cylindrical filaments found in the cytoskeleton of plant and animal cells. They are composed of the protein tubulin. [NIH]

Migration: The systematic movement of genes between populations of the same species, geographic race, or variety. [NIH]

Milliliter: A measure of volume for a liquid. A milliliter is approximately 950-times smaller than a quart and 30-times smaller than a fluid ounce. A milliliter of liquid and a cubic centimeter (cc) of liquid are the same. [NIH]

Mineralocorticoids: A group of corticosteroids primarily associated with the regulation of water and electrolyte balance. This is accomplished through the effect on ion transport in renal tubules, resulting in retention of sodium and loss of potassium. Mineralocorticoid secretion is itself regulated by plasma volume, serum potassium, and angiotensin II. [NIH]

Minor Histocompatibility Loci: Genetic loci responsible for the encoding of histocompatibility antigens other than those encoded by the major histocompatibility complex. The antigens encoded by these genes are often responsible for graft rejection in cases where histocompatibility has been established by standard tests. The location of some of these loci on the X and Y chromosomes explains why grafts from males to females may be rejected while grafts from females to males are accepted. In the mouse roughly 30 minor histocompatibility loci have been recognized, comprising more than 500 genes. [NIH]

Miotic: 1. Pertaining to, characterized by, or producing miosis : contraction of the pupil. 2. An agent that causes the pupil to contract. 3. Meiotic: characterized by cell division. [EU]

Mitochondrial Swelling: Increase in volume of mitochondria due to an influx of fluid; it occurs in hypotonic solutions due to osmotic pressure and in isotonic solutions as a result of altered permeability of the membranes of respiring mitochondria. [NIH]

Mitogen-Activated Protein Kinase Kinases: A serine-threonine protein kinase family whose members are components in protein kinase cascades activated by diverse stimuli. These MAPK kinases phosphorylate mitogen-activated protein kinases and are themselves phosphorylated by MAP kinase kinase kinases. JNK kinases (also known as SAPK kinases) are a subfamily. EC 2.7.10.- [NIH]

Mitogen-Activated Protein Kinases: A superfamily of protein-serine-threonine kinases that are activated by diverse stimuli via protein kinase cascades. They are the final components of the cascades, activated by phosphorylation by mitogen-activated protein kinase kinases which in turn are activated by mitogen-activated protein kinase kinase kinases (MAP kinase kinase kinases). Families of these mitogen-activated protein kinases (MAPKs) include extracellular signal-regulated kinases (ERKs), stress-activated protein kinases (SAPKs) (also known as c-jun terminal kinases (JNKs)), and p38-mitogen-activated protein kinases. EC 2,7,1.- [NIH]

Mitosis: A method of indirect cell division by means of which the two daughter nuclei normally receive identical complements of the number of chromosomes of the somatic cells of the species. [NIH]

Mitotic: Cell resulting from mitosis. [NIH]

Mitotic inhibitors: Drugs that kill cancer cells by interfering with cell division (mitostis). [NIH]

Mixed Connective Tissue Disease: A syndrome with overlapping clinical features of systemic lupus erythematosus, scleroderma, polymyositis, and Raynaud's phenomenon. The disease is differentially characterized by high serum titers of antibodies to ribonuclease-sensitive extractable (saline soluble) nuclear antigen and a "speckled" epidermal nuclear staining pattern on direct immunofluorescence. [NIH]

Mobility: Capability of movement, of being moved, or of flowing freely. [EU]

Modeling: A treatment procedure whereby the therapist presents the target behavior which the learner is to imitate and make part of his repertoire. [NIH]

Modification: A change in an organism, or in a process in an organism, that is acquired from its own activity or environment. [NIH]

Molecular: Of, pertaining to, or composed of molecules : a very small mass of matter. [EU]

Molecular Probes: A group of atoms or molecules attached to other molecules or cellular structures and used in studying the properties of these molecules and structures. Radioactive DNA or RNA sequences are used in molecular genetics to detect the presence of a complementary sequence by molecular hybridization. [NIH]

Molecule: A chemical made up of two or more atoms. The atoms in a molecule can be the same (an oxygen molecule has two oxygen atoms) or different (a water molecule has two hydrogen atoms and one oxygen atom). Biological molecules, such as proteins and DNA, can be made up of many thousands of atoms. [NIH]

Monitor: An apparatus which automatically records such physiological signs as respiration, pulse, and blood pressure in an anesthetized patient or one undergoing surgical or other procedures. [NIH]

Monoclonal: An antibody produced by culturing a single type of cell. It therefore consists of a single species of immunoglobulin molecules. [NIH]

Monoclonal antibodies: Laboratory-produced substances that can locate and bind to cancer cells wherever they are in the body. Many monoclonal antibodies are used in cancer detection or therapy; each one recognizes a different protein on certain cancer cells. Monoclonal antibodies can be used alone, or they can be used to deliver drugs, toxins, or radioactive material directly to a tumor. [NIH]

Monocyte: A type of white blood cell. [NIH]

Monocyte Chemoattractant Protein-1: A chemokine that is a chemoattractant for human monocytes and may also cause cellular activation of specific functions related to host defense. It is produced by leukocytes of both monocyte and lymphocyte lineage and by fibroblasts during tissue injury. [NIH]

Mononuclear: A cell with one nucleus. [NIH]

Morphological: Relating to the configuration or the structure of live organs. [NIH]

Morphology: The science of the form and structure of organisms (plants, animals, and other forms of life). [NIH]

Motility: The ability to move spontaneously. [EU]

Motion Sickness: Sickness caused by motion, as sea sickness, train sickness, car sickness, and air sickness. [NIH]

Motor Activity: The physical activity of an organism as a behavioral phenomenon. [NIH]

Mucins: A secretion containing mucopolysaccharides and protein that is the chief constituent of mucus. [NIH]

Mucolytic: Destroying or dissolving mucin; an agent that so acts : a mucopolysaccharide or glycoprotein, the chief constituent of mucus. [EU]

Mucosa: A mucous membrane, or tunica mucosa. [EU]

Mucus: The viscous secretion of mucous membranes. It contains mucin, white blood cells, water, inorganic salts, and exfoliated cells. [NIH]

Multidrug resistance: Adaptation of tumor cells to anticancer drugs in ways that make the drugs less effective. [NIH]

Multiple Myeloma: A malignant tumor of plasma cells usually arising in the bone marrow; characterized by diffuse involvement of the skeletal system, hyperglobulinemia, Bence-Jones proteinuria, and anemia. [NIH]

Multiple sclerosis: A disorder of the central nervous system marked by weakness, numbness, a loss of muscle coordination, and problems with vision, speech, and bladder control. Multiple sclerosis is thought to be an autoimmune disease in which the body's immune system destroys myelin. Myelin is a substance that contains both protein and fat (lipid) and serves as a nerve insulator and helps in the transmission of nerve signals. [NIH]

Muscle Fibers: Large single cells, either cylindrical or prismatic in shape, that form the basic unit of muscle tissue. They consist of a soft contractile substance enclosed in a tubular sheath. [NIH]

Muscular Atrophy: Derangement in size and number of muscle fibers occurring with aging, reduction in blood supply, or following immobilization, prolonged weightlessness, malnutrition, and particularly in denervation. [NIH]

Muscular Dystrophies: A general term for a group of inherited disorders which are characterized by progressive degeneration of skeletal muscles. [NIH]

Mutagenesis: Process of generating genetic mutations. It may occur spontaneously or be induced by mutagens. [NIH]

Mutagens: Chemical agents that increase the rate of genetic mutation by interfering with the function of nucleic acids. A clastogen is a specific mutagen that causes breaks in chromosomes. [NIH]

Myasthenia: Muscular debility; any constitutional anomaly of muscle. [EU]

Mycophenolate mofetil: A drug that is being studied for its effectiveness in preventing graft-versus-host disease and autoimmune disorders. [NIH]

Mydriatic: 1. Dilating the pupil. 2. Any drug that dilates the pupil. [EU]

Myelin: The fatty substance that covers and protects nerves. [NIH]

Myeloma: Cancer that arises in plasma cells, a type of white blood cell. [NIH]

Myocardial infarction: Gross necrosis of the myocardium as a result of interruption of the blood supply to the area; it is almost always caused by atherosclerosis of the coronary arteries, upon which coronary thrombosis is usually superimposed. [NIH]

Myocardial Ischemia: A disorder of cardiac function caused by insufficient blood flow to the muscle tissue of the heart. The decreased blood flow may be due to narrowing of the coronary arteries (coronary arteriosclerosis), to obstruction by a thrombus (coronary thrombosis), or less commonly, to diffuse narrowing of arterioles and other small vessels within the heart. Severe interruption of the blood supply to the myocardial tissue may result in necrosis of cardiac muscle (myocardial infarction). [NIH]

Myocardial Reperfusion: Generally, restoration of blood supply to heart tissue which is ischemic due to decrease in normal blood supply. The decrease may result from any source including atherosclerotic obstruction, narrowing of the artery, or surgical clamping. Reperfusion can be induced to treat ischemia. Methods include chemical dissolution of an occluding thrombus, administration of vasodilator drugs, angioplasty, catheterization, and artery bypass graft surgery. However, it is thought that reperfusion can itself further damage the ischemic tissue, causing myocardial reperfusion injury. [NIH]

Myocardial Reperfusion Injury: Functional, metabolic, or structural changes in ischemic heart muscle thought to result from reperfusion to the ischemic areas. Changes can be fatal to muscle cells and may include edema with explosive cell swelling and disintegration, sarcolemma disruption, fragmentation of mitochondria, contraction band necrosis, enzyme washout, and calcium overload. Other damage may include hemorrhage and ventricular arrhythmias. One possible mechanism of damage is thought to be oxygen free radicals. Treatment currently includes the introduction of scavengers of oxygen free radicals, and injury is thought to be prevented by warm blood cardioplegic infusion prior to reperfusion. [NIH]

Myocardium: The muscle tissue of the heart composed of striated, involuntary muscle known as cardiac muscle. [NIH]

Myopathy: Any disease of a muscle. [EU]

Myopia: That error of refraction in which rays of light entering the eye parallel to the optic axis are brought to a focus in front of the retina, as a result of the eyeball being too long from front to back (axial m.) or of an increased strength in refractive power of the media of the eye (index m.). Called also nearsightedness, because the near point is less distant than it is in emmetropia with an equal amplitude of accommodation. [EU]

Myositis: Inflammation of a voluntary muscle. [EU]

Myotonic Dystrophy: A condition presenting muscle weakness and wasting which may be progressive. [NIH]

Natriuresis: The excretion of abnormal amounts of sodium in the urine. [EU]

Natural selection: A part of the evolutionary process resulting in the survival and reproduction of the best adapted individuals. [NIH]

Nausea: An unpleasant sensation in the stomach usually accompanied by the urge to vomit. Common causes are early pregnancy, sea and motion sickness, emotional stress, intense pain, food poisoning, and various enteroviruses. [NIH]

NCI: National Cancer Institute. NCI, part of the National Institutes of Health of the United States Department of Health and Human Services, is the federal government's principal agency for cancer research. NCI conducts, coordinates, and funds cancer research, training, health information dissemination, and other programs with respect to the cause, diagnosis, prevention, and treatment of cancer. Access the NCI Web site at http://cancer.gov. [NIH]

Necrolysis: Separation or exfoliation of tissue due to necrosis. [EU]

Necrosis: A pathological process caused by the progressive degradative action of enzymes that is generally associated with severe cellular trauma. It is characterized by mitochondrial swelling, nuclear flocculation, uncontrolled cell lysis, and ultimately cell death. [NIH]

Need: A state of tension or dissatisfaction felt by an individual that impels him to action toward a goal he believes will satisfy the impulse. [NIH]

Neonatal: Pertaining to the first four weeks after birth. [EU]

Neoplasia: Abnormal and uncontrolled cell growth. [NIH]

Neoplasms: New abnormal growth of tissue. Malignant neoplasms show a greater degree of anaplasia and have the properties of invasion and metastasis, compared to benign neoplasms. [NIH]

Neoplastic: Pertaining to or like a neoplasm (= any new and abnormal growth); pertaining to neoplasia (= the formation of a neoplasm). [EU]

Nephritis: Inflammation of the kidney; a focal or diffuse proliferative or destructive process which may involve the glomerulus, tubule, or interstitial renal tissue. [EU]

Nephropathy: Disease of the kidneys. [EU]

Nerve: A cordlike structure of nervous tissue that connects parts of the nervous system with other tissues of the body and conveys nervous impulses to, or away from, these tissues. [NIH]

Nervous System: The entire nerve apparatus composed of the brain, spinal cord, nerves and ganglia. [NIH]

Networks: Pertaining to a nerve or to the nerves, a meshlike structure of interlocking fibers or strands. [NIH]

Neural: 1. Pertaining to a nerve or to the nerves. 2. Situated in the region of the spinal axis, as the neutral arch. [EU]

Neuralgia: Intense or aching pain that occurs along the course or distribution of a peripheral or cranial nerve. [NIH]

Neurogenic: Loss of bladder control caused by damage to the nerves controlling the bladder. [NIH]

Neurologic: Having to do with nerves or the nervous system. [NIH]

Neuromuscular: Pertaining to muscles and nerves. [EU]

Neuromuscular Junction: The synapse between a neuron and a muscle. [NIH]

Neuronal: Pertaining to a neuron or neurons (= conducting cells of the nervous system). [EU]

Neurons: The basic cellular units of nervous tissue. Each neuron consists of a body, an axon, and dendrites. Their purpose is to receive, conduct, and transmit impulses in the nervous system. [NIH]

Neuropathy: A problem in any part of the nervous system except the brain and spinal cord. Neuropathies can be caused by infection, toxic substances, or disease. [NIH]

Neuropeptides: Peptides released by neurons as intercellular messengers. Many neuropeptides are also hormones released by non-neuronal cells. [NIH]

Neurotransmitters: Endogenous signaling molecules that alter the behavior of neurons or effector cells. Neurotransmitter is used here in its most general sense, including not only messengers that act directly to regulate ion channels, but also those that act through second messenger systems, and those that act at a distance from their site of release. Included are neuromodulators, neuroregulators, neuromediators, and neurohumors, whether or not acting at synapses. [NIH]

Neutrons: Electrically neutral elementary particles found in all atomic nuclei except light hydrogen; the mass is equal to that of the proton and electron combined and they are unstable when isolated from the nucleus, undergoing beta decay. Slow, thermal, epithermal, and fast neutrons refer to the energy levels with which the neutrons are ejected from heavier nuclei during their decay. [NIH]

Neutrophils: Granular leukocytes having a nucleus with three to five lobes connected by slender threads of chromatin, and cytoplasm containing fine inconspicuous granules and stainable by neutral dyes. [NIH]

Niacin: Water-soluble vitamin of the B complex occurring in various animal and plant tissues. Required by the body for the formation of coenzymes NAD and NADP. Has pellagra-curative, vasodilating, and antilipemic properties. [NIH]

Nicardipine: 1,4-Dihydro-2,6-dimethyl-4-(3-nitrophenyl) methyl 2-(methyl(phenylmethyl)amino)-3,5-pyridinecarboxylic acid ethyl ester. A potent calcium channel blockader with marked vasodilator action. It has antihypertensive properties and is effective in the treatment of angina and coronary spasms without showing cardiodepressant effects. It has also been used in the treatment of asthma and enhances the action of specific antineoplastic agents. [NIH]

Nifedipine: A potent vasodilator agent with calcium antagonistic action. It is a useful anti-anginal agent that also lowers blood pressure. The use of nifedipine as a tocolytic is being investigated. [NIH]

Nimodipine: A calcium channel blockader with preferential cerebrovascular activity. It has marked cerebrovascular dilating effects and lowers blood pressure. [NIH]

Nisoldipine: 1,4-Dihydro-2,6-dimethyl-4 (2-nitrophenyl)-3,5-pyridinedicarboxylic acid methyl 2-methylpropyl ester. Nisoldipine is a dihydropyridine calcium channel antagonist that acts as a potent arterial vasodilator and antihypertensive agent. It is also effective in patients with cardiac failure and angina. [NIH]

Nitrates: Inorganic or organic salts and esters of nitric acid. These compounds contain the NO3- radical. [NIH]

Nitrendipine: Ethyl methyl 2,4-dihydro-2,6-dimethyl-4- (3-nitrophenyl)-3,5-pyridinedicarboxylate. A calcium channel blocker with marked vasodilator action. It is an effective antihypertensive agent and differs from other calcium channel blockers in that it does not reduce glomerular filtration rate and is mildly natriuretic, rather than sodium retentive. [NIH]

Nitric acid: A toxic, corrosive, colorless liquid used to make fertilizers, dyes, explosives, and other chemicals. [NIH]

Nitric Oxide: A free radical gas produced endogenously by a variety of mammalian cells. It is synthesized from arginine by a complex reaction, catalyzed by nitric oxide synthase. Nitric oxide is endothelium-derived relaxing factor. It is released by the vascular endothelium and mediates the relaxation induced by some vasodilators such as acetylcholine and bradykinin. It also inhibits platelet aggregation, induces disaggregation of aggregated platelets, and inhibits platelet adhesion to the vascular endothelium. Nitric oxide activates cytosolic guanylate cyclase and thus elevates intracellular levels of cyclic GMP. [NIH]

Nitrogen: An element with the atomic symbol N, atomic number 7, and atomic weight 14. Nitrogen exists as a diatomic gas and makes up about 78% of the earth's atmosphere by volume. It is a constituent of proteins and nucleic acids and found in all living cells. [NIH]

Nonoxynol: Nonionic surfactant mixtures varying in the number of repeating ethoxy (oxy-1,2-ethanediyl) groups. They are used as detergents, emulsifiers, wetting agents, defoaming agents, etc. Nonoxynol-9, the compound with 9 repeating ethoxy groups, is a spermatocide, formulated primarily as a component of vaginal foams and creams. [NIH]

Norepinephrine: Precursor of epinephrine that is secreted by the adrenal medulla and is a widespread central and autonomic neurotransmitter. Norepinephrine is the principal transmitter of most postganglionic sympathetic fibers and of the diffuse projection system in the brain arising from the locus ceruleus. It is also found in plants and is used pharmacologically as a sympathomimetic. [NIH]

Nuclear: A test of the structure, blood flow, and function of the kidneys. The doctor injects a mildly radioactive solution into an arm vein and uses x-rays to monitor its progress through the kidneys. [NIH]

Nuclear Family: A family composed of spouses and their children. [NIH]

Nuclear Proteins: Proteins found in the nucleus of a cell. Do not confuse with nucleoproteins which are proteins conjugated with nucleic acids, that are not necessarily present in the nucleus. [NIH]

Nuclei: A body of specialized protoplasm found in nearly all cells and containing the chromosomes. [NIH]

Nucleic acid: Either of two types of macromolecule (DNA or RNA) formed by polymerization of nucleotides. Nucleic acids are found in all living cells and contain the information (genetic code) for the transfer of genetic information from one generation to the next. [NIH]

Nucleic Acid Hybridization: The process whereby two single-stranded polynucleotides form a double-stranded molecule, with hydrogen bonding between the complementary bases in the two strains. [NIH]

Nucleoli: A small dense body (sub organelle) within the nucleus of eukaryotic cells, visible by phase contrast and interference microscopy in live cells throughout interphase. Contains RNA and protein and is the site of synthesis of ribosomal RNA. [NIH]

Nucleolus: A small dense body (sub organelle) within the nucleus of eukaryotic cells, visible by phase contrast and interference microscopy in live cells throughout interphase. Contains RNA and protein and is the site of synthesis of ribosomal RNA. [NIH]

Nucleolus Organizer Region: The chromosome region which is active in nucleolus formation and which functions in the synthesis of ribosomal RNA. [NIH]

Nucleoproteins: Proteins conjugated with nucleic acids. [NIH]

Nucleus: A body of specialized protoplasm found in nearly all cells and containing the chromosomes. [NIH]

Nutritional Status: State of the body in relation to the consumption and utilization of nutrients. [NIH]

Observational study: An epidemiologic study that does not involve any intervention, experimental or otherwise. Such a study may be one in which nature is allowed to take its course, with changes in one characteristic being studied in relation to changes in other characteristics. Analytical epidemiologic methods, such as case-control and cohort study designs, are properly called observational epidemiology because the investigator is observing without intervention other than to record, classify, count, and statistically analyze results. [NIH]

Octreotide: A potent, long-acting somatostatin octapeptide analog which has a wide range of physiological actions. It inhibits growth hormone secretion, is effective in the treatment of hormone-secreting tumors from various organs, and has beneficial effects in the management of many pathological states including diabetes mellitus, orthostatic hypertension, hyperinsulinism, hypergastrinemia, and small bowel fistula. [NIH]

Ocular: 1. Of, pertaining to, or affecting the eye. 2. Eyepiece. [EU]

Odds Ratio: The ratio of two odds. The exposure-odds ratio for case control data is the ratio of the odds in favor of exposure among cases to the odds in favor of exposure among noncases. The disease-odds ratio for a cohort or cross section is the ratio of the odds in favor of disease among the exposed to the odds in favor of disease among the unexposed. The prevalence-odds ratio refers to an odds ratio derived cross-sectionally from studies of prevalent cases. [NIH]

Odour: A volatile emanation that is perceived by the sense of smell. [EU]

Oedema: The presence of abnormally large amounts of fluid in the intercellular tissue spaces of the body; usually applied to demonstrable accumulation of excessive fluid in the subcutaneous tissues. Edema may be localized, due to venous or lymphatic obstruction or to increased vascular permeability, or it may be systemic due to heart failure or renal disease. Collections of edema fluid are designated according to the site, e.g. ascites (peritoneal cavity), hydrothorax (pleural cavity), and hydropericardium (pericardial sac). Massive generalized edema is called anasarca. [EU]

Ointments: Semisolid preparations used topically for protective emollient effects or as a vehicle for local administration of medications. Ointment bases are various mixtures of fats, waxes, animal and plant oils and solid and liquid hydrocarbons. [NIH]

Oligopeptides: Peptides composed of between two and twelve amino acids. [NIH]

Oligoribonucleotides: A group of ribonucleotides (up to 12) in which the phosphate residues of each ribonucleotide act as bridges in forming diester linkages between the ribose moieties. [NIH]

Oliguria: Clinical manifestation of the urinary system consisting of a decrease in the amount of urine secreted. [NIH]

Oncogene: A gene that normally directs cell growth. If altered, an oncogene can promote or allow the uncontrolled growth of cancer. Alterations can be inherited or caused by an environmental exposure to carcinogens. [NIH]

Oncogenic: Chemical, viral, radioactive or other agent that causes cancer; carcinogenic. [NIH]

Opacity: Degree of density (area most dense taken for reading). [NIH]

Open Reading Frames: Reading frames where successive nucleotide triplets can be read as codons specifying amino acids and where the sequence of these triplets is not interrupted by stop codons. [NIH]

Ophthalmologic: Pertaining to ophthalmology (= the branch of medicine dealing with the eye). [EU]

Ophthalmology: A surgical specialty concerned with the structure and function of the eye and the medical and surgical treatment of its defects and diseases. [NIH]

Opsin: A protein formed, together with retinene, by the chemical breakdown of meta-rhodopsin. [NIH]

Optic Disk: The portion of the optic nerve seen in the fundus with the ophthalmoscope. It is formed by the meeting of all the retinal ganglion cell axons as they enter the optic nerve. [NIH]

Oral Health: The optimal state of the mouth and normal functioning of the organs of the mouth without evidence of disease. [NIH]

Oral Hygiene: The practice of personal hygiene of the mouth. It includes the maintenance of oral cleanliness, tissue tone, and general preservation of oral health. [NIH]

Organelles: Specific particles of membrane-bound organized living substances present in eukaryotic cells, such as the mitochondria; the golgi apparatus; endoplasmic reticulum; lysomomes; plastids; and vacuoles. [NIH]

Orthostatic: Pertaining to or caused by standing erect. [EU]

Osmotic: Pertaining to or of the nature of osmosis (= the passage of pure solvent from a solution of lesser to one of greater solute concentration when the two solutions are separated by a membrane which selectively prevents the passage of solute molecules, but is permeable to the solvent). [EU]

Osteoarthritis: A progressive, degenerative joint disease, the most common form of arthritis, especially in older persons. The disease is thought to result not from the aging process but from biochemical changes and biomechanical stresses affecting articular cartilage. In the foreign literature it is often called osteoarthrosis deformans. [NIH]

Osteolysis: Dissolution of bone that particularly involves the removal or loss of calcium. [NIH]

Osteonectin: Non-collagenous, calcium-binding glycoprotein of developing bone. It links collagen to mineral in the bone matrix. In the synonym SPARC glycoprotein, the acronym stands for secreted protein, acidic and rich in cysteine. [NIH]

Osteoporosis: Reduction of bone mass without alteration in the composition of bone, leading to fractures. Primary osteoporosis can be of two major types: postmenopausal osteoporosis and age-related (or senile) osteoporosis. [NIH]

Outpatient: A patient who is not an inmate of a hospital but receives diagnosis or treatment in a clinic or dispensary connected with the hospital. [NIH]

Ovarian Follicle: Spheroidal cell aggregation in the ovary containing an ovum. It consists of an external fibro-vascular coat, an internal coat of nucleated cells, and a transparent, albuminous fluid in which the ovum is suspended. [NIH]

Ovaries: The pair of female reproductive glands in which the ova, or eggs, are formed. The ovaries are located in the pelvis, one on each side of the uterus. [NIH]

Ovary: Either of the paired glands in the female that produce the female germ cells and secrete some of the female sex hormones. [NIH]

Overexpress: An excess of a particular protein on the surface of a cell. [NIH]

Ovum: A female germ cell extruded from the ovary at ovulation. [NIH]

Oxidation: The act of oxidizing or state of being oxidized. Chemically it consists in the increase of positive charges on an atom or the loss of negative charges. Most biological oxidations are accomplished by the removal of a pair of hydrogen atoms (dehydrogenation) from a molecule. Such oxidations must be accompanied by reduction of an acceptor molecule. Univalent o. indicates loss of one electron; divalent o., the loss of two electrons. [EU]

Oxidative metabolism: A chemical process in which oxygen is used to make energy from carbohydrates (sugars). Also known as aerobic respiration, cell respiration, or aerobic metabolism. [NIH]

Oxidative Stress: A disturbance in the prooxidant-antioxidant balance in favor of the former, leading to potential damage. Indicators of oxidative stress include damaged DNA bases, protein oxidation products, and lipid peroxidation products (Sies, Oxidative Stress, 1991, pxv-xvi). [NIH]

Paclitaxel: Antineoplastic agent isolated from the bark of the Pacific yew tree, Taxus brevifolia. Paclitaxel stabilizes microtubules in their polymerized form and thus mimics the action of the proto-oncogene proteins c-mos. [NIH]

Palliative: 1. Affording relief, but not cure. 2. An alleviating medicine. [EU]

Pallor: A clinical manifestation consisting of an unnatural paleness of the skin. [NIH]

Pancreas: A mixed exocrine and endocrine gland situated transversely across the posterior abdominal wall in the epigastric and hypochondriac regions. The endocrine portion is comprised of the Islets of Langerhans, while the exocrine portion is a compound acinar gland that secretes digestive enzymes. [NIH]

Pancreatic: Having to do with the pancreas. [NIH]

Pancreatic cancer: Cancer of the pancreas, a salivary gland of the abdomen. [NIH]

Panniculitis: General term for inflammation of adipose tissue, usually of the skin, characterized by reddened subcutaneous nodules. [NIH]

Papillary: Pertaining to or resembling papilla, or nipple. [EU]

Paraffin: A mixture of solid hydrocarbons obtained from petroleum. It has a wide range of uses including as a stiffening agent in ointments, as a lubricant, and as a topical anti-inflammatory. It is also commonly used as an embedding material in histology. [NIH]

Paralysis: Loss of ability to move all or part of the body. [NIH]

Parathyroid: 1. Situated beside the thyroid gland. 2. One of the parathyroid glands. 3. A sterile preparation of the water-soluble principle(s) of the parathyroid glands, ad-ministered parenterally as an antihypocalcaemic, especially in the treatment of acute hypoparathyroidism with tetany. [EU]

Parathyroid hormone: A substance made by the parathyroid gland that helps the body store and use calcium. Also called parathormone, parathyrin, or PTH. [NIH]

Parenteral: Not through the alimentary canal but rather by injection through some other route, as subcutaneous, intramuscular, intraorbital, intracapsular, intraspinal, intrasternal, intravenous, etc. [EU]

Parietal: 1. Of or pertaining to the walls of a cavity. 2. Pertaining to or located near the parietal bone, as the parietal lobe. [EU]

Parietal Cells: Cells in the stomach wall that make hydrochloric acid. [NIH]

Parietal Lobe: Upper central part of the cerebral hemisphere. [NIH]

Parkinsonism: A group of neurological disorders characterized by hypokinesia, tremor, and muscular rigidity. [EU]

Parotid: The space that contains the parotid gland, the facial nerve, the external carotid artery, and the retromandibular vein. [NIH]

Paroxysmal: Recurring in paroxysms (= spasms or seizures). [EU]

Particle: A tiny mass of material. [EU]

Parturition: The act or process of given birth to a child. [EU]

Patch: A piece of material used to cover or protect a wound, an injured part, etc.: a patch over the eye. [NIH]

Pathogen: Any disease-producing microorganism. [EU]

Pathogenesis: The cellular events and reactions that occur in the development of disease. [NIH]

Pathologic: 1. Indicative of or caused by a morbid condition. 2. Pertaining to pathology (= branch of medicine that treats the essential nature of the disease, especially the structural and functional changes in tissues and organs of the body caused by the disease). [EU]

Pathologic Processes: The abnormal mechanisms and forms involved in the dysfunctions of tissues and organs. [NIH]

Pathologies: The study of abnormality, especially the study of diseases. [NIH]

Pathophysiology: Altered functions in an individual or an organ due to disease. [NIH]

Patient Compliance: Voluntary cooperation of the patient in following a prescribed regimen. [NIH]

Patient Education: The teaching or training of patients concerning their own health needs. [NIH]

Pelvic: Pertaining to the pelvis. [EU]

Pemphigus: Group of chronic blistering diseases characterized histologically by acantholysis and blister formation within the epidermis. [NIH]

Penicillamine: 3-Mercapto-D-valine. The most characteristic degradation product of the penicillin antibiotics. It is used as an antirheumatic and as a chelating agent in Wilson's disease. [NIH]

Penicillin: An antibiotic drug used to treat infection. [NIH]

Penis: The external reproductive organ of males. It is composed of a mass of erectile tissue enclosed in three cylindrical fibrous compartments. Two of the three compartments, the corpus cavernosa, are placed side-by-side along the upper part of the organ. The third compartment below, the corpus spongiosum, houses the urethra. [NIH]

Peptide: Any compound consisting of two or more amino acids, the building blocks of proteins. Peptides are combined to make proteins. [NIH]

Peptide Fragments: Partial proteins formed by partial hydrolysis of complete proteins. [NIH]

Peptide T: N-(N-(N(2)-(N-(N-(N-(N-D-Alanyl L-seryl)-L-threonyl)-L-threonyl) L-threonyl)-

L-asparaginyl)-L-tyrosyl) L-threonine. Octapeptide sharing sequence homology with HIV envelope protein gp120. It is potentially useful as antiviral agent in AIDS therapy. The core pentapeptide sequence, TTNYT, consisting of amino acids 4-8 in peptide T, is the HIV envelope sequence required for attachment to the CD4 receptor. [NIH]

Percutaneous: Performed through the skin, as injection of radiopacque material in radiological examination, or the removal of tissue for biopsy accomplished by a needle. [EU]

Perforation: 1. The act of boring or piercing through a part. 2. A hole made through a part or substance. [EU]

Perfusion: Bathing an organ or tissue with a fluid. In regional perfusion, a specific area of the body (usually an arm or a leg) receives high doses of anticancer drugs through a blood vessel. Such a procedure is performed to treat cancer that has not spread. [NIH]

Pericardium: The fibroserous sac surrounding the heart and the roots of the great vessels. [NIH]

Periodontitis: Inflammation of the periodontal membrane; also called periodontitis simplex. [NIH]

Peripheral blood: Blood circulating throughout the body. [NIH]

Peripheral Nervous System: The nervous system outside of the brain and spinal cord. The peripheral nervous system has autonomic and somatic divisions. The autonomic nervous system includes the enteric, parasympathetic, and sympathetic subdivisions. The somatic nervous system includes the cranial and spinal nerves and their ganglia and the peripheral sensory receptors. [NIH]

Peripheral Neuropathy: Nerve damage, usually affecting the feet and legs; causing pain, numbness, or a tingling feeling. Also called "somatic neuropathy" or "distal sensory polyneuropathy." [NIH]

Peripheral stem cells: Immature cells found circulating in the bloodstream. New blood cells develop from peripheral stem cells. [NIH]

Peripheral Vascular Disease: Disease in the large blood vessels of the arms, legs, and feet. People who have had diabetes for a long time may get this because major blood vessels in their arms, legs, and feet are blocked and these limbs do not receive enough blood. The signs of PVD are aching pains in the arms, legs, and feet (especially when walking) and foot sores that heal slowly. Although people with diabetes cannot always avoid PVD, doctors say they have a better chance of avoiding it if they take good care of their feet, do not smoke, and keep both their blood pressure and diabetes under good control. [NIH]

Peritoneal: Having to do with the peritoneum (the tissue that lines the abdominal wall and covers most of the organs in the abdomen). [NIH]

Peritoneal Cavity: The space enclosed by the peritoneum. It is divided into two portions, the greater sac and the lesser sac or omental bursa, which lies behind the stomach. The two sacs are connected by the foramen of Winslow, or epiploic foramen. [NIH]

Perivascular: Situated around a vessel. [EU]

Petroleum: Naturally occurring complex liquid hydrocarbons which, after distillation, yield combustible fuels, petrochemicals, and lubricants. [NIH]

PH: The symbol relating the hydrogen ion (H+) concentration or activity of a solution to that of a given standard solution. Numerically the pH is approximately equal to the negative logarithm of H+ concentration expressed in molarity. pH 7 is neutral; above it alkalinity increases and below it acidity increases. [EU]

Phallic: Pertaining to the phallus, or penis. [EU]

Pharmaceutical Preparations: Drugs intended for human or veterinary use, presented in their finished dosage form. Included here are materials used in the preparation and/or formulation of the finished dosage form. [NIH]

Pharmacodynamic: Is concerned with the response of living tissues to chemical stimuli, that is, the action of drugs on the living organism in the absence of disease. [NIH]

Pharmacokinetic: The mathematical analysis of the time courses of absorption, distribution, and elimination of drugs. [NIH]

Pharmacologic: Pertaining to pharmacology or to the properties and reactions of drugs. [EU]

Phenotype: The outward appearance of the individual. It is the product of interactions between genes and between the genotype and the environment. This includes the killer phenotype, characteristic of yeasts. [NIH]

Phenyl: Ingredient used in cold and flu remedies. [NIH]

Phenylalanine: An aromatic amino acid that is essential in the animal diet. It is a precursor of melanin, dopamine, noradrenalin, and thyroxine. [NIH]

Phosphodiesterase: Effector enzyme that regulates the levels of a second messenger, the cyclic GMP. [NIH]

Phospholipases: A class of enzymes that catalyze the hydrolysis of phosphoglycerides or glycerophosphatidates. EC 3.1.-. [NIH]

Phosphorus: A non-metallic element that is found in the blood, muscles, nevers, bones, and teeth, and is a component of adenosine triphosphate (ATP; the primary energy source for the body's cells.) [NIH]

Phosphorylated: Attached to a phosphate group. [NIH]

Phosphorylates: Attached to a phosphate group. [NIH]

Phosphorylating: Attached to a phosphate group. [NIH]

Phosphorylation: The introduction of a phosphoryl group into a compound through the formation of an ester bond between the compound and a phosphorus moiety. [NIH]

Photochemotherapy: Therapy using oral or topical photosensitizing agents with subsequent exposure to light. [NIH]

Photopheresis: A process in which peripheral blood is exposed in an extracorporeal flow system to photoactivated 8-methoxypsoralen (methoxsalen) and ultraviolet light - a procedure known as PUVA therapy. Photopheresis is at present a standard therapy for advanced cutaneous T-cell lymphoma; it shows promise in the treatment of autoimmune diseases. [NIH]

Photosensitizing Agents: Drugs that are pharmacologically inactive but when exposed to ultraviolet radiation or sunlight are converted to their active metabolite to produce a beneficial reaction affecting the diseased tissue. These compounds can be administered topically or systemically and have been used therapeutically to treat psoriasis and various types of neoplasms. [NIH]

Phototherapy: Treatment of disease by exposure to light, especially by variously concentrated light rays or specific wavelengths. [NIH]

Physical Examination: Systematic and thorough inspection of the patient for physical signs of disease or abnormality. [NIH]

Physical Therapy: The restoration of function and the prevention of disability following disease or injury with the use of light, heat, cold, water, electricity, ultrasound, and exercise. [NIH]

Physiologic: Having to do with the functions of the body. When used in the phrase "physiologic age," it refers to an age assigned by general health, as opposed to calendar age. [NIH]

Physiology: The science that deals with the life processes and functions of organismus, their cells, tissues, and organs. [NIH]

Pigment: A substance that gives color to tissue. Pigments are responsible for the color of skin, eyes, and hair. [NIH]

Pigmentation: Coloration or discoloration of a part by a pigment. [NIH]

Pilocarpine: A slowly hydrolyzed muscarinic agonist with no nicotinic effects. Pilocarpine is used as a miotic and in the treatment of glaucoma. [NIH]

Pilot Projects: Small-scale tests of methods and procedures to be used on a larger scale if the pilot study demonstrates that these methods and procedures can work. [NIH]

Pilot study: The initial study examining a new method or treatment. [NIH]

Pituitary Gland: A small, unpaired gland situated in the sella turcica tissue. It is connected to the hypothalamus by a short stalk. [NIH]

Plants: Multicellular, eukaryotic life forms of the kingdom Plantae. They are characterized by a mainly photosynthetic mode of nutrition; essentially unlimited growth at localized regions of cell divisions (meristems); cellulose within cells providing rigidity; the absence of organs of locomotion; absense of nervous and sensory systems; and an alteration of haploid and diploid generations. [NIH]

Plaque: A clear zone in a bacterial culture grown on an agar plate caused by localized destruction of bacterial cells by a bacteriophage. The concentration of infective virus in a fluid can be estimated by applying the fluid to a culture and counting the number of. [NIH]

Plasma: The clear, yellowish, fluid part of the blood that carries the blood cells. The proteins that form blood clots are in plasma. [NIH]

Plasma cells: A type of white blood cell that produces antibodies. [NIH]

Plasma Exchange: Removal of plasma and replacement with various fluids, e.g., fresh frozen plasma, plasma protein fractions (PPF), albumin preparations, dextran solutions, saline. Used in treatment of autoimmune diseases, immune complex diseases, diseases of excess plasma factors, and other conditions. [NIH]

Plasma protein: One of the hundreds of different proteins present in blood plasma, including carrier proteins (such albumin, transferrin, and haptoglobin), fibrinogen and other coagulation factors, complement components, immunoglobulins, enzyme inhibitors, precursors of substances such as angiotension and bradykinin, and many other types of proteins. [EU]

Plasmin: A product of the lysis of plasminogen (profibrinolysin) by plasminogen activators. It is composed of two polypeptide chains, light (B) and heavy (A), with a molecular weight of 75,000. It is the major proteolytic enzyme involved in blood clot retraction or the lysis of fibrin and quickly inactivated by antiplasmins. EC 3.4.21.7. [NIH]

Plasminogen: Precursor of fibrinolysin (plasmin). It is a single-chain beta-globulin of molecular weight 80-90,000 found mostly in association with fibrinogen in plasma; plasminogen activators change it to fibrinolysin. It is used in wound debriding and has been investigated as a thrombolytic agent. [NIH]

Plasminogen Activator Inhibitor 1: A member of the serpin family of proteins. It inhibits both the tissue-type and urokinase-type plasminogen activators. [NIH]

Plasminogen Activators: A heterogeneous group of proteolytic enzymes that convert plasminogen to plasmin. They are concentrated in the lysosomes of most cells and in the vascular endothelium, particularly in the vessels of the microcirculation. EC 3.4.21.-. [NIH]

Plasticity: In an individual or a population, the capacity for adaptation: a) through gene changes (genetic plasticity) or b) through internal physiological modifications in response to changes of environment (physiological plasticity). [NIH]

Platelet Activation: A series of progressive, overlapping events triggered by exposure of the platelets to subendothelial tissue. These events include shape change, adhesiveness, aggregation, and release reactions. When carried through to completion, these events lead to the formation of a stable hemostatic plug. [NIH]

Platelet Aggregation: The attachment of platelets to one another. This clumping together can be induced by a number of agents (e.g., thrombin, collagen) and is part of the mechanism leading to the formation of a thrombus. [NIH]

Platelet-Derived Growth Factor: Mitogenic peptide growth hormone carried in the alpha-granules of platelets. It is released when platelets adhere to traumatized tissues. Connective tissue cells near the traumatized region respond by initiating the process of replication. [NIH]

Platelets: A type of blood cell that helps prevent bleeding by causing blood clots to form. Also called thrombocytes. [NIH]

Platinum: Platinum. A heavy, soft, whitish metal, resembling tin, atomic number 78, atomic weight 195.09, symbol Pt. (From Dorland, 28th ed) It is used in manufacturing equipment for laboratory and industrial use. It occurs as a black powder (platinum black) and as a spongy substance (spongy platinum) and may have been known in Pliny's time as "alutiae". [NIH]

Pleural: A circumscribed area of hyaline whorled fibrous tissue which appears on the surface of the parietal pleura, on the fibrous part of the diaphragm or on the pleura in the interlobar fissures. [NIH]

Pleural cavity: A space enclosed by the pleura (thin tissue covering the lungs and lining the interior wall of the chest cavity). It is bound by thin membranes. [NIH]

Pneumoconiosis: Condition characterized by permanent deposition of substantial amounts of particulate matter in the lungs, usually of occupational or environmental origin, and by the tissue reaction to its presence. [NIH]

Point Mutation: A mutation caused by the substitution of one nucleotide for another. This results in the DNA molecule having a change in a single base pair. [NIH]

Poisoning: A condition or physical state produced by the ingestion, injection or inhalation of, or exposure to a deleterious agent. [NIH]

Polyarthritis: An inflammation of several joints together. [EU]

Polycystic: An inherited disorder characterized by many grape-like clusters of fluid-filled cysts that make both kidneys larger over time. These cysts take over and destroy working kidney tissue. PKD may cause chronic renal failure and end-stage renal disease. [NIH]

Polymerase: An enzyme which catalyses the synthesis of DNA using a single DNA strand as a template. The polymerase copies the template in the 5'-3'direction provided that sufficient quantities of free nucleotides, dATP and dTTP are present. [NIH]

Polymorphism: The occurrence together of two or more distinct forms in the same population. [NIH]

Polypeptide: A peptide which on hydrolysis yields more than two amino acids; called tripeptides, tetrapeptides, etc. according to the number of amino acids contained. [EU]

Polysaccharide: A type of carbohydrate. It contains sugar molecules that are linked together chemically. [NIH]

Posterior: Situated in back of, or in the back part of, or affecting the back or dorsal surface of the body. In lower animals, it refers to the caudal end of the body. [EU]

Postmenopausal: Refers to the time after menopause. Menopause is the time in a woman's life when menstrual periods stop permanently; also called "change of life." [NIH]

Postnatal: Occurring after birth, with reference to the newborn. [EU]

Postsynaptic: Nerve potential generated by an inhibitory hyperpolarizing stimulation. [NIH]

Potassium: An element that is in the alkali group of metals. It has an atomic symbol K, atomic number 19, and atomic weight 39.10. It is the chief cation in the intracellular fluid of muscle and other cells. Potassium ion is a strong electrolyte and it plays a significant role in the regulation of fluid volume and maintenance of the water-electrolyte balance. [NIH]

Potentiates: A degree of synergism which causes the exposure of the organism to a harmful substance to worsen a disease already contracted. [NIH]

Potentiation: An overall effect of two drugs taken together which is greater than the sum of the effects of each drug taken alone. [NIH]

Practicability: A non-standard characteristic of an analytical procedure. It is dependent on the scope of the method and is determined by requirements such as sample throughout and costs. [NIH]

Practice Guidelines: Directions or principles presenting current or future rules of policy for the health care practitioner to assist him in patient care decisions regarding diagnosis, therapy, or related clinical circumstances. The guidelines may be developed by government agencies at any level, institutions, professional societies, governing boards, or by the convening of expert panels. The guidelines form a basis for the evaluation of all aspects of health care and delivery. [NIH]

Precursor: Something that precedes. In biological processes, a substance from which another, usually more active or mature substance is formed. In clinical medicine, a sign or symptom that heralds another. [EU]

Predisposition: A latent susceptibility to disease which may be activated under certain conditions, as by stress. [EU]

Prednisolone: A glucocorticoid with the general properties of the corticosteroids. It is the drug of choice for all conditions in which routine systemic corticosteroid therapy is indicated, except adrenal deficiency states. [NIH]

Prednisone: A synthetic anti-inflammatory glucocorticoid derived from cortisone. It is biologically inert and converted to prednisolone in the liver. [NIH]

Presynaptic: Situated proximal to a synapse, or occurring before the synapse is crossed. [EU]

Prevalence: The total number of cases of a given disease in a specified population at a designated time. It is differentiated from incidence, which refers to the number of new cases in the population at a given time. [NIH]

Prickle: Several layers of the epidermis where the individual cells are connected by cell bridges. [NIH]

Primary Biliary Cirrhosis: A chronic liver disease. Slowly destroys the bile ducts in the liver. This prevents release of bile. Long-term irritation of the liver may cause scarring and cirrhosis in later stages of the disease. [NIH]

Probe: An instrument used in exploring cavities, or in the detection and dilatation of strictures, or in demonstrating the potency of channels; an elongated instrument for exploring or sounding body cavities. [NIH]

Procollagen: A biosynthetic precursor of collagen containing additional amino acid sequences at the amino-terminal ends of the three polypeptide chains. Protocollagen, a precursor of procollagen consists of procollagen peptide chains in which proline and lysine have not yet been hydroxylated. [NIH]

Progeny: The offspring produced in any generation. [NIH]

Progeria: An abnormal congenital condition characterized by premature aging in children, where all the changes of cell senescence occur. It is manifested by premature greying, hair loss, hearing loss, cataracts, arthritis,osteoporosis, diabetes mellitus, atrophy of subcutaneous fat, skeletal hypoplasia, and accelerated atherosclerosis. Many affected individuals develop malignant tumors, especially sarcomas. [NIH]

Progesterone: Pregn-4-ene-3,20-dione. The principal progestational hormone of the body, secreted by the corpus luteum, adrenal cortex, and placenta. Its chief function is to prepare the uterus for the reception and development of the fertilized ovum. It acts as an antiovulatory agent when administered on days 5-25 of the menstrual cycle. [NIH]

Progression: Increase in the size of a tumor or spread of cancer in the body. [NIH]

Progressive: Advancing; going forward; going from bad to worse; increasing in scope or severity. [EU]

Progressive disease: Cancer that is increasing in scope or severity. [NIH]

Projection: A defense mechanism, operating unconsciously, whereby that which is emotionally unacceptable in the self is rejected and attributed (projected) to others. [NIH]

Proline: A non-essential amino acid that is synthesized from glutamic acid. It is an essential component of collagen and is important for proper functioning of joints and tendons. [NIH]

Promoter: A chemical substance that increases the activity of a carcinogenic process. [NIH]

Promotor: In an operon, a nucleotide sequence located at the operator end which contains all the signals for the correct initiation of genetic transcription by the RNA polymerase holoenzyme and determines the maximal rate of RNA synthesis. [NIH]

Prophase: The first phase of cell division, in which the chromosomes become visible, the nucleus starts to lose its identity, the spindle appears, and the centrioles migrate toward opposite poles. [NIH]

Prophylaxis: An attempt to prevent disease. [NIH]

Proportional: Being in proportion : corresponding in size, degree, or intensity, having the same or a constant ratio; of, relating to, or used in determining proportions. [EU]

Propylene Glycol: A clear, colorless, viscous organic solvent and diluent used in pharmaceutical preparations. [NIH]

Prostaglandin: Any of a group of components derived from unsaturated 20-carbon fatty acids, primarily arachidonic acid, via the cyclooxygenase pathway that are extremely potent mediators of a diverse group of physiologic processes. The abbreviation for prostaglandin is PG; specific compounds are designated by adding one of the letters A through I to indicate the type of substituents found on the hydrocarbon skeleton and a subscript (1, 2 or 3) to indicate the number of double bonds in the hydrocarbon skeleton e.g., PGE2. The predominant naturally occurring prostaglandins all have two double bonds and are synthesized from arachidonic acid (5,8,11,14-eicosatetraenoic acid) by the pathway shown in the illustration. The 1 series and 3 series are produced by the same pathway with fatty acids having one fewer double bond (8,11,14-eicosatrienoic acid or one more double bond (5,8,11,14,17-eicosapentaenoic acid) than arachidonic acid. The subscript a or ß indicates the configuration at C-9 (a denotes a substituent below the plane of the ring, ß, above the plane). The naturally occurring PGF's have the a configuration, e.g., PGF2a. All of the prostaglandins act by binding to specific cell-surface receptors causing an increase in the level of the intracellular second messenger cyclic AMP (and in some cases cyclic GMP also). The effect produced by the cyclic AMP increase depends on the specific cell type. In some cases there is also a positive feedback effect. Increased cyclic AMP increases prostaglandin synthesis leading to further increases in cyclic AMP. [EU]

Prostaglandin Endoperoxides: Precursors in the biosynthesis of prostaglandins and thromboxanes from arachidonic acid. They are physiologically active compounds, having effect on vascular and airway smooth muscles, platelet aggregation, etc. [NIH]

Prostaglandins A: (13E,15S)-15-Hydroxy-9-oxoprosta-10,13-dien-1-oic acid (PGA(1)); (5Z,13E,15S)-15-hydroxy-9-oxoprosta-5,10,13-trien-1-oic acid (PGA(2)); (5Z,13E,15S,17Z)-15-hydroxy-9-oxoprosta-5,10,13,17-tetraen-1-oic acid (PGA(3)). A group of naturally occurring secondary prostaglandins derived from PGE. PGA(1) and PGA(2) as well as their 19-hydroxy derivatives are found in many organs and tissues. [NIH]

Prostaglandins D: Physiologically active prostaglandins found in many tissues and organs. They show pressor activity, are mediators of inflammation, and have potential antithrombotic effects. [NIH]

Prostate: A gland in males that surrounds the neck of the bladder and the urethra. It secretes a substance that liquifies coagulated semen. It is situated in the pelvic cavity behind the lower part of the pubic symphysis, above the deep layer of the triangular ligament, and rests upon the rectum. [NIH]

Protease: Proteinase (= any enzyme that catalyses the splitting of interior peptide bonds in a protein). [EU]

Protective Agents: Synthetic or natural substances which are given to prevent a disease or disorder or are used in the process of treating a disease or injury due to a poisonous agent. [NIH]

Protein C: A vitamin-K dependent zymogen present in the blood, which, upon activation by thrombin and thrombomodulin exerts anticoagulant properties by inactivating factors Va and VIIIa at the rate-limiting steps of thrombin formation. [NIH]

Protein Conformation: The characteristic 3-dimensional shape of a protein, including the secondary, supersecondary (motifs), tertiary (domains) and quaternary structure of the peptide chain. Quaternary protein structure describes the conformation assumed by multimeric proteins (aggregates of more than one polypeptide chain). [NIH]

Protein Kinase C: An enzyme that phosphorylates proteins on serine or threonine residues in the presence of physiological concentrations of calcium and membrane phospholipids. The additional presence of diacylglycerols markedly increases its sensitivity to both calcium and phospholipids. The sensitivity of the enzyme can also be increased by phorbol esters and it is believed that protein kinase C is the receptor protein of tumor-promoting phorbol esters. EC 2.7.1.-. [NIH]

Protein S: The vitamin K-dependent cofactor of activated protein C. Together with protein C, it inhibits the action of factors VIIIa and Va. A deficiency in protein S can lead to recurrent venous and arterial thrombosis. [NIH]

Proteins: Polymers of amino acids linked by peptide bonds. The specific sequence of amino acids determines the shape and function of the protein. [NIH]

Protein-Serine-Threonine Kinases: A group of enzymes that catalyzes the phosphorylation of serine or threonine residues in proteins, with ATP or other nucleotides as phosphate donors. EC 2.7.10. [NIH]

Proteinuria: The presence of protein in the urine, indicating that the kidneys are not working properly. [NIH]

Proteoglycans: Glycoproteins which have a very high polysaccharide content. [NIH]

Proteolytic: 1. Pertaining to, characterized by, or promoting proteolysis. 2. An enzyme that promotes proteolysis (= the splitting of proteins by hydrolysis of the peptide bonds with formation of smaller polypeptides). [EU]

Prothrombin: A plasma protein that is the inactive precursor of thrombin. It is converted to thrombin by a prothrombin activator complex consisting of factor Xa, factor V, phospholipid, and calcium ions. Deficiency of prothrombin leads to hypoprothrombinemia. [NIH]

Protocol: The detailed plan for a clinical trial that states the trial's rationale, purpose, drug or vaccine dosages, length of study, routes of administration, who may participate, and other aspects of trial design. [NIH]

Protons: Stable elementary particles having the smallest known positive charge, found in the nuclei of all elements. The proton mass is less than that of a neutron. A proton is the nucleus of the light hydrogen atom, i.e., the hydrogen ion. [NIH]

Proto-Oncogene Proteins: Products of proto-oncogenes. Normally they do not have oncogenic or transforming properties, but are involved in the regulation or differentiation of cell growth. They often have protein kinase activity. [NIH]

Proto-Oncogene Proteins c-mos: Cellular proteins encoded by the c-mos genes. They function in the cell cycle to maintain maturation promoting factor in the active state and have protein-serine/threonine kinase activity. Oncogenic transformation can take place when c-mos proteins are expressed at the wrong time. [NIH]

Proximal: Nearest; closer to any point of reference; opposed to distal. [EU]

Pruritic: Pertaining to or characterized by pruritus. [EU]

Pruritus: An intense itching sensation that produces the urge to rub or scratch the skin to obtain relief. [NIH]

Psoralen: A substance that binds to the DNA in cells and stops them from multiplying. It is being studied in the treatment of graft-versus-host disease and is used in the treatment of psoriasis and vitiligo. [NIH]

Psoriasis: A common genetically determined, chronic, inflammatory skin disease characterized by rounded erythematous, dry, scaling patches. The lesions have a predilection for nails, scalp, genitalia, extensor surfaces, and the lumbosacral region. Accelerated epidermopoiesis is considered to be the fundamental pathologic feature in psoriasis. [NIH]

Psychiatry: The medical science that deals with the origin, diagnosis, prevention, and treatment of mental disorders. [NIH]

Psychosis: A mental disorder characterized by gross impairment in reality testing as evidenced by delusions, hallucinations, markedly incoherent speech, or disorganized and agitated behaviour without apparent awareness on the part of the patient of the incomprehensibility of his behaviour; the term is also used in a more general sense to refer to mental disorders in which mental functioning is sufficiently impaired as to interfere grossly with the patient's capacity to meet the ordinary demands of life. Historically, the term has been applied to many conditions, e.g. manic-depressive psychosis, that were first described in psychotic patients, although many patients with the disorder are not judged psychotic. [EU]

Psychotherapy: A generic term for the treatment of mental illness or emotional disturbances primarily by verbal or nonverbal communication. [NIH]

Public Policy: A course or method of action selected, usually by a government, from among alternatives to guide and determine present and future decisions. [NIH]

Publishing: "The business or profession of the commercial production and issuance of literature" (Webster's 3d). It includes the publisher, publication processes, editing and editors. Production may be by conventional printing methods or by electronic publishing. [NIH]

Pulmonary: Relating to the lungs. [NIH]

Pulmonary Artery: The short wide vessel arising from the conus arteriosus of the right ventricle and conveying unaerated blood to the lungs. [NIH]

Pulmonary Circulation: The circulation of blood through the lungs. [NIH]

Pulmonary Edema: An accumulation of an excessive amount of watery fluid in the lungs, may be caused by acute exposure to dangerous concentrations of irritant gasses. [NIH]

Pulmonary Embolism: Embolism in the pulmonary artery or one of its branches. [NIH]

Pulmonary Fibrosis: Chronic inflammation and progressive fibrosis of the pulmonary alveolar walls, with steadily progressive dyspnea, resulting finally in death from oxygen lack or right heart failure. [NIH]

Pulmonary hypertension: Abnormally high blood pressure in the arteries of the lungs. [NIH]

Pulse: The rhythmical expansion and contraction of an artery produced by waves of pressure caused by the ejection of blood from the left ventricle of the heart as it contracts. [NIH]

Pupil: The aperture in the iris through which light passes. [NIH]

Purifying: Respiratory equipment whose function is to remove contaminants from otherwise wholesome air. [NIH]

Purines: A series of heterocyclic compounds that are variously substituted in nature and are known also as purine bases. They include adenine and guanine, constituents of nucleic acids, as well as many alkaloids such as caffeine and theophylline. Uric acid is the metabolic end product of purine metabolism. [NIH]

Purpura: Purplish or brownish red discoloration, easily visible through the epidermis, caused by hemorrhage into the tissues. [NIH]

Pustular: Pertaining to or of the nature of a pustule; consisting of pustules (= a visible collection of pus within or beneath the epidermis). [EU]

Pyridoxal: 3-Hydroxy-5-(hydroxymethyl)-2-methyl-4- pyridinecarboxaldehyde. [NIH]

Pyridoxal Phosphate: 3-Hydroxy-2-methyl-5-((phosphonooxy)methyl)-4-pyridinecarboxaldehyde. An enzyme co-factor vitamin. [NIH]

Pyruvate Dehydrogenase Complex: An organized assembly of three kinds of enzymes; catalyzes the oxidative decarboxylation of pyruvate. [NIH]

Quality of Life: A generic concept reflecting concern with the modification and enhancement of life attributes, e.g., physical, political, moral and social environment. [NIH]

Quiescent: Marked by a state of inactivity or repose. [EU]

Race: A population within a species which exhibits general similarities within itself, but is both discontinuous and distinct from other populations of that species, though not sufficiently so as to achieve the status of a taxon. [NIH]

Radiation: Emission or propagation of electromagnetic energy (waves/rays), or the waves/rays themselves; a stream of electromagnetic particles (electrons, neutrons, protons, alpha particles) or a mixture of these. The most common source is the sun. [NIH]

Radiation therapy: The use of high-energy radiation from x-rays, gamma rays, neutrons, and other sources to kill cancer cells and shrink tumors. Radiation may come from a machine outside the body (external-beam radiation therapy), or it may come from radioactive material placed in the body in the area near cancer cells (internal radiation therapy, implant radiation, or brachytherapy). Systemic radiation therapy uses a radioactive substance, such as a radiolabeled monoclonal antibody, that circulates throughout the body. Also called radiotherapy. [NIH]

Radioactive: Giving off radiation. [NIH]

Radiolabeled: Any compound that has been joined with a radioactive substance. [NIH]

Radiological: Pertaining to radiodiagnostic and radiotherapeutic procedures, and interventional radiology or other planning and guiding medical radiology. [NIH]

Radiotherapy: The use of ionizing radiation to treat malignant neoplasms and other benign conditions. The most common forms of ionizing radiation used as therapy are x-rays, gamma rays, and electrons. A special form of radiotherapy, targeted radiotherapy, links a cytotoxic radionuclide to a molecule that targets the tumor. When this molecule is an antibody or other immunologic molecule, the technique is called radioimmunotherapy. [NIH]

Randomized: Describes an experiment or clinical trial in which animal or human subjects are assigned by chance to separate groups that compare different treatments. [NIH]

Rarefaction: The reduction of the density of a substance; the attenuation of a gas. [NIH]

Reactivation: The restoration of activity to something that has been inactivated. [EU]

Reactive Oxygen Species: Reactive intermediate oxygen species including both radicals and non-radicals. These substances are constantly formed in the human body and have been shown to kill bacteria and inactivate proteins, and have been implicated in a number of diseases. Scientific data exist that link the reactive oxygen species produced by inflammatory phagocytes to cancer development. [NIH]

Reagent: A substance employed to produce a chemical reaction so as to detect, measure, produce, etc., other substances. [EU]

Reality Testing: The individual's objective evaluation of the external world and the ability to differentiate adequately between it and the internal world; considered to be a primary ego function. [NIH]

Reassurance: A procedure in psychotherapy that seeks to give the client confidence in a favorable outcome. It makes use of suggestion, of the prestige of the therapist. [NIH]

Receptor: A molecule inside or on the surface of a cell that binds to a specific substance and causes a specific physiologic effect in the cell. [NIH]

Receptors, Serotonin: Cell-surface proteins that bind serotonin and trigger intracellular changes which influence the behavior of cells. Several types of serotonin receptors have been recognized which differ in their pharmacology, molecular biology, and mode of action. [NIH]

Recombinant: A cell or an individual with a new combination of genes not found together in either parent; usually applied to linked genes. [EU]

Recombination: The formation of new combinations of genes as a result of segregation in crosses between genetically different parents; also the rearrangement of linked genes due to crossing-over. [NIH]

Reconstitution: 1. A type of regeneration in which a new organ forms by the rearrangement of tissues rather than from new formation at an injured surface. 2. The restoration to original form of a substance previously altered for preservation and storage, as the restoration to a liquid state of blood serum or plasma that has been dried and stored. [EU]

Rectum: The last 8 to 10 inches of the large intestine. [NIH]

Recur: To occur again. Recurrence is the return of cancer, at the same site as the original (primary) tumor or in another location, after the tumor had disappeared. [NIH]

Recurrence: The return of a sign, symptom, or disease after a remission. [NIH]

Red blood cells: RBCs. Cells that carry oxygen to all parts of the body. Also called erythrocytes. [NIH]

Red Nucleus: A pinkish-yellow portion of the midbrain situated in the rostral mesencephalic tegmentum. It receives a large projection from the contralateral half of the cerebellum via the superior cerebellar peduncle and a projection from the ipsilateral motor cortex. [NIH]

Reductase: Enzyme converting testosterone to dihydrotestosterone. [NIH]

Refer: To send or direct for treatment, aid, information, de decision. [NIH]

Reflex: An involuntary movement or exercise of function in a part, excited in response to a stimulus applied to the periphery and transmitted to the brain or spinal cord. [NIH]

Refraction: A test to determine the best eyeglasses or contact lenses to correct a refractive error (myopia, hyperopia, or astigmatism). [NIH]

Refractory: Not readily yielding to treatment. [EU]

Regeneration: The natural renewal of a structure, as of a lost tissue or part. [EU]

Regimen: A treatment plan that specifies the dosage, the schedule, and the duration of treatment. [NIH]

Regurgitation: A backward flowing, as the casting up of undigested food, or the backward flowing of blood into the heart, or between the chambers of the heart when a valve is incompetent. [EU]

Relapse: The return of signs and symptoms of cancer after a period of improvement. [NIH]

Relative risk: The ratio of the incidence rate of a disease among individuals exposed to a specific risk factor to the incidence rate among unexposed individuals; synonymous with risk ratio. Alternatively, the ratio of the cumulative incidence rate in the exposed to the cumulative incidence rate in the unexposed (cumulative incidence ratio). The term relative risk has also been used synonymously with odds ratio. This is because the odds ratio and relative risk approach each other if the disease is rare (5 percent of population) and the number of subjects is large. [NIH]

Relaxin: Hormone produced by the ovaries during pregnancy that loosens ligaments that hold the hip bones together. [NIH]

Reliability: Used technically, in a statistical sense, of consistency of a test with itself, i. e. the extent to which we can assume that it will yield the same result if repeated a second time. [NIH]

Remission: A decrease in or disappearance of signs and symptoms of cancer. In partial remission, some, but not all, signs and symptoms of cancer have disappeared. In complete remission, all signs and symptoms of cancer have disappeared, although there still may be cancer in the body. [NIH]

Renal Artery: A branch of the abdominal aorta which supplies the kidneys, adrenal glands and ureters. [NIH]

Renal failure: Progressive renal insufficiency and uremia, due to irreversible and progressive renal glomerular tubular or interstitial disease. [NIH]

Renin: An enzyme which is secreted by the kidney and is formed from prorenin in plasma and kidney. The enzyme cleaves the Leu-Leu bond in angiotensinogen to generate angiotensin I. EC 3.4.23.15. (Formerly EC 3.4.99.19). [NIH]

Renin-Angiotensin System: A system consisting of renin, angiotensin-converting enzyme, and angiotensin II. Renin, an enzyme produced in the kidney, acts on angiotensinogen, an alpha-2 globulin produced by the liver, forming angiotensin I. The converting enzyme contained in the lung acts on angiotensin I in the plasma converting it to angiotensin II, the most powerful directly pressor substance known. It causes contraction of the arteriolar smooth muscle and has other indirect actions mediated through the adrenal cortex. [NIH]

Reperfusion: Restoration of blood supply to tissue which is ischemic due to decrease in normal blood supply. The decrease may result from any source including atherosclerotic obstruction, narrowing of the artery, or surgical clamping. It is primarily a procedure for treating infarction or other ischemia, by enabling viable ischemic tissue to recover, thus limiting further necrosis. However, it is thought that reperfusion can itself further damage the ischemic tissue, causing reperfusion injury. [NIH]

Reperfusion Injury: Functional, metabolic, or structural changes, including necrosis, in ischemic tissues thought to result from reperfusion to ischemic areas of the tissue. The most common instance is myocardial reperfusion injury. [NIH]

Research Support: Financial support of research activities. [NIH]

Reserpine: An alkaloid found in the roots of Rauwolfia serpentina and R. vomitoria. Reserpine inhibits the uptake of norepinephrine into storage vesicles resulting in depletion of catecholamines and serotonin from central and peripheral axon terminals. It has been used as an antihypertensive and an antipsychotic as well as a research tool, but its adverse effects limit its clinical use. [NIH]

Resorption: The loss of substance through physiologic or pathologic means, such as loss of dentin and cementum of a tooth, or of the alveolar process of the mandible or maxilla. [EU]

Respiration: The act of breathing with the lungs, consisting of inspiration, or the taking into the lungs of the ambient air, and of expiration, or the expelling of the modified air which contains more carbon dioxide than the air taken in (Blakiston's Gould Medical Dictionary, 4th ed.). This does not include tissue respiration (= oxygen consumption) or cell respiration (= cell respiration). [NIH]

Respiratory distress syndrome: A lung disease that occurs primarily in premature infants; the newborn must struggle for each breath and blueing of its skin reflects the baby's inability to get enough oxygen. [NIH]

Respiratory failure: Inability of the lungs to conduct gas exchange. [NIH]

Response Elements: Nucleotide sequences, usually upstream, which are recognized by specific regulatory transcription factors, thereby causing gene response to various regulatory agents. These elements may be found in both promotor and enhancer regions. [NIH]

Restoration: Broad term applied to any inlay, crown, bridge or complete denture which restores or replaces loss of teeth or oral tissues. [NIH]

Retina: The ten-layered nervous tissue membrane of the eye. It is continuous with the optic nerve and receives images of external objects and transmits visual impulses to the brain. Its outer surface is in contact with the choroid and the inner surface with the vitreous body. The outer-most layer is pigmented, whereas the inner nine layers are transparent. [NIH]

Retinal: 1. Pertaining to the retina. 2. The aldehyde of retinol, derived by the oxidative enzymatic splitting of absorbed dietary carotene, and having vitamin A activity. In the retina, retinal combines with opsins to form visual pigments. One isomer, 11-cis retinal combines with opsin in the rods (scotopsin) to form rhodopsin, or visual purple. Another, all-trans retinal (trans-r.); visual yellow; xanthopsin) results from the bleaching of rhodopsin by light, in which the 11-cis form is converted to the all-trans form. Retinal also combines with opsins in the cones (photopsins) to form the three pigments responsible for colour vision. Called also retinal, and retinene1. [EU]

Retinal Detachment: Separation of the inner layers of the retina (neural retina) from the pigment epithelium. Retinal detachment occurs more commonly in men than in women, in eyes with degenerative myopia, in aging and in aphakia. It may occur after an uncomplicated cataract extraction, but it is seen more often if vitreous humor has been lost during surgery. (Dorland, 27th ed; Newell, Ophthalmology: Principles and Concepts, 7th ed, p310-12). [NIH]

Retinoblastoma: An eye cancer that most often occurs in children younger than 5 years. It occurs in hereditary and nonhereditary (sporadic) forms. [NIH]

Retinoid: Vitamin A or a vitamin A-like compound. [NIH]

Retinol: Vitamin A. It is essential for proper vision and healthy skin and mucous membranes. Retinol is being studied for cancer prevention; it belongs to the family of drugs called retinoids. [NIH]

Retroviral vector: RNA from a virus that is used to insert genetic material into cells. [NIH]

Retrovirus: A member of a group of RNA viruses, the RNA of which is copied during viral replication into DNA by reverse transcriptase. The viral DNA is then able to be integrated into the host chromosomal DNA. [NIH]

Rheumatic Diseases: Disorders of connective tissue, especially the joints and related structures, characterized by inflammation, degeneration, or metabolic derangement. [NIH]

Rheumatism: A group of disorders marked by inflammation or pain in the connective tissue structures of the body. These structures include bone, cartilage, and fat. [NIH]

Rheumatoid: Resembling rheumatism. [EU]

Rheumatoid arthritis: A form of arthritis, the cause of which is unknown, although infection, hypersensitivity, hormone imbalance and psychologic stress have been suggested as possible causes. [NIH]

Rheumatology: A subspecialty of internal medicine concerned with the study of inflammatory or degenerative processes and metabolic derangement of connective tissue structures which pertain to a variety of musculoskeletal disorders, such as arthritis. [NIH]

Rhinitis: Inflammation of the mucous membrane of the nose. [NIH]

Ribonuclease: RNA-digesting enzyme. [NIH]

Ribonucleic acid: RNA. One of the two nucleic acids found in all cells. The other is deoxyribonucleic acid (DNA). Ribonucleic acid transfers genetic information from DNA to proteins produced by the cell. [NIH]

Ribonucleoproteins: Proteins conjugated with ribonucleic acids (RNA) or specific RNA. Many viruses are ribonucleoproteins. [NIH]

Ribose: A pentose active in biological systems usually in its D-form. [NIH]

Ribosome: A granule of protein and RNA, synthesized in the nucleolus and found in the cytoplasm of cells. Ribosomes are the main sites of protein synthesis. Messenger RNA attaches to them and there receives molecules of transfer RNA bearing amino acids. [NIH]

Risk factor: A habit, trait, condition, or genetic alteration that increases a person's chance of developing a disease. [NIH]

Rod: A reception for vision, located in the retina. [NIH]

Saline: A solution of salt and water. [NIH]

Saliva: The clear, viscous fluid secreted by the salivary glands and mucous glands of the mouth. It contains mucins, water, organic salts, and ptylin. [NIH]

Salivary: The duct that convey saliva to the mouth. [NIH]

Salivary glands: Glands in the mouth that produce saliva. [NIH]

Saponins: Sapogenin glycosides. A type of glycoside widely distributed in plants. Each consists of a sapogenin as the aglycon moiety, and a sugar. The sapogenin may be a steroid or a triterpene and the sugar may be glucose, galactose, a pentose, or a methylpentose. Sapogenins are poisonous towards the lower forms of life and are powerful hemolytics when injected into the blood stream able to dissolve red blood cells at even extreme dilutions. [NIH]

Sarcoidosis: An idiopathic systemic inflammatory granulomatous disorder comprised of epithelioid and multinucleated giant cells with little necrosis. It usually invades the lungs with fibrosis and may also involve lymph nodes, skin, liver, spleen, eyes, phalangeal bones, and parotid glands. [NIH]

Scans: Pictures of structures inside the body. Scans often used in diagnosing, staging, and monitoring disease include liver scans, bone scans, and computed tomography (CT) or computerized axial tomography (CAT) scans and magnetic resonance imaging (MRI) scans. In liver scanning and bone scanning, radioactive substances that are injected into the bloodstream collect in these organs. A scanner that detects the radiation is used to create pictures. In CT scanning, an x-ray machine linked to a computer is used to produce detailed pictures of organs inside the body. MRI scans use a large magnet connected to a computer to create pictures of areas inside the body. [NIH]

Scatter: The extent to which relative success and failure are divergently manifested in qualitatively different tests. [NIH]

Sclera: The tough white outer coat of the eyeball, covering approximately the posterior five-sixths of its surface, and continuous anteriorly with the cornea and posteriorly with the external sheath of the optic nerve. [EU]

Scleritis: Refers to any inflammation of the sclera including episcleritis, a benign condition affecting only the episclera, which is generally short-lived and easily treated. Classic scleritis, on the other hand, affects deeper tissue and is characterized by higher rates of visual acuity loss and even mortality, particularly in necrotizing form. Its characteristic symptom is severe and general head pain. Scleritis has also been associated with systemic collagen disease. Etiology is unknown but is thought to involve a local immune response. Treatment is difficult and includes administration of anti-inflammatory and immunosuppressive agents such as corticosteroids. Inflammation of the sclera may also be secondary to inflammation of adjacent tissues, such as the conjunctiva. [NIH]

Scleroderma: A chronic disorder marked by hardening and thickening of the skin. Scleroderma can be localized or it can affect the entire body (systemic). [NIH]

Scleroderma, Systemic: A chronic, progressive dermatosis characterized by boardlike hardening and immobility of the affected skin, with visceral involvement, especially of lungs, esophagus, kidneys and heart. It may be accompanied by calcinosis, Raynaud's phenomenon, and telangiectasis (CREST syndrome). It includes acrosclerosis and sclerodactyly. [NIH]

Sclerosis: A pathological process consisting of hardening or fibrosis of an anatomical structure, often a vessel or a nerve. [NIH]

Sclerotic: Pertaining to the outer coat of the eye; the sclera; hard, indurated or sclerosed. [NIH]

Screening: Checking for disease when there are no symptoms. [NIH]

Sebaceous: Gland that secretes sebum. [NIH]

Sebaceous gland: Gland that secretes sebum. [NIH]

Sebum: The oily substance secreted by sebaceous glands. It is composed of keratin, fat, and cellular debris. [NIH]

Second Messenger Systems: Systems in which an intracellular signal is generated in response to an intercellular primary messenger such as a hormone or neurotransmitter. They are intermediate signals in cellular processes such as metabolism, secretion, contraction, phototransduction, and cell growth. Examples of second messenger systems are the adenyl cyclase-cyclic AMP system, the phosphatidylinositol diphosphate-inositol triphosphate system, and the cyclic GMP system. [NIH]

Secretion: 1. The process of elaborating a specific product as a result of the activity of a gland; this activity may range from separating a specific substance of the blood to the elaboration of a new chemical substance. 2. Any substance produced by secretion. [EU]

Secretory: Secreting; relating to or influencing secretion or the secretions. [NIH]

Sediment: A precipitate, especially one that is formed spontaneously. [EU]

Segregation: The separation in meiotic cell division of homologous chromosome pairs and their contained allelomorphic gene pairs. [NIH]

Seizures: Clinical or subclinical disturbances of cortical function due to a sudden, abnormal, excessive, and disorganized discharge of brain cells. Clinical manifestations include abnormal motor, sensory and psychic phenomena. Recurrent seizures are usually referred to as epilepsy or "seizure disorder." [NIH]

Selective estrogen receptor modulator: SERM. A drug that acts like estrogen on some tissues, but blocks the effect of estrogen on other tissues. Tamoxifen and raloxifene are SERMs. [NIH]

Self Care: Performance of activities or tasks traditionally performed by professional health care providers. The concept includes care of oneself or one's family and friends. [NIH]

Self Tolerance: The normal lack of the ability to produce an immunological response to autologous (self) antigens. A breakdown of self tolerance leads to autoimmune diseases. The ability to recognize the difference between self and non-self is the prime function of the immune system. [NIH]

Sella: A deep depression in the shape of a Turkish saddle in the upper surface of the body of the sphenoid bone in the deepest part of which is lodged the hypophysis cerebri. [NIH]

Semen: The thick, yellowish-white, viscid fluid secretion of male reproductive organs discharged upon ejaculation. In addition to reproductive organ secretions, it contains spermatozoa and their nutrient plasma. [NIH]

Semisynthetic: Produced by chemical manipulation of naturally occurring substances. [EU]

Senescence: The bodily and mental state associated with advancing age. [NIH]

Senile: Relating or belonging to old age; characteristic of old age; resulting from infirmity of old age. [NIH]

Sequence Homology: The degree of similarity between sequences. Studies of amino acid and nucleotide sequences provide useful information about the genetic relatedness of certain species. [NIH]

Sequencing: The determination of the order of nucleotides in a DNA or RNA chain. [NIH]

Serine: A non-essential amino acid occurring in natural form as the L-isomer. It is synthesized from glycine or threonine. It is involved in the biosynthesis of purines, pyrimidines, and other amino acids. [NIH]

Serologic: Analysis of a person's serum, especially specific immune or lytic serums. [NIH]

Serotonin: A biochemical messenger and regulator, synthesized from the essential amino acid L-tryptophan. In humans it is found primarily in the central nervous system, gastrointestinal tract, and blood platelets. Serotonin mediates several important physiological functions including neurotransmission, gastrointestinal motility, hemostasis, and cardiovascular integrity. Multiple receptor families (receptors, serotonin) explain the broad physiological actions and distribution of this biochemical mediator. [NIH]

Serous: Having to do with serum, the clear liquid part of blood. [NIH]

Serum: The clear liquid part of the blood that remains after blood cells and clotting proteins have been removed. [NIH]

Sex Characteristics: Those characteristics that distinguish one sex from the other. The primary sex characteristics are the ovaries and testes and their related hormones. Secondary sex characteristics are those which are masculine or feminine but not directly related to reproduction. [NIH]

Sex Determination: The biological characteristics which distinguish human beings as female or male. [NIH]

Sexual Partners: Married or single individuals who share sexual relations. [NIH]

Shock: The general bodily disturbance following a severe injury; an emotional or moral upset occasioned by some disturbing or unexpected experience; disruption of the circulation, which can upset all body functions: sometimes referred to as circulatory shock. [NIH]

Sicca: Failure of lacrimal secretion, keratoconjunctivitis sicca, failure of secretion of the salivary glands and mucous glands of the upper respiratory tract and polyarthritis. [NIH]

Side effect: A consequence other than the one(s) for which an agent or measure is used, as the adverse effects produced by a drug, especially on a tissue or organ system other than the one sought to be benefited by its administration. [EU]

Signal Transduction: The intercellular or intracellular transfer of information (biological activation/inhibition) through a signal pathway. In each signal transduction system, an activation/inhibition signal from a biologically active molecule (hormone, neurotransmitter) is mediated via the coupling of a receptor/enzyme to a second messenger system or to an ion channel. Signal transduction plays an important role in activating cellular functions, cell differentiation, and cell proliferation. Examples of signal transduction systems are the GABA-postsynaptic receptor-calcium ion channel system, the receptor-mediated T-cell activation pathway, and the receptor-mediated activation of phospholipases. Those coupled to membrane depolarization or intracellular release of calcium include the receptor-mediated activation of cytotoxic functions in granulocytes and the synaptic potentiation of protein kinase activation. Some signal transduction pathways may be part of larger signal transduction pathways; for example, protein kinase activation is part of the platelet activation signal pathway. [NIH]

Signs and Symptoms: Clinical manifestations that can be either objective when observed by a physician, or subjective when perceived by the patient. [NIH]

Silicosis: A type of pneumoconiosis caused by inhalation of particles of silica, quartz, ganister or slate. [NIH]

Skeletal: Having to do with the skeleton (boney part of the body). [NIH]

Skeleton: The framework that supports the soft tissues of vertebrate animals and protects many of their internal organs. The skeletons of vertebrates are made of bone and/or cartilage. [NIH]

Skin Aging: The process of aging due to changes in the structure and elasticity of the skin over time. It may be a part of physiological aging or it may be due to the effects of ultraviolet radiation, usually through exposure to sunlight. [NIH]

Skin graft: Skin that is moved from one part of the body to another. [NIH]

Skin Physiology: The functions of the skin in the human and animal body. It includes the pigmentation of the skin and its appendages. [NIH]

Skin Pigmentation: Coloration of the skin. [NIH]

Small intestine: The part of the digestive tract that is located between the stomach and the large intestine. [NIH]

Smooth muscle: Muscle that performs automatic tasks, such as constricting blood vessels. [NIH]

Soaps: Sodium or potassium salts of long chain fatty acids. These detergent substances are obtained by boiling natural oils or fats with caustic alkali. Sodium soaps are harder and are used as topical anti-infectives and vehicles in pills and liniments; potassium soaps are soft, used as vehicles for ointments and also as topical antimicrobials. [NIH]

Social Environment: The aggregate of social and cultural institutions, forms, patterns, and processes that influence the life of an individual or community. [NIH]

Social Support: Support systems that provide assistance and encouragement to individuals with physical or emotional disabilities in order that they may better cope. Informal social support is usually provided by friends, relatives, or peers, while formal assistance is provided by churches, groups, etc. [NIH]

Sodium: An element that is a member of the alkali group of metals. It has the atomic symbol Na, atomic number 11, and atomic weight 23. With a valence of 1, it has a strong affinity for oxygen and other nonmetallic elements. Sodium provides the chief cation of the extracellular body fluids. Its salts are the most widely used in medicine. (From Dorland, 27th ed) Physiologically the sodium ion plays a major role in blood pressure regulation, maintenance of fluid volume, and electrolyte balance. [NIH]

Soft tissue: Refers to muscle, fat, fibrous tissue, blood vessels, or other supporting tissue of the body. [NIH]

Solid tumor: Cancer of body tissues other than blood, bone marrow, or the lymphatic system. [NIH]

Solvent: 1. Dissolving; effecting a solution. 2. A liquid that dissolves or that is capable of dissolving; the component of a solution that is present in greater amount. [EU]

Soma: The body as distinct from the mind; all the body tissue except the germ cells; all the axial body. [NIH]

Somatic: 1. Pertaining to or characteristic of the soma or body. 2. Pertaining to the body wall in contrast to the viscera. [EU]

Somatic cells: All the body cells except the reproductive (germ) cells. [NIH]

Somatostatin: A polypeptide hormone produced in the hypothalamus, and other tissues and organs. It inhibits the release of human growth hormone, and also modulates important physiological functions of the kidney, pancreas, and gastrointestinal tract. Somatostatin receptors are widely expressed throughout the body. Somatostatin also acts as a neurotransmitter in the central and peripheral nervous systems. [NIH]

Spasm: An involuntary contraction of a muscle or group of muscles. Spasms may involve skeletal muscle or smooth muscle. [NIH]

Spatial disorientation: Loss of orientation in space where person does not know which way is up. [NIH]

Specialist: In medicine, one who concentrates on 1 special branch of medical science. [NIH]

Species: A taxonomic category subordinate to a genus (or subgenus) and superior to a subspecies or variety, composed of individuals possessing common characters distinguishing them from other categories of individuals of the same taxonomic level. In taxonomic nomenclature, species are designated by the genus name followed by a Latin or Latinized adjective or noun. [EU]

Specificity: Degree of selectivity shown by an antibody with respect to the number and types of antigens with which the antibody combines, as well as with respect to the rates and the extents of these reactions. [NIH]

Spectrum: A charted band of wavelengths of electromagnetic vibrations obtained by refraction and diffraction. By extension, a measurable range of activity, such as the range of bacteria affected by an antibiotic (antibacterial s.) or the complete range of manifestations of a disease. [EU]

Sperm: The fecundating fluid of the male. [NIH]

Spermatocyte: An early stage in the development of a spermatozoon. [NIH]

Spermatozoa: Mature male germ cells that develop in the seminiferous tubules of the testes. Each consists of a head, a body, and a tail that provides propulsion. The head consists mainly of chromatin. [NIH]

Spermatozoon: The mature male germ cell. [NIH]

Spermicide: An agent that is destructive to spermatozoa. [EU]

Sphincter: A ringlike band of muscle fibres that constricts a passage or closes a natural orifice; called also musculus sphincter. [EU]

Spinal cord: The main trunk or bundle of nerves running down the spine through holes in the spinal bone (the vertebrae) from the brain to the level of the lower back. [NIH]

Spinous: Like a spine or thorn in shape; having spines. [NIH]

Spleen: An organ that is part of the lymphatic system. The spleen produces lymphocytes, filters the blood, stores blood cells, and destroys old blood cells. It is located on the left side of the abdomen near the stomach. [NIH]

Splint: A rigid appliance used for the immobilization of a part or for the correction of deformity. [NIH]

Spondylitis: Inflammation of the vertebrae. [EU]

Sporadic: Neither endemic nor epidemic; occurring occasionally in a random or isolated manner. [EU]

Squamous: Scaly, or platelike. [EU]

Squamous Epithelium: Tissue in an organ such as the esophagus. Consists of layers of flat, scaly cells. [NIH]

Stabilization: The creation of a stable state. [EU]

Staging: Performing exams and tests to learn the extent of the cancer within the body, especially whether the disease has spread from the original site to other parts of the body. [NIH]

Standard therapy: A currently accepted and widely used treatment for a certain type of cancer, based on the results of past research. [NIH]

Stasis: A word termination indicating the maintenance of (or maintaining) a constant level; preventing increase or multiplication. [EU]

Stem cell transplantation: A method of replacing immature blood-forming cells that were destroyed by cancer treatment. The stem cells are given to the person after treatment to help the bone marrow recover and continue producing healthy blood cells. [NIH]

Stem Cells: Relatively undifferentiated cells of the same lineage (family type) that retain the ability to divide and cycle throughout postnatal life to provide cells that can become specialized and take the place of those that die or are lost. [NIH]

Stents: Devices that provide support for tubular structures that are being anastomosed or for body cavities during skin grafting. [NIH]

Sterility: 1. The inability to produce offspring, i.e., the inability to conceive (female s.) or to induce conception (male s.). 2. The state of being aseptic, or free from microorganisms. [EU]

Steroid: A group name for lipids that contain a hydrogenated cyclopentanoperhydrophenanthrene ring system. Some of the substances included in this group are progesterone, adrenocortical hormones, the gonadal hormones, cardiac aglycones, bile acids, sterols (such as cholesterol), toad poisons, saponins, and some of the carcinogenic hydrocarbons. [EU]

Stimulant: 1. Producing stimulation; especially producing stimulation by causing tension on muscle fibre through the nervous tissue. 2. An agent or remedy that produces stimulation. [EU]

Stimulus: That which can elicit or evoke action (response) in a muscle, nerve, gland or other excitable issue, or cause an augmenting action upon any function or metabolic process. [NIH]

Stomach: An organ of digestion situated in the left upper quadrant of the abdomen between the termination of the esophagus and the beginning of the duodenum. [NIH]

Stool: The waste matter discharged in a bowel movement; feces. [NIH]

Strand: DNA normally exists in the bacterial nucleus in a helix, in which two strands are coiled together. [NIH]

Stress: Forcibly exerted influence; pressure. Any condition or situation that causes strain or tension. Stress may be either physical or psychologic, or both. [NIH]

Stress management: A set of techniques used to help an individual cope more effectively with difficult situations in order to feel better emotionally, improve behavioral skills, and often to enhance feelings of control. Stress management may include relaxation exercises, assertiveness training, cognitive restructuring, time management, and social support. It can be delivered either on a one-to-one basis or in a group format. [NIH]

Stroke: Sudden loss of function of part of the brain because of loss of blood flow. Stroke may be caused by a clot (thrombosis) or rupture (hemorrhage) of a blood vessel to the brain. [NIH]

Stromal: Large, veil-like cell in the bone marrow. [NIH]

Subacute: Somewhat acute; between acute and chronic. [EU]

Subarachnoid: Situated or occurring between the arachnoid and the pia mater. [EU]

Subclinical: Without clinical manifestations; said of the early stage(s) of an infection or other disease or abnormality before symptoms and signs become apparent or detectable by clinical examination or laboratory tests, or of a very mild form of an infection or other disease or abnormality. [EU]

Subcutaneous: Beneath the skin. [NIH]

Submaxillary: Four to six lymph glands, located between the lower jaw and the submandibular salivary gland. [NIH]

Subspecies: A category intermediate in rank between species and variety, based on a smaller number of correlated characters than are used to differentiate species and generally conditioned by geographical and/or ecological occurrence. [NIH]

Substance P: An eleven-amino acid neurotransmitter that appears in both the central and peripheral nervous systems. It is involved in transmission of pain, causes rapid contractions of the gastrointestinal smooth muscle, and modulates inflammatory and immune responses. [NIH]

Substrate: A substance upon which an enzyme acts. [EU]

Substrate Specificity: A characteristic feature of enzyme activity in relation to the kind of substrate on which the enzyme or catalytic molecule reacts. [NIH]

Sulfates: Inorganic salts of sulfuric acid. [NIH]

Sulfur: An element that is a member of the chalcogen family. It has an atomic symbol S, atomic number 16, and atomic weight 32.066. It is found in the amino acids cysteine and methionine. [NIH]

Sulfuric acid: A strong acid that, when concentrated is extemely corrosive to the skin and mucous membranes. It is used in making fertilizers, dyes, electroplating, and industrial explosives. [NIH]

Sunburn: An injury to the skin causing erythema, tenderness, and sometimes blistering and resulting from excessive exposure to the sun. The reaction is produced by the ultraviolet radiation in sunlight. [NIH]

Superoxide: Derivative of molecular oxygen that can damage cells. [NIH]

Support group: A group of people with similar disease who meet to discuss how better to cope with their cancer and treatment. [NIH]

Supportive care: Treatment given to prevent, control, or relieve complications and side effects and to improve the comfort and quality of life of people who have cancer. [NIH]

Suppression: A conscious exclusion of disapproved desire contrary with repression, in which the process of exclusion is not conscious. [NIH]

Supraventricular: Situated or occurring above the ventricles, especially in an atrium or atrioventricular node. [EU]

Surfactant: A fat-containing protein in the respiratory passages which reduces the surface tension of pulmonary fluids and contributes to the elastic properties of pulmonary tissue. [NIH]

Sympathectomy: The removal or interruption of some part of the sympathetic nervous system for therapeutic or research purposes. [NIH]

Sympathetic Nervous System: The thoracolumbar division of the autonomic nervous system. Sympathetic preganglionic fibers originate in neurons of the intermediolateral column of the spinal cord and project to the paravertebral and prevertebral ganglia, which in turn project to target organs. The sympathetic nervous system mediates the body's response to stressful situations, i.e., the fight or flight reactions. It often acts reciprocally to the parasympathetic system. [NIH]

Sympathomimetic: 1. Mimicking the effects of impulses conveyed by adrenergic postganglionic fibres of the sympathetic nervous system. 2. An agent that produces effects similar to those of impulses conveyed by adrenergic postganglionic fibres of the sympathetic nervous system. Called also adrenergic. [EU]

Symphysis: A secondary cartilaginous joint. [NIH]

Symptomatic: Having to do with symptoms, which are signs of a condition or disease. [NIH]

Synapses: Specialized junctions at which a neuron communicates with a target cell. At classical synapses, a neuron's presynaptic terminal releases a chemical transmitter stored in synaptic vesicles which diffuses across a narrow synaptic cleft and activates receptors on the postsynaptic membrane of the target cell. The target may be a dendrite, cell body, or axon of another neuron, or a specialized region of a muscle or secretory cell. Neurons may also communicate through direct electrical connections which are sometimes called electrical synapses; these are not included here but rather in gap junctions. [NIH]

Synapsis: The pairing between homologous chromosomes of maternal and paternal origin during the prophase of meiosis, leading to the formation of gametes. [NIH]

Synaptic: Pertaining to or affecting a synapse (= site of functional apposition between neurons, at which an impulse is transmitted from one neuron to another by electrical or chemical means); pertaining to synapsis (= pairing off in point-for-point association of homologous chromosomes from the male and female pronuclei during the early prophase of meiosis). [EU]

Synaptic Transmission: The communication from a neuron to a target (neuron, muscle, or secretory cell) across a synapse. In chemical synaptic transmission, the presynaptic neuron releases a neurotransmitter that diffuses across the synaptic cleft and binds to specific synaptic receptors. These activated receptors modulate ion channels and/or second-messenger systems to influence the postsynaptic cell. Electrical transmission is less common in the nervous system, and, as in other tissues, is mediated by gap junctions. [NIH]

Synaptonemal Complex: The three-part structure of ribbon-like proteinaceous material that serves to align and join the paired homologous chromosomes during the pachytene stage of meiotic division. It is a prerequisite for crossing-over. [NIH]

Synergistic: Acting together; enhancing the effect of another force or agent. [EU]

Synovial: Of pertaining to, or secreting synovia. [EU]

Synovial Fluid: The clear, viscous fluid secreted by the synovial membrane. It contains mucin, albumin, fat, and mineral salts and serves to lubricate joints. [NIH]

Synovial Membrane: The inner membrane of a joint capsule surrounding a freely movable joint. It is loosely attached to the external fibrous capsule and secretes synovial fluid. [NIH]

Synovitis: Inflammation of a synovial membrane. It is usually painful, particularly on motion, and is characterized by a fluctuating swelling due to effusion within a synovial sac. Synovitis is qualified as fibrinous, gonorrhoeal, hyperplastic, lipomatous, metritic, puerperal, rheumatic, scarlatinal, syphilitic, tuberculous, urethral, etc. [EU]

Systemic: Affecting the entire body. [NIH]

Systemic disease: Disease that affects the whole body. [NIH]

Systemic lupus erythematosus: SLE. A chronic inflammatory connective tissue disease marked by skin rashes, joint pain and swelling, inflammation of the kidneys, inflammation of the fibrous tissue surrounding the heart (i.e., the pericardium), as well as other problems. Not all affected individuals display all of these problems. May be referred to as lupus. [NIH]

Systolic: Indicating the maximum arterial pressure during contraction of the left ventricle of the heart. [EU]

Tamoxifen: A first generation selective estrogen receptor modulator (SERM). It acts as an agonist for bone tissue and cholesterol metabolism but is an estrogen antagonist in mammary and uterine. [NIH]

Telangiectasia: The permanent enlargement of blood vessels, causing redness in the skin or mucous membranes. [NIH]

Teratogenic: Tending to produce anomalies of formation, or teratism (= anomaly of formation or development : condition of a monster). [EU]

Testosterone: A hormone that promotes the development and maintenance of male sex characteristics. [NIH]

Tetracycline: An antibiotic originally produced by Streptomyces viridifaciens, but used mostly in synthetic form. It is an inhibitor of aminoacyl-tRNA binding during protein synthesis. [NIH]

Thalamic: Cell that reaches the lateral nucleus of amygdala. [NIH]

Thalamic Diseases: Disorders of the centrally located thalamus, which integrates a wide range of cortical and subcortical information. Manifestations include sensory loss, movement disorders; ataxia, pain syndromes, visual disorders, a variety of neuropsychological conditions, and coma. Relatively common etiologies include cerebrovascular disorders; craniocerebral trauma; brain neoplasms; brain hypoxia; intracranial hemorrhages; and infectious processes. [NIH]

Thalidomide: A pharmaceutical agent originally introduced as a non-barbiturate hypnotic, but withdrawn from the market because of its known tetratogenic effects. It has been reintroduced and used for a number of immunological and inflammatory disorders. Thalidomide displays immunosuppresive and anti-angiogenic activity. It inhibits release of tumor necrosis factor alpha from monocytes, and modulates other cytokine action. [NIH]

Theophylline: Alkaloid obtained from Thea sinensis (tea) and others. It stimulates the heart and central nervous system, dilates bronchi and blood vessels, and causes diuresis. The drug is used mainly in bronchial asthma and for myocardial stimulation. Among its more prominent cellular effects are inhibition of cyclic nucleotide phosphodiesterases and antagonism of adenosine receptors. [NIH]

Therapeutics: The branch of medicine which is concerned with the treatment of diseases, palliative or curative. [NIH]

Thermal: Pertaining to or characterized by heat. [EU]

Thermography: Measurement of the regional temperature of the body or an organ by infrared sensing devices, based on self-emanating infrared radiation. [NIH]

Thigh: A leg; in anatomy, any elongated process or part of a structure more or less comparable to a leg. [NIH]

Threonine: An essential amino acid occurring naturally in the L-form, which is the active form. It is found in eggs, milk, gelatin, and other proteins. [NIH]

Threshold: For a specified sensory modality (e. g. light, sound, vibration), the lowest level (absolute threshold) or smallest difference (difference threshold, difference limen) or intensity of the stimulus discernible in prescribed conditions of stimulation. [NIH]

Thrombin: An enzyme formed from prothrombin that converts fibrinogen to fibrin. (Dorland, 27th ed) EC 3.4.21.5. [NIH]

Thrombocytes: Blood cells that help prevent bleeding by causing blood clots to form. Also called platelets. [NIH]

Thrombolytic: 1. Dissolving or splitting up a thrombus. 2. A thrombolytic agent. [EU]

Thrombomodulin: A cell surface glycoprotein of endothelial cells that binds thrombin and serves as a cofactor in the activation of protein C and its regulation of blood coagulation. [NIH]

Thrombosis: The formation or presence of a blood clot inside a blood vessel. [NIH]

Thrombus: An aggregation of blood factors, primarily platelets and fibrin with entrapment of cellular elements, frequently causing vascular obstruction at the point of its formation. Some authorities thus differentiate thrombus formation from simple coagulation or clot formation. [EU]

Thymus: An organ that is part of the lymphatic system, in which T lymphocytes grow and multiply. The thymus is in the chest behind the breastbone. [NIH]

Thyroid: A gland located near the windpipe (trachea) that produces thyroid hormone, which helps regulate growth and metabolism. [NIH]

Thyroid Gland: A highly vascular endocrine gland consisting of two lobes, one on either side of the trachea, joined by a narrow isthmus; it produces the thyroid hormones which are concerned in regulating the metabolic rate of the body. [NIH]

Thyroiditis: Inflammation of the thyroid gland. [NIH]

Thyroxine: An amino acid of the thyroid gland which exerts a stimulating effect on thyroid metabolism. [NIH]

Time Management: Planning and control of time to improve efficiency and effectiveness. [NIH]

Tin: A trace element that is required in bone formation. It has the atomic symbol Sn, atomic number 50, and atomic weight 118.71. [NIH]

Tissue: A group or layer of cells that are alike in type and work together to perform a specific function. [NIH]

Tolerance: 1. The ability to endure unusually large doses of a drug or toxin. 2. Acquired drug tolerance; a decreasing response to repeated constant doses of a drug or the need for increasing doses to maintain a constant response. [EU]

Tomography: Imaging methods that result in sharp images of objects located on a chosen plane and blurred images located above or below the plane. [NIH]

Topical: On the surface of the body. [NIH]

Toxemia: A generalized intoxication produced by toxins and other substances elaborated by an infectious agent. [NIH]

Toxic: Having to do with poison or something harmful to the body. Toxic substances usually cause unwanted side effects. [NIH]

Toxicity: The quality of being poisonous, especially the degree of virulence of a toxic microbe or of a poison. [EU]

Toxicokinetics: Study of the absorption, distribution, metabolism, and excretion of test substances. [NIH]

Toxicology: The science concerned with the detection, chemical composition, and pharmacologic action of toxic substances or poisons and the treatment and prevention of toxic manifestations. [NIH]

Toxins: Specific, characterizable, poisonous chemicals, often proteins, with specific biological properties, including immunogenicity, produced by microbes, higher plants, or animals. [NIH]

Trachea: The cartilaginous and membranous tube descending from the larynx and branching into the right and left main bronchi. [NIH]

Transcriptase: An enzyme which catalyses the synthesis of a complementary mRNA molecule from a DNA template in the presence of a mixture of the four ribonucleotides (ATP, UTP, GTP and CTP). [NIH]

Transcription Factors: Endogenous substances, usually proteins, which are effective in the initiation, stimulation, or termination of the genetic transcription process. [NIH]

Transcutaneous: Transdermal. [EU]

Transdermal: Entering through the dermis, or skin, as in administration of a drug applied to the skin in ointment or patch form. [EU]

Transduction: The transfer of genes from one cell to another by means of a viral (in the case of bacteria, a bacteriophage) vector or a vector which is similar to a virus particle (pseudovirion). [NIH]

Transfection: The uptake of naked or purified DNA into cells, usually eukaryotic. It is analogous to bacterial transformation. [NIH]

Transfer Factor: Factor derived from leukocyte lysates of immune donors which can transfer both local and systemic cellular immunity to nonimmune recipients. [NIH]

Transferases: Transferases are enzymes transferring a group, for example, the methyl group or a glycosyl group, from one compound (generally regarded as donor) to another compound (generally regarded as acceptor). The classification is based on the scheme "donor:acceptor group transferase". (Enzyme Nomenclature, 1992) EC 2. [NIH]

Transforming Growth Factor beta: A factor synthesized in a wide variety of tissues. It acts synergistically with TGF-alpha in inducing phenotypic transformation and can also act as a negative autocrine growth factor. TGF-beta has a potential role in embryonal development, cellular differentiation, hormone secretion, and immune function. TGF-beta is found mostly as homodimer forms of separate gene products TGF-beta1, TGF-beta2 or TGF-beta3. Heterodimers composed of TGF-beta1 and 2 (TGF-beta1.2) or of TGF-beta2 and 3 (TGF-beta2.3) have been isolated. The TGF-beta proteins are synthesized as precursor proteins. [NIH]

Transgenes: Genes that are introduced into an organism using gene transfer techniques. [NIH]

Translation: The process whereby the genetic information present in the linear sequence of ribonucleotides in mRNA is converted into a corresponding sequence of amino acids in a protein. It occurs on the ribosome and is unidirectional. [NIH]

Translational: The cleavage of signal sequence that directs the passage of the protein through a cell or organelle membrane. [NIH]

Translocation: The movement of material in solution inside the body of the plant. [NIH]

Transmitter: A chemical substance which effects the passage of nerve impulses from one cell to the other at the synapse. [NIH]

Transplantation: Transference of a tissue or organ, alive or dead, within an individual, between individuals of the same species, or between individuals of different species. [NIH]

Trauma: Any injury, wound, or shock, must frequently physical or structural shock, producing a disturbance. [NIH]

Treatment Outcome: Evaluation undertaken to assess the results or consequences of management and procedures used in combating disease in order to determine the efficacy, effectiveness, safety, practicability, etc., of these interventions in individual cases or series. [NIH]

Trophic: Of or pertaining to nutrition. [EU]

Tryptophan: An essential amino acid that is necessary for normal growth in infants and for nitrogen balance in adults. It is a precursor serotonin and niacin. [NIH]

Tuberculosis: Any of the infectious diseases of man and other animals caused by species of Mycobacterium. [NIH]

Tuberous Sclerosis: A rare congenital disease in which the essential pathology is the appearance of multiple tumors in the cerebrum and in other organs, such as the heart or kidneys. [NIH]

Tumor marker: A substance sometimes found in an increased amount in the blood, other body fluids, or tissues and which may mean that a certain type of cancer is in the body. Examples of tumor markers include CA 125 (ovarian cancer), CA 15-3 (breast cancer), CEA (ovarian, lung, breast, pancreas, and gastrointestinal tract cancers), and PSA (prostate cancer). Also called biomarker. [NIH]

Tumor Necrosis Factor: Serum glycoprotein produced by activated macrophages and other mammalian mononuclear leukocytes which has necrotizing activity against tumor cell lines and increases ability to reject tumor transplants. It mimics the action of endotoxin but differs from it. It has a molecular weight of less than 70,000 kDa. [NIH]

Tumor suppressor gene: Genes in the body that can suppress or block the development of cancer. [NIH]

Tyrosine: A non-essential amino acid. In animals it is synthesized from phenylalanine. It is also the precursor of epinephrine, thyroid hormones, and melanin. [NIH]

Ulcerative colitis: Chronic inflammation of the colon that produces ulcers in its lining. This condition is marked by abdominal pain, cramps, and loose discharges of pus, blood, and mucus from the bowel. [NIH]

Unconscious: Experience which was once conscious, but was subsequently rejected, as the "personal unconscious". [NIH]

Uracil: An anticancer drug that belongs to the family of drugs called alkylating agents. [NIH]

Urea: A compound (CO(NH2)2), formed in the liver from ammonia produced by the deamination of amino acids. It is the principal end product of protein catabolism and constitutes about one half of the total urinary solids. [NIH]

Uremia: The illness associated with the buildup of urea in the blood because the kidneys are not working effectively. Symptoms include nausea, vomiting, loss of appetite, weakness, and mental confusion. [NIH]

Ureters: Tubes that carry urine from the kidneys to the bladder. [NIH]

Urethra: The tube through which urine leaves the body. It empties urine from the bladder. [NIH]

Urinalysis: Examination of urine by chemical, physical, or microscopic means. Routine urinalysis usually includes performing chemical screening tests, determining specific gravity, observing any unusual color or odor, screening for bacteriuria, and examining the sediment microscopically. [NIH]

Urinary: Having to do with urine or the organs of the body that produce and get rid of urine. [NIH]

Urine: Fluid containing water and waste products. Urine is made by the kidneys, stored in the bladder, and leaves the body through the urethra. [NIH]

Urokinase: A drug that dissolves blood clots or prevents them from forming. [NIH]

Ursodeoxycholic Acid: An epimer of chenodeoxycholic acid. It is a mammalian bile acid found first in the bear and is apparently either a precursor or a product of chenodeoxycholate. Its administration changes the composition of bile and may dissolve gallstones. It is used as a cholagogue and choleretic. [NIH]

Urticaria: A vascular reaction of the skin characterized by erythema and wheal formation due to localized increase of vascular permeability. The causative mechanism may be allergy, infection, or stress. [NIH]

Uterus: The small, hollow, pear-shaped organ in a woman's pelvis. This is the organ in which a fetus develops. Also called the womb. [NIH]

Vaccine: A substance or group of substances meant to cause the immune system to respond to a tumor or to microorganisms, such as bacteria or viruses. [NIH]

Vagina: The muscular canal extending from the uterus to the exterior of the body. Also called the birth canal. [NIH]

Vaginal: Of or having to do with the vagina, the birth canal. [NIH]

Vaginitis: Inflammation of the vagina characterized by pain and a purulent discharge. [NIH]

Valine: A branched-chain essential amino acid that has stimulant activity. It promotes muscle growth and tissue repair. It is a precursor in the penicillin biosynthetic pathway. [NIH]

Vascular: Pertaining to blood vessels or indicative of a copious blood supply. [EU]

Vascular endothelial growth factor: VEGF. A substance made by cells that stimulates new blood vessel formation. [NIH]

Vasculitis: Inflammation of a blood vessel. [NIH]

Vasoactive: Exerting an effect upon the calibre of blood vessels. [EU]

Vasoconstriction: Narrowing of the blood vessels without anatomic change, for which constriction, pathologic is used. [NIH]

Vasodilation: Physiological dilation of the blood vessels without anatomic change. For dilation with anatomic change, dilatation, pathologic or aneurysm (or specific aneurysm) is used. [NIH]

Vasodilator: An agent that widens blood vessels. [NIH]

Vector: Plasmid or other self-replicating DNA molecule that transfers DNA between cells in nature or in recombinant DNA technology. [NIH]

Vein: Vessel-carrying blood from various parts of the body to the heart. [NIH]

Venous: Of or pertaining to the veins. [EU]

Venous Thrombosis: The formation or presence of a thrombus within a vein. [NIH]

Ventricle: One of the two pumping chambers of the heart. The right ventricle receives oxygen-poor blood from the right atrium and pumps it to the lungs through the pulmonary artery. The left ventricle receives oxygen-rich blood from the left atrium and pumps it to the body through the aorta. [NIH]

Ventricular: Pertaining to a ventricle. [EU]

Ventricular Dysfunction: A condition in which the ventricles of the heart exhibit a decreased functionality. [NIH]

Venules: The minute vessels that collect blood from the capillary plexuses and join together to form veins. [NIH]

Verapamil: A calcium channel blocker that is a class IV anti-arrhythmia agent. [NIH]

Vertebrae: A bony unit of the segmented spinal column. [NIH]

Vertigo: An illusion of movement; a sensation as if the external world were revolving around the patient (objective vertigo) or as if he himself were revolving in space (subjective vertigo). The term is sometimes erroneously used to mean any form of dizziness. [EU]

Vesicular: 1. Composed of or relating to small, saclike bodies. 2. Pertaining to or made up of vesicles on the skin. [EU]

Veterinary Medicine: The medical science concerned with the prevention, diagnosis, and treatment of diseases in animals. [NIH]

Viral: Pertaining to, caused by, or of the nature of virus. [EU]

Virulence: The degree of pathogenicity within a group or species of microorganisms or viruses as indicated by case fatality rates and/or the ability of the organism to invade the tissues of the host. [NIH]

Virus: Submicroscopic organism that causes infectious disease. In cancer therapy, some viruses may be made into vaccines that help the body build an immune response to, and kill, tumor cells. [NIH]

Virus Diseases: A general term for diseases produced by viruses. [NIH]

Viscera: Any of the large interior organs in any one of the three great cavities of the body, especially in the abdomen. [NIH]

Visceral: , from viscus a viscus) pertaining to a viscus. [EU]

Visual Acuity: Acuteness or clearness of vision, especially of form vision, which is dependent mainly on the sharpness of the retinal focus. [NIH]

Vital Capacity: The volume of air that is exhaled by a maximal expiration following a maximal inspiration. [NIH]

Vitiligo: A disorder consisting of areas of macular depigmentation, commonly on extensor aspects of extremities, on the face or neck, and in skin folds. Age of onset is often in young adulthood and the condition tends to progress gradually with lesions enlarging and extending until a quiescent state is reached. [NIH]

Vitreous Hemorrhage: Hemorrhage into the vitreous body. [NIH]

Vitreous Humor: The transparent, colorless mass of gel that lies behind the lens and in front of the retina and fills the center of the eyeball. [NIH]

Vitro: Descriptive of an event or enzyme reaction under experimental investigation occurring outside a living organism. Parts of an organism or microorganism are used together with artificial substrates and/or conditions. [NIH]

Vivo: Outside of or removed from the body of a living organism. [NIH]

Vocal cord: The vocal folds of the larynx. [NIH]

Vulgaris: An affection of the skin, especially of the face, the back and the chest, due to chronic inflammation of the sebaceous glands and the hair follicles. [NIH]

Warfarin: An anticoagulant that acts by inhibiting the synthesis of vitamin K-dependent coagulation factors. Warfarin is indicated for the prophylaxis and/or treatment of venous thrombosis and its extension, pulmonary embolism, and atrial fibrillation with embolization. It is also used as an adjunct in the prophylaxis of systemic embolism after myocardial infarction. Warfarin is also used as a rodenticide. [NIH]

Wetting Agents: A surfactant that renders a surface wettable by water or enhances the spreading of water over the surface; used in foods and cosmetics; important in contrast media; also with contact lenses, dentures, and some prostheses. Synonyms: humectants; hydrating agents. [NIH]

White blood cell: A type of cell in the immune system that helps the body fight infection and disease. White blood cells include lymphocytes, granulocytes, macrophages, and others. [NIH]

Windpipe: A rigid tube, 10 cm long, extending from the cricoid cartilage to the upper border of the fifth thoracic vertebra. [NIH]

Wound Healing: Restoration of integrity to traumatized tissue. [NIH]

Xenograft: The cells of one species transplanted to another species. [NIH]

Xerostomia: Decreased salivary flow. [NIH]

X-ray: High-energy radiation used in low doses to diagnose diseases and in high doses to treat cancer. [NIH]

X-ray therapy: The use of high-energy radiation from x-rays to kill cancer cells and shrink tumors. Radiation may come from a machine outside the body (external-beam radiation therapy) or from materials called radioisotopes. Radioisotopes produce radiation and can be placed in or near the tumor or in the area near cancer cells. This type of radiation treatment is called internal radiation therapy, implant radiation, interstitial radiation, or brachytherapy. Systemic radiation therapy uses a radioactive substance, such as a radiolabeled monoclonal antibody, that circulates throughout the body. X-ray therapy is also called radiation therapy, radiotherapy, and irradiation. [NIH]

Yeasts: A general term for single-celled rounded fungi that reproduce by budding. Brewers' and bakers' yeasts are Saccharomyces cerevisiae; therapeutic dried yeast is dried yeast. [NIH]

Zymogen: Inactive form of an enzyme which can then be converted to the active form, usually by excision of a polypeptide, e. g. trypsinogen is the zymogen of trypsin. [NIH]

INDEX

Printed in the United States
30326LVS00001B/151

9 780597 842993